PRAISE FOR *THE EMPEROR OF SCENT*

"[An] engaging, picaresque account of Turin's scientific journey."
—*The New York Times Book Review*

"Elegant . . . an illustration of what happens when a maverick scientific theory threatens conventional wisdom."
—*Forbes*

"Exciting . . . Burr does a nice job of laying bare the jealousies and vested interests that the "vibration theory" challenged. Otherwise, it is Burr's genius to step out of the way and let his dynamic, unorthodox scientist subject do most of the talking."
—*Time Out New York*

"A gem of a book; I challenge any curious mind not to tumble into this story and become immediately engrossed. I fell in love with Luca Turin. He is . . . imaginative, determined, elitist without a trace of snobbery, and, above all, a creative genius. And Chandler Burr is a magician himself: I was mesmerized and enlightened by the many perfect asides woven into the main body of this incredible true tale."

—ALEXANDRA FULLER, author of *Don't Let's Go to the Dogs Tonight*

"Professional perfume critic, obsessive collector of rare fragrances, academic-bad-boy biochemist and world-class eccentric, Luca Turin would be the worthy subject of a book even if he hadn't come up with a revolutionary scientific theory. Written with skill and verve, *The Emperor of Scent* is an engrossing intellectual detective story about one iconoclast's quest to solve a centuries-old mystery—how smell works."

—MILES HARVEY, author of *The Island of Lost Maps*

"[Burr's] clear-eyed enthusiasm is one of the joys of *The Emperor of Scent*. . . . Burr has a knack for apt metaphor and telling detail, as well as an allegiance not so much to his subject as to a fair story. . . . The only disappointing thing about *The Emperor of Scent* is that it doesn't come with a scratch-and-sniff page."

—*The Oregonian*

"Burr's book is part scientific report, part detective story, part biography. . . . [It throws light] on the workings of the scientific community and the surprising . . . resistance a new idea gets when it goes against vested interests. . . . [*The Emperor of Scent*] is that rare book that will appeal both to the aesthete and to the average reader."

—*The Plain Dealer*

"[Burr's] peek behind the secretive walls of the perfume industry is plain old fun. . . . Science dilettantes and others of a thoughtful bent who prefer some intellectual kick to their thrillers will find much to enjoy here."

—*St. Petersburg Times*

ABOUT THE AUTHOR

CHANDLER BURR is the author of *A Separate Creation: The Search for the Biological Origins of Sexual Orientation*. He has contributed to *The Atlantic* and written for *The New York Times Magazine, The Washington Post*, the *Los Angeles Times,* and other publications.

www.chandlerburr.com

ALSO BY CHANDLER BURR

A Separate Creation

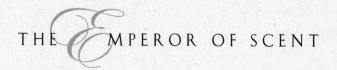

THE EMPEROR OF SCENT

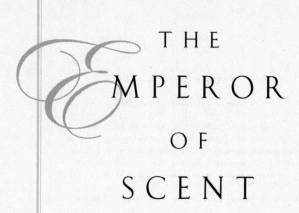

THE
EMPEROR
OF
SCENT

✦

A TRUE STORY OF PERFUME

AND OBSESSION

CHANDLER BURR

RANDOM HOUSE TRADE PAPERBACKS

NEW YORK

Grateful acknowledgment is made to Rutgers University Press for permission to
reprint excerpts from *Ignition,* by John D. Clark. Copyright © 1972 by Rutgers,
The State University. Reprinted by permission of Rutgers University Press.

All the illustrations in this work were drawn by Marie Guibert, excluding the
drawings of musical notes on page 26, which were done by Christopher J. Mossey,
and the drawing of the molecular shapes of ferrocene and nickelocene
on page 106, which was done by Luca Turin. All illustrations
are used by permission of the individual artists.

Library of Congress Cataloging-in-Publication Data

Burr, Chandler.
The emperor of scent : a true story of perfume and obsession / Chandler Burr.
p.   cm.
ISBN 0-375-75981-6
1. Turin, Luca.   2. Smell.   3. Nose.
4. Biophysicists—Great Britain—Biography.
I. Title.

QP458 .B83   2002
612.8'6—dc21   2002023697

Random House website address: www.atrandom.com
Printed in the United States of America
2 4 6 8 9 7 5 3
Book design by JoAnne Metsch

This one is to my family,

Devon, Nancy, Ralph and Ginny,

Marjorie, and David.

I should think that we might fairly gauge the future of biological science, centuries ahead, by estimating the time it will take to reach a complete comprehensive understanding of odor. It . . . contains, piece by piece, all the mysteries.

—Lewis Thomas

ACKNOWLEDGMENTS

MY GRATITUDE GOES to Walter Stewart, Giovanni Galizia, Barbara Talamo, John Kauer, Martin Heisenberg, Obaid Siddiqi, Leslie Vosshal, Peter Mombaerts, Nirao Shah, Randy Reed, Richard L. Doty, Tibor Krenacs, Geoffrey Webster, Upi Bhalla, Linda Buck, Barbara Banks, Heidi Hamm, Veronica Rodrigues, Philippe Béhé, Glenis Scadding, Tim Pearce, Alison Baum, and John Lynch. And to all those who helped.

In particular, I thank John Stephen for the flying lessons; Jane Brock, Tim Arnett, Martin Rosendaal, and Marshall Stoneham for recollection and analysis; the simply delightful Janet Rippard; Christopher Sheldrake for both molecules and Vietnamese food; Charles Sell and Karen Rossiter, despite how it turned out; Quraysh Aziz; and Manisha Nair, Aditya Kapil, Arjun Guha, Vinisha Khemani, and Mohinish "Mo!" Shukla for, along with everything else, picking us up at three in the morning. Mike Strong and Nick Moore ran my Department of Housing on West Ninety-first Street.

To my readers, thanks to Jay Marcus, Anne Lester Trevisan, Mark Lester, John Rowell, the über-diplomatic Bill McIlhenny (my future Italian landlord), Aileen Cheatham, and my ever-faithful supporter and reader, Devon Burr, who took the time from her Ph.D.

in geophysics and interplanetary remote sensing. And to Norman Carlin and Richard Pillard, two men possessed of awe-inspiring incisiveness and powers of perception which they use for good, not for evil.

Because Scott thinks I draw *like an eighth grader,* I'm happy and relieved that Christopher Mossey and Marie Guibert came through so beautifully. So is Scott.

This book was, in what is becoming a habit for me, incubated at *The Atlantic* by Cullen Murphy in the leading role, with Bill Whitworth, Amy Meeker, and Michael Kelly supporting. At Random House—what a great home it is!—my gratitude goes to Sunshine Lucas, Ann Godoff, Carol Schneider, Tom Perry, Sybil Pincus, Bonnie Thompson, James Lambert, Carole Lowenstein, and Ivan Held.

And last, to three:

I could never have done it without Joe Tomkiewicz (which is, absurdly enough, how you actually spell his name). He was a rock.

To the home team: Eric Simonoff (Tranquility Base) and Eadie Klemm (Base Manager), Scott Moyers (Force of Nature), and Elena Schneider (HQ). Thanks, Scott, for seeing, and for believing, and after that for sticking the course. You the man.

And to Luca Turin, Desa Philippi, and Adela Turin. It was not easy, in all sorts of ways, and Luca's efforts were herculean. And also to Eurostar for being twenty minutes late leaving for London on the morning of January 5, 1998, although they're now welcome to stop that.

CONTENTS

For the sake of scientific and narrative clarity, I have edited certain e-mails and correspondence and presented some events out of order. Some names and details have been changed to protect privacy.

PART I

CREATION

I

✦

MYSTERY

*S*TART WITH THE deepest mystery of smell. No one knows how we do it.

Despite everything, despite the billions the secretive giant corporations of smell have riding on it and the powerful computers they throw at it, despite the sorcery of their legions of chemists and the years of toiling in the labs and all the famous neurowizardry aimed at mastering it, the exact way we smell things—anything, crushed raspberry and mint, the subway at West Fourteenth and Eighth, a newborn infant—remains a mystery. Luca Turin began with that mystery.

Or perhaps he began further back, with the perfumes. "The reason I got *into* this," Turin will say, "is that I started collecting perfume. I've loved perfume from when I was a kid in Paris and Italy."

Or maybe (he'll tell you another day, considering it from a different angle), maybe it was "because I'm French, at least by upbringing. Frenchmen will do things Anglo men won't, and France is a country of smells. There's something called *pourriture noble*. Noble rot. It's a fungus. It grows on grapes, draws the water out, concentrates the juice wonderfully, adds its own fungal flavor, and then you make wines like the sweet Sauternes. Paradise. From rotten grapes."

The idea that things should be slightly dirty, overripe, slightly fecal is everywhere in France. They like rotten cheese and dirty sheets and unwashed women. Guy Robert is about seventy, a third-generation perfumer, lives in the south of France, used to work for International Flavors & Fragrances, created *Calèche* for Hermès. One day he asked me, '*Est-ce que vous avez senti* some molecule or other?' And I said no, I'd never smelled it, what'd it smell like? And he considered this gravely and replied, '*Ça sent la femme qui se néglige.*' " (It smells of the woman who neglects herself.)

This makes him remember something, and he leans forward enthusiastically. "One of the stories I heard when I started meeting the perfumers and was let into their tightly closed world involves Jean Carles, one of the greatest perfume makers in Paris—he used to work for Roure in Grasse, near Nice, where all perfumes used to be made. He became anosmic, lost his sense of smell, and he simply carried on from memory, creating perfumes. Like Beethoven after his deafness. Jean Carles went on to create the great *Ma Griffe* for Carven, a result of pure imagination in the complete absence of the relevant physical sense. Carles's condition was known only to him and his son. When a client came in, he'd go through the motions, make a big show of smelling various ingredients and, finally, the perfume he had created, which he would present with great gravity to the client, smelling it and waving its odor around the room. And he couldn't smell anything!" Turin smiles, thinking about it.

The perfume obsession led Turin to write the perfume guide, which out of the blue cracked open for him doors into the vast, secret world in which perfumes are created, and there he started noticing little things that didn't make sense. A weird warp in official reality. Plus there were the other clues, the small pockets of strangeness he bumped into in the scientific literature, carefully fitting these into the puzzle without even realizing it, without (as he'd be the first to admit) really understanding what he was doing. And somewhere along the line, between scouring the French Riviera for bottles of hidden fragrances, pursuing (in his own very particular way) the strange triplets of biology and chemistry and physics, and prowling the library's remotest stacks, randomly sliding into things he found there—something that due to his intellectual promiscuity he does a lot of—somewhere Luca Turin got the idea of cracking smell. But it started with the mystery at smell's heart, which is not only that we don't know *how* we do it. We actually shouldn't be able to smell at all.

◆   ◆   ◆

FROM EVERYTHING WE know about evolution and molecular biology, smell does the impossible. Look at two other systems inside your body, and you'll understand.

First, digestion. Human beings have evolved over millennia while eating certain molecules—lipids and carbohydrates and proteins in the roots and berries and various unlucky animals we've gotten our hands on. The tiny carbs and proteins are made of tinier atoms and molecules, and for your body to burn them as various fuels, evolution has engineered a digestive system for you. The system's first task is to recognize *which* raw fuel it's dealing with, so it can send out the right enzymes to break that fuel down, process it for us. (Enzymes are catalysts, molecule wranglers, and every enzyme in every one of our cells—and there are tens of thousands of different enzymes—binds to a molecule and processes it. Some break molecules down, scrapping them to use their dismantled parts, some zip them together, and some rearrange them for the body's own purposes.) But in every case the enzyme "recognizes" its molecule by that molecule's particular shape. Fat, thin, lumpy, rounded, oblong, rectangular. The enzyme feels some cleft in some molecule, fits its special fingers into it like a key fits into a lock. And if the shape of the lock and the shape of the key conform, bingo: Recognition! By shape.

And what gives a molecule its shape? We think of atoms as these perfectly symmetrical spheres, shining and frozen on labels of "Super-Strong!" kitchen cleaners, their electrons zipping around their nuclei like perfectly spherical stainless-steel bracelets. Since electrons move at close to the speed of light, if you filmed those cartoon atoms in motion you'd see a round electron membrane, a solid, buzzing sphere made of blisteringly fast-moving electrons.

But that's kitchen-cleaner labels. The skins of atoms *are* actually made of the paths of their outermost electrons, but not only don't they zip around in perfectly circular orbits, they carve an almost infinite variety of 3-D orbital grooves around their nuclei. If that's not enough, atoms get shoved against and glued to one another in molecules, forming bulbous structures, or nonspherical structures with disks and oblongs. Imagine taking the giant inflatable balloons in the Macy's parade, each one shaped differently, and pushing them against one another; their skins smoosh and warp, their bulbs and crevices contract and expand. So the electrons zip along in these new configurations, in elongated ellipses and valleys and sharp peaks and strange arcs. Which means that each molecule creates a unique shape that an enzyme can recognize as precisely as a retinal scan.

In fact, molecular recognition is arguably the fundamental mechanism of all life, and it is based on this single, universal principle: Shape. Receptor cells from your head to your glands and skin recognize enzymes, hormones, and neurotransmitters by their molecular shapes. The only variable is time.

The thing about enzymes is that evolution has learned over millennia that you're going to need to digest (break down, make up, or molecularly rearrange) certain things—wild almonds and crab apples and dead squirrels (sugars, fats, and proteins)—and not others—raw petroleum or sand or silicate (fluorocarbons and borazines). So evolution has by now selected for you a complete, fixed genetic library of enzymes that will bind to and deal with a fixed list of molecules. (It's not an exact one-to-one enzyme-to-foodstuff ratio, but it's precise enough that it's why your dog famously can't digest chocolate, a culinary product his wolf ancestors never ate: evolution never selected for dogs an enzyme that recognized the shape of chocolate's molecules, so if you feed them these molecules, they get sick.) And if just one enzyme is missing, you end up with nasty, sometimes lethal, diseases and disorders. You can dump the squirrels for *terrine de lapin et petits légumes,* it doesn't matter: it's the same lipids and proteins in your library, and as long as you don't eat, say, plastic, for which you have no enzyme, your digestive system happily recognizes the molecules you consume, be it McDonald's or the fifth course at the Clifton Inn. The thing to remember here, however, is *time:* enzymes stand ready to identify the right molecule *instantly.*

For contrast, take the immune system. Antibodies are designed (they have to be) to bind to things that *weren't* around our ancestors, unknown bacteria and foreign parasites and each year's new, nastier, mutated viruses we've never seen before. Your visual system can recognize things that weren't in *Homo sapiens*'s evolutionary environment, like Ferraris and *Star Wars* and Barbra Streisand, and so can your immune system, but your visual system deciphers photon wavelengths while your immune system is feeling out molecules' shapes. Here's the difference. When it encounters a new virus, the immune system starts rapidly rearranging genes at random, spewing out antibodies until it hits on one that fits the invader's shape, binds to it, and destroys it. (It's the exact opposite of a "fixed library" idea; Susumu Tonegawa of MIT won a 1987 Nobel Prize for figuring this out.) So that's why you're at home for a few days with the flu. Your immune system needs time to break the invader's shape code and produce the shape weapon to fight it. Where the digestive system is limited but instant, the immune system is unlimited—it "takes all comers"; but it also takes time.

But here is the problem. Someone hands you a molecule called a borane. You lift it to your nose. And without fail, you smell it. There's just one catch: boranes were created by inorganic chemists at the beginning of the twentieth century and never existed in the ancestral environment of any human being. Yet we smell them. This is impossible.

The fact is that we have never found any molecule in the smellable size range that we could not smell instantly. This is the mystery of smell. You smell boranes instantly, not in a few days or weeks, even though you cannot have an evolutionarily selected receptor molecule for their unique shape. Smell is unlimited, like the immune system, and yet it is instant, like the digestive system. And everything we know about Shape and molecular recognition says this should be impossible.

We understand the human sense of vision intimately, down to exactly which vibration of a particle of light caught in the vision receptor in the retina will make us see exactly which color (a 1967 Nobel given for vision). We know hearing in exquisite detail, can predict with absolute accuracy which air vibration in the cochlea will create what tone (a 1961 Nobel for hearing). But of smell, we do not know, cannot predict. This is why smell is the object of two cut-throat races.

The first is scientific. This all-out race is being run in some of the most powerful labs (by the most competitive researchers with the biggest egos). The prize is the unscrambling of one of the most important secrets of biology, not to mention (everyone is betting on this) a Nobel Prize. An astounding 1 percent of human genes, we recently discovered, are devoted to olfaction. "So smell must be incredibly important for us," notes NIH geneticist Dean Hamer, "to devote so much of our DNA to it. The only comparable system— and this was the big surprise to everyone—is the immune system, and we all know why it's important to fight off invaders. This says smell was central in our evolution in a way that, presently, we don't really understand."

The other race is for money. Approximately $20 billion is generated every year by industrially manufactured smells, and virtually all these smells are made by only seven companies, the Big Boys, which split the billions among themselves. The Big Boys shroud themselves in secrecy to protect the public brand image of their clients. They make the molecules that you associate with the smells of Tide laundry detergent, Clorox bleach, and Palmolive soap, but they are also the actual creators of the superexpensive fragrances sold under the rarefied labels Calvin Klein and Chanel and L'Oréal, Miyake and Armani. The creation of a single commercially successful fragrance molecule represents tens of millions of dollars, and the Big Boys employ an army of chemists tasked with creating them. The *way* to create them is the magic formula.

This is why Luca Turin's theory is as important as it is unknown. It is not only a new theory of smell. Financially, it implies a technology that threatens thousands of engineers and corporate executives, the investment of billions of dollars, and the industrial structures of massive corporations in North America, Europe, and Japan. Scientifically, it is a wildly revolutionary proposal contradicting a universal, bedrock assumption of biology—Shape—and positing an astounding, microscopic electrical mechanism that operates inside the human body and is made of human flesh. You might as well, fumed one furious scientist who heard about Turin's idea, propose a new theory of digestion through tiny nuclear reactors in people's stomachs. Perhaps the only thing odder than the theory is the story of how Turin actually came up with it, and then of what happened to him when he did, which is what this book is about.

II

✦

CREATION

*I*F LUCA TURIN collected you at London's Euston Square tube station, he would lead the way enthusiastically down Gower Street to the biology building at University College London. If this was back when he was teaching there, when things were simpler, he'd take you up a large wooden stairwell and into his old office. The office, during his occupancy, looked like a hand-grenade test site. Transistors, wires, tubes, plane tickets, bottles of perfume, obscure scientific journals and copies of *Vogue* and magazines about airplanes, gadgets of every size and design, and God knows what else, and, everywhere, vials and vials and vials. Turin would dive in and begin selecting vials from among the hundreds spread out chaotically on counters. Each would contain a single kind of molecule. Each would have a single smell.

Turin can nail any odor descriptively in a few words. He's generally not only exactly spot on, he gets incredible torque from the most recherché nouns. (His descriptions are almost entirely in the nominative; he uses adjectives rarely to never.) He screws off a cap, pushes over a molecule, and you look at the label: "cis-3-hexenol." Cautiously your nose goes to the tiny opening of the dark, little bottle, shoulders tensed as if rounding a corner in a tight, dark space, eyes narrowed. "Cut grass," says Turin, watching you. Two words, definitive. You sniff. The molecule cis-3-hexenol happens to smell —it is impossible to describe it any other way—exactly like cut grass, and very strongly. He picks up benzonitrile. "Shoe polish." This structure of atoms smells overwhelmingly reminiscent of round metal tins of Kiwi shoe polish. He stands a foot away, looking intently down at you—he's around six foot three, gangly frame, looks paradigmatically northern Italian (which he is), light brown hair receding in wisps from a Gianni Versace face that's large and open and animated—and as you gingerly draw some molecule from the vial up into your nose states, "Scrambled egg, gasoline." You're smelling the smell, it's filling your mind with a vague, inchoate presence. And the instant he says the words the smell snaps into concreteness, into realness, and the smell of scrambled eggs with gasoline is *precisely,* bizarrely, the smell filling you. (Turin speaks a grammatically perfect, highly inflected English, quite rapidly, with a totally American accent although he learned English in Britain and lives in London. So why the American accent. "I don't know." He shrugs. "I guess because I'd've had to decide *which* English accent, which is a major pain in the ass, given what that means here. The hell with it." On the other hand, he uses British syllabic emphasis on words like *laboratory*—accent on the second syllable—and *aluminium*—the third—which, combined with the American accent, can produce an odd effect. Words in French and Italian, his two native languages, he invariably renders with their native pronunciations, as he does with Russian, which he speaks a little. Every so often, the faintest foreignness will appear in his English, generally as a slightly swallowed consonant; when he says "Fantastic!" which he does often, it sounds Dutch.)

"It makes everyone nervous, smelling," he says re the vial, "because smell is such a strong sense." Turin gives talks on smell to scientific audiences, and the squeamish reaction pisses him off. The intellectual squeamishness, too. "People will say, 'But isn't smell totally subjective?' And I'll say 'What the hell does *that* mean?' It's not more subjective than color or sound. Real men and scientists feel slightly ridiculous smelling something. I'll say 'Let me show you some smells,' and I start passing out vials and everyone titters, like I've just asked them to take off their *clothes* or something. It's at the heart of the research problem, because experts on the biology of smell will put vanillin under 'herbal.' *God.* When I wrote the perfume guide, most of my readers were gay men, and most of my acquaintances assumed I was gay, which I'm not, not that I give a damn. Real men don't smell things. It's a female thing.

"For a perfumer there is no bad smell. All the great French perfumes, every last one, has some ingredient in it that is repulsive, like civet, this hideous and ferociously powerful extract from the butt-hole of a Chinese tomcat. Beaver pelt oil. Something. Americans dedicate their lives to the notion that shit shouldn't stink. American perfumery is really, well . . . Americans have an obsessional neurosis about being clean. What do you call that?"

He thinks of something strange, mulls it over. "You know, there's an aspect of smell that seems to be missing from the other senses. When you hear a piece of music, you can identify the composer, or if it is derivative, the composer's main influences, by name. 'That's Bizet, that's Glass.' When you see a painting, you can do the same. 'Oh, Miró.' But when you experience a famous work of smell—*Chanel No. 5, Shalimar, Charlie, CK One, Opium*—though a number of them have actually been designed by the same perfumer, you can never identify their creator. There is no 'signature' in perfumes."

He picks up a group of vials. "OK, these are great. Oxane." He pauses and says, "Sweaty mango." You smell it. It is, exactly, hot sweat on ripe mango. He grins, goes on, "That's a single synthetic molecule they manufactured in a lab, a six-membered ring with an Oxygen and a Sulfur: phenomenal power. I heard the Quest chemists once accidentally dropped a hundred grams down the drain, and all of Kent smelled of mango for a few hours. The odor is a shimmering mixture of sweat and tropical fruit, with a 'green' marijuana-like note. Used in perfumery much as trombones in the orchestra, imparting an edge and rich bloom to virtually any composition.

"Vertelon: mushroom liqueur. Again, this complex odor you're smelling is *a single molecule*. Mushrooms are at once clean and dirty;

it's a creature freshly born of decay. Vertelon *clears* a perfume, like when you pour paraffin oil on an opaque sheet of paper and watch as the paper becomes translucent. I am at present working on a mushroom-Oriental that will smell of sex, but clean sex.

"Gardamide: grapefruit and hot horses. This is the horse you get from removing the saddle after riding.

"Violet nitrile: steel cucumber. Aldehyde $HC=O$ groups can be replaced with nitriles, which are CNs." He sniffs this for himself, just to see. Thinks about it. Sets it aside and opens the next one.

"Cashmeran, a pure synthetic. Technically classed as a musk, it is actually a peculiar combination of a transparent sweet note with no precise character, a musty, wet-concrete note with camphorlike feel, and a fruity, blackberries note that pops in and out of focus. You just cannot believe that a single molecule has so many features. The musty, wet-concrete. The camphor. The fruit. The velvet. Smell that? Getting this molecule in your nose is like coming up close to a beautiful face and finding it's made of independently 'wrong' features that add up to a fine harmony.

"Tuberose: black rubber flower. This is a natural oil, a complex mixture. This one's smell evolves. The rubber is kinky, dusted with talcum. Then an almost meaty bloodlike smell reminiscent of carnations, and finally a 'white flower.'" He pauses. Smiles. "Decorous but unquestionably poisonous. *Fracas,* the classic Piguet fragrance created by Germaine Cellier, was very close but made of different pieces. Bear in mind," he notes, "this is several hundred molecules flying in tight formation."

◆　　◆　　◆

LUCA TURIN'S MOTHER, ignoring the flow of Western History as she would more or less ignore all strictures life might try to place on her, emigrated from the New World back to the Old.

Adela Mandelli was born in the center of Milan, though just barely. The Mandellis were a tenth-century Milan family possessed of one of the city's oldest names, as well as great wealth. (Adela never told Luca any of this; he discovered it one day, by accident, while nosing around the British Museum.) Her father was born in

1899, a diabetic. Not expecting their eldest son to live long, his parents indulged him, and by adulthood he had become a cultured aristocrat who had studied letters at several estimable European universities and such a compulsive and inveterate gambler that his father gave him a last lump of money and sent him to seek his fortune in South America. There, it was sincerely hoped, he would finally cease decimating the family fortune. He gambled the money away on the ship and arrived in the New World penniless, where he soon met the daughter of an anarchist who had been exiled from Lombardy for various political reasons. He married her and took her back to Milan, where they had three children, Adela the third, and where he attempted a decreasingly successful series of business affairs between Milan and Paris. His anti-Fascist political views were getting him into trouble, and just ahead of the ignition of World War II, when Adela was four, the family returned to Argentina, where his diabetes finally caught up with him. He died, just after the war, blinded by the disease, at forty-five.

Adela grew up in Buenos Aires and studied art history and in 1950 returned definitively to her father's continent, where she finished her studies in Milan and then Paris. One evening in Turin, at a party of the architects and designers who orbited the prestigious magazine *Urbanistica* and its founder, Adriano Olivetti, some friends introduced her to a young man named Duccio Turin. She had something in common with the young architect, her friends pointed out: he was another Italian-Argentine who had gone against the current.

Duccio had been born in Italy into a family of Waldensians, an ancient, tiny Protestant minority. His father had married into a Jewish family, and when in 1936 his wife lost her teaching job under Mussolini's anti-Jewish laws, the family emigrated to western Argentina. Professionally Duccio occupied the somewhat singular position of having trained as an architect, which he loved, but not particularly as a means to building things. What did intrigue him on a practical level was economics. He wound up fusing the two into a passion for the industry of architecture: how did one create building industries in impoverished countries and—particularly—how did rich countries impose inappropriate architecture on poor ones.

He got a job with the United Nations Refugee Welfare Association as a young architect and town planner, which led to a position with the United Nations in 1951 as architect of a Palestinian camp, which is why Adela and Duccio's first and only son, Luca, was born in Lebanon, on November 20, 1953. They gave him their Italian nationality. (He still travels on an Italian passport.)

The family left Lebanon for Paris, where Duccio worked for the Centre Scientifique et Technique du Batiment in Paris. They had a Spanish maid, from Valencia, with whom Turin spoke Spanish with a vaguely Argentinian accent he'd gotten from his mother. "He learned to read at age four," Adela says, "because the Valenciana was *analphabète*, illiterate. She was about forty, and she couldn't travel alone because she couldn't read the metro signs. So I decided to teach her to read. Luca would wander in and watch us. And all of a sudden one day I found him reading headlines. I have an image of this small child holding a very big newspaper." She spreads her arms out, clenches her hands around an invisible paper, opens her eyes wide. His parents exposed him to classical music, his father favoring Mozart and earlier music, his mother Beethoven and the Romantics. That same year, Duccio got a job with the United Nations and moved the family to Geneva. Duccio and Adela divorced there.

Their son was miserable in Switzerland. "When he started school," says Adela, "he could already read, but in Switzerland one starts to learn at seven, and that's it. And he was just going crazy. He would come home from school hysterical, breaking things. I asked for *une dispense d'âge*, letting him skip two grades. It became a state affair. I took him to a place where they gave him all sorts of tests. The tests lasted three days. At the end, they had this big convocation, very formal, where a man from the Department of Schools told me he was the most brilliant child they'd ever seen. But when they finally gave me the *dispense d'âge*, it was only of one year, so he found himself just as bored as before.

"His teacher told me, 'In the teaching corps we don't like brilliant children.' I've always remembered her face when she told me that." Adela muses on this for a moment. "I never took his teachers' side. He would arrive home with the punishment of writing three hundred times '*Je ne dois pas bavarder en classe.*'" (I must not talk in class.) "My handwriting was very similar to his at the time, and we'd sit side by side and he would write '*Je ne dois pas*' and I'd write '*bavarder en classe.*' When he returned with bad notes in conduct, it made me laugh. When I was a girl and was bored I thought about other things."

After a few years Adela, who had been working as a designer for Lanvin Castillo in the 1950s and '60s, moved with him to Paris and became art director of an advertising agency. "Luca didn't have many friends." She says this frankly. "He's not someone who has lots of friends." She makes a dismissive moue, shakes her hands to indicate many, superficial people. But the boy fell in love with the Palais de la Découverte, the Paris science museum at the bottom of the Champs-Elysées. That was where he saw the first image he'd ever seen on a color TV, when color TV was still pretty much experimental, a fruit salad with the color turned up way too high. He was eleven. He and his mother were living in the Latin Quarter, at the corner of rue Dauphine and rue Saint André des Arts, and he was attending the Lycée Montaigne. "I couldn't accompany him everywhere, so he went off by himself. When he came back, he recounted to me what he'd seen. My head was elsewhere, but what thrilled and impressed me was his interest in absolutely everything. We lived like that. It was clear that I had my things and he had his, and he had total responsibility for his little existence." Luca used to spend entire days at the Palais. He knew the museum by heart. He was famous for boring everyone to death with useless, disconnected facts, like the distance between the earth and moon in Egyptian cubits. He picked up information like flypaper.

And then there were the smells. It was a little odd. Adela, not knowing what else to do, took it in stride. "I think the first time it really struck me was the summer we rented the house at the beach on the Côte d'Azur. He was seven. And the moment we arrived in this strange place he set about systematically analyzing the smell of the thyme that grew wild everywhere." She sits up straight, almost wary at the memory of it.

When she became manager of product and image design at the

Upim chain of department stores, she took him to Milan. Duccio always spoke to Luca in Italian, so he swam immediately in the language. (Adela spoke to him in French, which she'd learned in Argentina from some Russian aristocrats who had fallen on hard times.) In Milan she founded, in 1974, a feminist publishing house for children's books, Dalla Parte delle Bambine, which set itself the task of "denouncing society's sexism on behalf of children through illustrated books." It publishes today in Italian, French, and Spanish as Du Côté des Filles, "On the Side of the Girls." On moving back to Paris, she founded in 1994 an antisexist organization that creates educational material and runs a website: www.ducotedesfilles.org.

Her leftist politics are contrasted by the Darwinian rightism of her son, essentially molded by his instinctively scientific view of reality. Adela, who labels him "anarcho-conservative" (Turin, for his part, couldn't care less what political camp he falls in), attributes his political views "to his belief in genetics having a great deal to do with human nature."

Duccio, for his part, was developing a scientific theory about appropriate technology, essentially creating an entire field. He was noticed. University College London, which his son would eventually attend as a student, decided to create a professorship in building and so sought out Duccio. He was made a professor at thirty-nine. The United Nations called him back as a deputy secretary-general to organize the famous 1976 Habitat Conference in Vancouver, to which he devoted two years of his life. After the conference, poised for greatness if momentarily exhausted, he left in his car for a vacation in Italy. On a highway near Turin, about thirty miles from where his father was buried, Duccio got in an automobile accident and was killed.

◆　　◆　　◆

IN 1982 AT age twenty-eight, just after he'd finished his Ph.D. in physiology at University College London and moved to the south of France to research at the Villefranche Marine Station near Nice, Luca Turin began getting seriously into perfume.

Villefranche is on the Côte d'Azur just east of Nice and west of

Monte Carlo. It is an interesting hybrid of a place, an island of scientific research floating in a sun-drenched sea of aesthetic hedon-
ism. Turin had a tenured position inside the Centre National de
Recherche Scientifique (CNRS), the massive French scientific bureaucracy that runs most French scientists and, among myriad other
institutes, the Villefranche Marine Station. One could mistake the
marine station for a Club Med with test tubes. One of the many
attractions of the place is the stunning library of the Observatoire
de Nice, high in the hills above the Mediterranean, where observers
and scientists can go and gaze down through the library's wide glass
windows at the sailboats and the tourists in or out of swimsuits
lying far below on the beach, getting melanomas.

It was from this operational base that Turin launched a campaign
of perfume reconnaissances. He carried out these sorties in the
1956 Peugeot 203 of a biology grad student named Philippe Béhé.
Their boss indulged them. "We'd drive," says Turin, "talk, think, listen to classical music on France Musique, discuss everything and
nothing. We lived a completely separate existence." He started with
two fragrances from Caron, new editions of old perfumes, *En Avion*
and *Poivre*.

The collection grew. While he was scouring the perfume shops
of Nice, someone mentioned a Madame Pillaud of Menton, a
French town on the Italian border. So they went. The perfume store
turned out to be run with an iron hand by a woman of somewhere
between sixty and ninety named Madame Claudine Pillaud, who
appeared to be borderline psychotic and whose personal toilette—
makeup and dress—made her very closely resemble a prostitute.
She was both preternaturally suspicious—a paranoiac on a Lavrenty
Beria scale—and sensationally vulgar. "Everyone comes in here and
wants some cocksucking perfume!" she'd bellow, which was an interesting way for a perfume seller to view her clientele. At least she
was consistent: she ran her store according to the iconoclastic economic principle that her perfumes were to be sold to customers
only if she liked them. Should she decide at any given instant that
she didn't, she'd snatch the bottle from the counter, it would disappear into the store's shadowy bowels, and that would be that. There
was no appeal. The difficulty of actually completing a transaction

with Madame was spectacularly compounded by the fact that she was given to violent mood swings.

Many of her perfumes were mundane, but she also had treasures, things no one had seen for fifty years. (Turin was once astounded to realize he was looking at a whole shelf of bottles of Coty's *Chypre*.) She had been buying up the last cases of everything from everyone who had gone out of business and so in her basement had stockpiled the entire history of French perfumery.

Béhé and Turin regularly skipped out of the lab for the forty-five-minute drive to Madame's imperium. The first time he walked into the store, he saw a bunch of rotund sales assistants, like in a bakery. He said, "I'm looking for an old perfume." They said, "*Ah! ça c'est Madame Pillaud qui s'en occupe,*" and carefully stayed out of her territory. She materialized, looked him up and down. "*Oui, jeune homme,*" she said. Yes, young man.

"I'm looking for *Diorama,*" said Turin.

"Everyone's looking for *that,*" she snapped, and then immediately, like the Sphinx, hissed at him: "What is the principal note in *Bellodgia?*"

Turin said, "Carnation."

She blinked her viper lids, withdrew an inch. Well. She evaluated him with narrowed eyes. Reached her claw down into somewhere and slowly, slowly brought out the *Diorama.* "It was real *Diorama,*" says Turin, awed, "a one-ounce tester, the first postwar Dior perfume, not the crap you buy today for two hundred dollars on avenue Montaigne that bears no resemblance to the original fragrance." He paid her a hundred dollars for it.

Then she snapped, "That's nothing!" She disappeared into the depths and a moment later reemerged. He braced himself. She opened her hand, and he saw she was holding a bottle of Lucien Lelong's perfume, which famously contained two dancers inside the bottle, a man and a woman embracing and turning, swimming inside the liquid. She wound it up, and it made music. He moved, entranced, to touch it. She smacked his hand, the arm clutching the bottle snatched it back, and she whisked the Lelong back down into the depths of the store.

Turin tried to be friendly with her. He tried to show that he had a genuine interest in the perfumes. He brought roses to put her in a good mood. It didn't work. She had *real* collectors who came from far away. Who was *he?* Even Turin's considerable charm slid off her. As he put it, she held the knife by the handle. He'd say, "I'm looking for *Chypre.*" She'd say, "I don't have any." He'd say, "What about that?" He'd be pointing at four bottles of *Chypre* lined up on the shelf directly behind her. "I don't have any." "That, right there." She'd glare around at it, then turn back like a python curling its neck and state, "*Ce n'est pas à vendre.*" It's not for sale.

Other days, she was velvet and cream. Delteil's *Shaina* was unknown to Turin, and she simply offered it, spontaneously, as if it were her habit. "This is a good fragrance," she allowed. "I'll sell this one to you." She even let him smell it first. "Sensationally wonderful," he remembered. "Mystical. It was a great modern Oriental, up there with *Emeraude.*"

He drained the money from his salary and paid whatever she demanded.

And eventually, grudgingly, she began allowing him to buy some of her treasures, the classics from the 1800s to 1930s. She would drum her lacquered fingers on the counter, frown, and disappear to emerge with (you never knew what it would be) *Futur* by Piguet, Millot's *Crêpe de Chine* (Turin: "Utterly great! Very famous, from 1929, powdery and sweet with a strong wood"), Lentheric's *Shanghai,* Coty's *L'Origan.* He wore them sometimes, both the men's and the women's fragrances. He liked the unusual old ones like *Futur,* a dry woody chypre, and, every time he could possibly find one, the marvelous creations from Coty's glory days.

Béhé found two things odd about Turin. The first was that where he, Béhé, actually liked to keep the perfumes somewhat distant, mysterious, vaguely magical, Turin wanted to open the hood and get into the engine block, know exactly how they functioned. The second thing was that in all the time he spent with Turin, early mornings and late nights and long drives, he never, ever once saw him yawn.

Many houses were issuing new editions of their old fragrances. The reissues, which bore the names of their originals but frequently differed molecularly, were in part a matter of cost and in part a matter of law. No one dared use the magnificent ambergris tincture or iris of Florence anymore, as their prices per ounce had rocketed past the possible, if not the thinkable. Wonderful molecules called nitro musks—one was the molecule musk ambrette, a Swiss creation—had been used commonly for years, but the Big Boys and, more important, their regulators realized they were toxins and replaced them with other molecules, a trade-off that brought safer molecules but fewer smells. And then there was the adulteration of changing tastes. "Among the Caron reissues," says Turin, "until 1984 they were top level, and then you could tell they'd started slightly inflecting the formula to make them more palatable. *Tabac Blond* was the oddest of the greats, a profoundly strange fragrance, and was thus, of course, the first to be sacrificed."

Sometimes they would go to Paris. Walking down rue Dauphine in the Sixth Arrondissement they found a store specializing in old perfumes. Turin spent hours talking to the young man who ran it. "He was *mad* about perfume, crazy, totally, utterly obsessed. He died of AIDS. He wore *Shanghai,* a woman's fragrance. Ginger, very unusual. It's one of only three fragrances I know of that use ginger. I bought a bottle of Coty's *L'Origan* from him and gave it to a good friend of mine. She used it in two weeks and said, Have you got any more? I said, You have just used the last bottle of *L'Origan* in the known universe."

At the same time, Turin was pursuing his science. He was doing biology, at least officially, but up at the Observatoire de Nice he was dipping into chemistry, and also they had fantastic physics going on, so he started spending time browsing physics in the library. "I've always been interested in everything. I'm reading chemistry books at night for the heck of it, physics in the morning. I find that physics is like oysters—it's best first thing in the morning—so I always have these physics books in the loo."

✦   ✦   ✦

ONE DAY AROUND 1985, Turin was hanging out in the Villefranche library, the solar-heated cobalt-blue sheet of Mediterranean far below, rummaging through old scientific journals. For no particular reason he picked up one called *Chemistry and Industry.* Flipping the pages he noticed a paper on . . . smell. "Odor and Molecular Vibration." He flipped to the front for a second to check: 1977. He flipped back and read through the paper. It proposed a radical idea, one purporting to reveal the secret key to smell. He thought that the whole thing was, as he put it later, "complete crap." Its author, a Canadian named R. H. Wright, was basically just pushing an idea already proposed by an English scientist named Malcolm Dyson in 1938. And Dyson's idea was—to be polite about it—highly unusual.

Dyson had become conscious of a specific, amazing power of the human nose: we can smell and instantly identify the actual *atoms* hidden inside a molecule. A sniff, and we know: "Nitrogen atoms in here," "Sulfur atoms in here." And we never get it wrong. What's more, we can tell every molecule apart from every other. When you encounter "rotten egg" smell, you know there's Sulfur in there. No other atom smells like that, and you never misanalyze that atom. In 1938, Dyson had delivered a paper titled "The Scientific Basis of Odor" to the British Society for Chemistry and Industry. To those serious-minded fellows, peering down at him from the wooden benches of the Oxford amphitheater, he had said: It seems, gentlemen, that the human nose somehow houses some sort of spectroscope made of human flesh. At which point the eyebrows of the fellows of the British Society for Chemistry and Industry shot upward.

A spectroscope is a well-known scientific instrument that, alone in the world of all instruments, has an amazing power: give it some substance, and it can faultlessly identify the atoms inside—"Sulfur in here, Nitrogen in there"—and the molecules they make up, and it does this by measuring molecular vibrations. All molecules pulse with vibrations. They shimmer and wiggle and sing with the vibrations of the electron strings that hold them together, which means molecules are, oddly enough, a sort of musical instrument. Think of microscopic metal Calder mobiles, weighted clumps of atoms connected by springy electron bonds. Mobiles and wind chimes, when struck, usually move only one way: round and round or back and forth. Electron bonds move in and out or side to side, and the more there are in a single molecule, the more complex a wiggling, vibrating motion the molecule will have, and the more notes it will sing. Each molecule gives rise to its own unique set of vibrations, of notes. A spectroscope identifies a molecule by the song it sings.

An atom is a cloud of electrons frenetically orbiting a hard core of protons and neutrons. A molecule is just atoms glued to other atoms. Could be two atoms, could be two thousand. (There are 112 known types of atoms, but the vast majority of common smellable molecules are built of only five: Carbon, Hydrogen, Oxygen, Nitrogen, and Sulfur.) Atoms glue to each other by roping themselves together in cords of electrons. Somewhere in microspace, a Carbon atom approaches a Nitrogen atom. The Carbon's electrons zip around it in a ball, and the Nitrogen's as well, two buzzing spheres. The space between the two diminishes toward zero, their pulsating surfaces kiss—and suddenly one of the Carbon's outermost electrons arcs outward, encircles the Nitrogen, and tightly lassos it like an electric rope, smooshing it toward the Carbon. And the Nitrogen's outermost electron curves like some rogue meteor at lightning speed and envelops the Carbon. Each of these two tiny electrons now orbits both atoms, binding them together like taut double ropes. Which makes the two atoms now one molecule: C=N. (Read that "Carbon double bond Nitrogen.") Each of the ropes is called an electron bond.

The thing about these electron bonds is that they are elastic. Pull the atoms apart and release them. Depending on the strength of the spring and how much the atoms hanging off those springs weigh, each combination of atoms will sing a note just as a piano string, plucked and quivering, sounds its B flat, or its G. Some bonds vibrate lazily at a slow, deep bass, some quiver at slightly faster tenor notes, or brighter altos, or high-pitched sopranos. And like every piano string (a D string only plays a D), every combination of atom-and-bond is tuned to its *one* particular frequency, can only sing its own note. That note—that vibration—is what scientists call a "wave number." Look at a wave-number spectrum: there are only eighty-eight vibrations in a piano (eighty-eight keys from lowest to highest on the keyboard), but wave numbers run from 0 to 4000. Imagine a keyboard of four thousand keys. (Actually, on *this* instrument you can play notes between the keys, too, which means that you basically have an infinite number of notes.)

And if each atomic bond sings one note, every molecule is a fist-ful of these notes, in a unique combination, which means that each molecule is a chord. These bonds—these molecular chords—are what a spectroscope plays.

It plays them by using a familiar phenomenon: resonance. Stand at a piano with the lid open, hold down the sustain pedal, and sing a note. Then listen. You'll hear the piano softly singing your note back to you, because the piano strings matching the frequencies in your note will have been struck, will be resonating, responding. A spectroscope does exactly this: it shines light of thousands and thousands of frequencies at a molecule, and reports exactly which faint, atomic, vibrational echoes at exactly which frequencies are responding to its humming light. Light at frequency 1342.88 pours into the molecule, plucks the electron bonds tuned to 1342.88, and they must sing back. It dusts the mysterious molecule for an audible fingerprint.

Try another analogy. "Imagine," says Turin, "a large pendulum swinging back and forth. *De de de de de de.*" He moves his finger back and forth rhythmically. "A pendulum with a particular height and a particular weight inherently swings back and forth at a particular frequency. Fine. How do you add energy to the swing? You can only do it if you give pushes at the pendulum's natural frequency, when it's moving *away* from you at just the right intervals. *Do, do, do, do,* back and forth." (He hums the notes; the finger moves ever higher.) "Push at the wrong interval"—he pushes his hand jerkily, out of sync, and it crashes into the oncoming imaginary pendulum, which slams to a halt—"and you just counteract the energy."

The expression "We're on the same wavelength" captures it. The best way to sway a person emotionally or intellectually, to get them to say "Yes!," is by hitting them with ideas that correspond to their natural mental frequency: tell them what they already believe.

What is sort of confusing, incidentally, is that if you add energy by shooting in more photons, pouring in more light, the vibration doesn't speed up. It just "gets *bigger.*" But there's an example of this that everyone's experienced: Blow across the mouth of a Coke bot-tle; you get a pitch. Blow harder; the pitch gets louder, but it stays the same pitch. The Coke bottle's mouth has one innate pitch. Of course, it's the same with a piano string. G strings will always play G, struck softly or loudly. The string has an inherent G-ness. So do electron bonds.

It's why spectroscopes are the detective tools of the molecular world. They play the electron bonds together, listen to their chords, and because the vibrations reflect the weights and connecting bonds of the atoms, each molecule's song is a foolproof identity card, its wave-number fingerprint, allowing us to identify it with absolute precision. You come across some strange molecule. You have no idea what atoms are in it. You want to find out. You take the molecule, you put it in this machine, the spectroscope, and you turn it on. The spectroscope aims its laser at the molecules and cuts loose with a blast of photons, particles of light. Billions of photons slam into your molecule, and the spectroscope puts its ear to this humming glob of atoms, its vibrating electrons bonding Oxygen to Carbon. The O-C bonds sing their unique wave number, the spectroscope tells you what it's hearing—and you know: "Oh, there's Oxygen bonded to Carbon in here." Read all the vibrations, add them all up, and you know what the molecule is.

Take the simple ester named methyl acetate, CH_3-C(=O)-O-CH_3. (It's a molecule with a sweet smell, sort of ethereal and not very long lasting.) Like a musical chord with the vibrations C, E, and G—a combination of vibrations that any musician could, with dead certainty, identify: "Oh, C major"—methyl acetate's vibrations all form a specific chord. (The formula, by the way, for figuring out how many vibrational notes are in any molecule is simple: add up the total number of atoms in that molecule, multiply by three, and subtract six. So if your molecule has five atoms, it thus has $5 \times 3 - 6 = 9$ different vibrations. Which is to say the molecule plays its own unique nine-note chord on this keyboard of four thousand wave numbers.) Methyl acetate has eleven atoms, which means it has twenty-seven notes. Its lowest note happens to vibrate at wave number 97. Its top note, way up the scale, is at wave number 3004. Once you know the notes, you know with dead certainty that this is methyl acetate.

You write musical notes in standard musical notation, of course. A single note—say, F in the treble clef—is written like this:

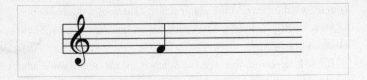

So how to write down just one electron note in a molecule's entire, complex chord? Write that one electron's wave number. Pick some electron string binding a Nitrogen atom to a Sulfur atom. Aim a photon gun at the string and pull the trigger. Wham. The photon slams into the string, making it rocket back and forth (let's say) twenty-five hundred times per second. You can write down that single wave number like this:

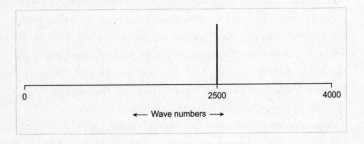

If you write the vibrations in a full chord of musical notes—F dominant seventh—this is what it looks like:

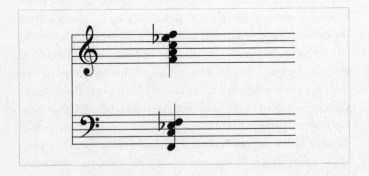

In microspace, a Boron atom and an Oxygen atom bond to each other, plastered together in a high-energy embrace. The embrace sings a note. Stuck onto the B-O by another electron (which sings its own note) are a Carbon and a Nitrogen, which are bound to each other by a tight smear of two electrons. The smear sings two more notes. Write all the notes of the vibrational chord of an entire molecule—say, methyl acetate—and this is what it looks like:

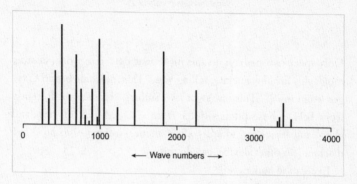

Only methyl acetate will have these notes. It's as clear as G major seventh.

It happens that molecular notes are spread very unevenly over the wave-number scale. From 0 up to around 1500 you find lots of bass and tenor electron bonds. But there aren't many altos, and there are very few electron sopranos; start looking for notes above 1500, and you find they're spread pretty thin, only one every hundred wave numbers or so. Nitrile groups are altos, singing at around 2100. And then there's nothing much until you reach 2500, which is the frenetic soprano of the S-H bond, Sulfur and Hydrogen. As far as Turin knew, nothing else in organic chemistry ever vibrated at precisely 2500 *except* the sulfurous, smelly S-H bond, "so if it's vibrating at twenty-five hundred, you know it's Sulfur, period, end of discussion." Then trudge through another four hundred or so wave numbers of empty desert in which nothing ever, ever vibrates, till at last, on the outermost horizon, the electrons that bond Carbon to Hydrogen vibrate, shrieking, at 2900 or so, with the OHs and the NHs (alcohols and amines) at the very upper limit.

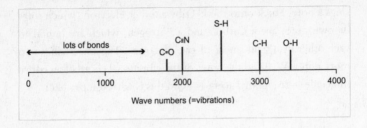

Only spectroscopes can do this molecular detective work, dusting molecules for fingerprints, telling you, "This molecule has an Oxygen atom in it!" "This one's got two Sulfurs!" H_2S sings differently from FeH, whose pitches differ from C_3O_2. A box of glass and metal and lasers can identify all of them. Nothing else, no other machine, no other device, can do this.

Except the human nose.

And this was Dyson's observation. Sniff something—a mango, an egg, a fizzing, just lit match—and you'll effortlessly smell *atoms,* Sulfur and Hydrogen and Oxygen atoms. Carbons that are bonded to Nitrogens we identify by smelling their metallic oily odor, and Nitrogen-Carbon-Sulfur bonds (called isothiocyanate groups) give a molecule a mustardy smell. Amine groups (NH_3) you can smell by the fishy odor they add to any molecule, and you smell nitro groups (NO_2) as a sweet ethereal—or etherlike—odor. AsH_2 (arsine groups) smell like cabbage. Wrinkling your nose at that "sulfur smell" *is an atomic analysis absolutely diagnostic of Sulfur and Hydrogen atoms.* Malcolm Dyson's 1938 theory—that the nose was operating like a spectroscope—explained this.

And it explained something else: the Mystery. It solved the paradox that smell is both instant and yet unlimited. If you say the nose is measuring Vibration, the mystery, which exists only because of Shape's well-understood limitations, disappears. With Vibration, smell could be instant *and* unlimited. Smell, said Malcolm Dyson, must therefore *not* be Shape. Smell must be Vibration. How else, he argued, how else in the world could human beings possibly smell molecules, all of them, instantly? The nose *must* be a spectroscope. The theory made eminent sense. It explained the facts, as all good theories are supposed to. It was logical, insightful, and ingenious. There was only one problem with it: it was absurd.

The absurdity was very simple: there was absolutely no way you were going to make a spectroscope out of meat, of human flesh. Spectroscopes have to generate infrared light, must have pockets that hold molecules, must be connected to energy sources, all of which adds up to a heavy, bulky, four-foot-long machine of glass and metal and wires that sits on your lab bench. It was ridiculous. Everyone told Dyson this in 1938, and they repeated it when Wright tried to revive the Vibrational theory in the 1960s.

This is what they said: It's Shape. Smell is Shape. Every molecule has a unique combination of bumps and grooves and curves, as singular as a fingerprint, and when a smell molecule flies into the receptor, the receptor feels its shape all over, and says, "Aha! It's *this!*" Shape (we know) is the way every other receptor works, from digestive enzymes to neurotransmitters to the immune system. So Shape must be smell. Smell is Shape.

Biologists split into Vibrationists and Shapists. The Shapists were led into battle against the Vibrationists by the English scientist John Amoore. Amoore had a powerful weapon, a strange pair of molecules called enantiomers.

Enantiomers are mirror-image molecules. Their shapes are exactly identical—except exactly reversed, literally reflections of each other, as if you were holding a model of one up to a mirror. But this means that smell receptors *feel* them as shaped differently, just as someone reaching out to shake your hand would feel a difference if you gave them first your right hand, then your left (even though your hands are virtually the same shape). That's why the mirror versions of enantiomers are called R (from the Latin *rectus,* or right-handed) and S (*sinister,* or left-handed). And since the Right and Left versions have the exact same electron bonds, they have the same vibrations, and so sing the exact same song. So enantiomers—like the ones called carvones—have (as far as the receptor is concerned) *different* shapes, but they have the *same* vibrations (both R and S carvones have ten atoms and thus fifty-four vibrations, or notes). So far, unremarkable. The huge problem enantiomers posed for the Vibrationists was this: Shapists pointed out, triumphantly and repeatedly, that no matter how pure you made them, R carvone smells of mint. But S smells like caraway seeds. Same vibrations. Different shapes. And different smells. Smell, therefore, must be Shape.

And so, as Turin put it, "you're screwed." And by 1980, with Amoore pointing out the absurdity of a flesh spectroscope and Shapists chanting "Carvones!," the Vibrational smell theory was.

Turin dropped the paper and went happily back to rummaging through old journals.

◆   ◆   ◆

THEN TURIN LEFT Nice and the observatory's views. It was 1988. He went to Paris and the Pasteur Institute, one of the more prestigious, high-powered science factories in the world and the center of the universe for French biology. "And of course I was bored," says Turin, "and looking for something different in my profession." One thing he decided to tackle, because he thought it would be fun, was a tiny mystery. It happened to involve something he hadn't much thought about before, called electron transfer.

In Nice, he'd happened upon a book on a thing called a polarograph, and he'd gotten interested. It's a machine that uses pearls of mercury to give you a perfectly smooth, creamy surface in a water bath. You throw a handful of molecules into the water, connect the droplet of mercury to a battery, and measure different currents as electrons jump from the mercury to the molecules. The weird thing was, people had noticed that when you cranked the battery up to a certain voltage, the mercury would sometimes begin to spin like molten lava in a washing machine. No one knew why, and very few people cared. Which meant that Turin got hooked. This wasn't his field at all, not biology at all, it was physics really, an alien realm that biologists didn't usually dare enter, but he wasn't intimidated, and he headed directly into it.

He was in bed—it was 1989—at 2:00 A.M. in his flat in Montmartre when the answer came to him suddenly in a single image. The details are complex; what mattered was that he was thinking about electrons, electron bonds, electrons moving places. He wrote up a paper and for the hell of it published it in the journal *Soviet Electrochemistry,* "because it was a cool journal." (Also because he was curious how they'd translate it from the English into Russian, and then back into English for the international version. He happily considered after the exercise that the paper had gained something in the translations.) Then instead of getting out, he dove into electrochemistry and solid-state electronics, reading everything he could get his hands on. He became totally obsessed with electrochemistry for a year. People said, "Turin, what the hell are you doing? You're a biologist." His cheerful response was "Screw you," and he kept on reading.

Because he was consuming these sorts of things, he found a paper by a scientist named Shinagawa called "The Semi-Conductive Nature of the Brdicka Current." And because he'd waded through enough electrochemistry, he understood it. The paper suggested something strange: that it was theoretically possible to make proteins carry electrons, conduct electricity. This, everyone figured, was (with all due respect to Shinagawa) garbage. They'd already tried it. They'd taken pure proteins. Dried them and made tablets, something like aspirin. They'd put two wires on either side of the tablets and asked if current flowed through them. Yes? No. Proteins didn't conduct. Everyone knew this.

Turin decided to see if he could make proteins conduct.

He wasn't, in trying to do what people thought couldn't be done, just being willfully perverse. Shinagawa's argument struck him as solid. Also, a person could find a nice little publishing niche by writing up a proof contradicting the literature and What Everyone Knew about proteins. And also, yes, for the hell of it. But mostly it was because he had noticed something.

While working with the polarograph, he'd found it really tricky, this business of squeezing out these little droplets of mercury; the droplets tended to glom on to each other instantly, but in the 1920s people had noticed that a little bit of protein would prevent this. The protein acted like a nonstick cooking spray on the mercury drops, covered them in a very thin layer, like a one-molecule-thick film of butter.

Sparked by Shinagawa, Turin now thought this over. What would happen if you took two of these mercury drops, covered each with this single layer of nonstick protein, squeezed them up next to each other, stuck a wire in them, and sent an electrical current through both droplets and their protein layer? Would electrons flow across the protein? Because now you were no longer measuring thousands of densely layered proteins like in the aspirin tablet. You were measuring exactly two, an electron jumping from one layer of protein a single molecule deep to another.

He tried it. The electrons flowed. Proteins did indeed conduct electrons. Turin realized that everyone else had been wrong because this was the first time anyone had tried to make electrons flow between only one layer of proteins so that the electrons needed to jump only once. And so—now this was *really* fun—he set out to make a diode, a device that conducts electrons in only one direction, out of protein. Which protein? Well, how about albumin— egg white—because, he figured, it's the cheapest protein you can buy. Egg white is a big protein, 50,000 daltons (atomic mass units). He made the diode. It worked. It was, in fact, quite stable. No one else had ever made a diode out of protein, animal cells, bits of biological material, so he got it patented. The patent title is "A Semiconductor Device with Protein as Its Active Element," U.S. Patent No. 5258627. It's listed on a webpage that someone keeps on weird diodes.

So he was spending a lot of time thinking about how proteins transferred electrons. And—in no obviously connected way— because of his perfume habit he also happened to be thinking a lot about smell. Which was perhaps why an American colleague approached him: Hey, Turin, the U.S. Navy is funding a project on olfaction, you should go for some DOD money. The navy wanted, it turned out, to smell submarines. Specifically, they wanted to make sensors that could smell the odors that spent ordnance, or the enemy subs themselves, left behind, the trail of their scent as they slid through the waters. So Turin put together an application to the U.S. Navy and sent it in.

Then something nasty happened. The incident forced a profound change in Turin's life. He won't talk about it. It happened in 1990, and it involved his chancing upon someone's major scientific fraud (the someone being, unfortunately for Turin, a very important and powerful French scientist). This was followed by the bitter leveling of accusations, some hurried behind-the-scenes deal making, and the strong suggestion by the top people in the CNRS that Turin find another lab within a week. After which Turin made a few grim international phone calls.

One call Turin made was to an American neurophysiologist, a friend of his named Mark Dearborn. They'd met in England at University College London. Dearborn was now at the National Institutes of Health in North Carolina. Was there, Turin wondered, a visiting position for him at the NIH? It would (his bosses at the CNRS had indicated) be convenient to have an ocean approximately the size of the Atlantic between him and France. I'm on it, said Dearborn.

Turin moved to North Carolina in June of 1990 to set up shop at the NIH.

✦　　✦　　✦

HE ADAPTED EASILY to the move with the help of Dearborn and his wife, Anna. The Dearborns had a screened porch on their house, and most quiet Carolina evenings they ate dinner there together. Turin tagged along with them and their infant son on various trips, looking around interestedly at America and enjoying the South. It was in North Carolina in 1991 that two things happened, completely unrelated. Luca learned about the first at breakfast one morning on the porch, when Mark handed him the *New York Times* Science Times section over the table and pointed apologetically at an article about smell.

All biologists knew that people who researched smell had faced, for what seemed like forever, a galling, embarassingly fundamental problem: despite all efforts, no biologist had ever managed to find the receptor proteins for smell in the nose, the most basic parts of the smell machine, the pieces that actually grabbed the smell molecules. You couldn't really work on the sense without them. Scientists had long ago turned up the receptors that received photons for vision, not to mention those handling digestion, the immune system, the reception of neurotransmitters, and on and on. But not, bizarrely, smell. They had to be there. There was even a forest of proteins people were hunting in, a huge, generic class of multipurpose receptors (they were called G-protein-coupled receptors because they used little things called G-proteins as their bike messengers to other enzymes inside the cell). These receptors had been worked out molecularly—a Nobel Prize in Physiology and Medicine for this—and everyone assumed the olfactory receptors were hidden, somewhere in the foliage of this vast class. For years several labs had been sending expeditions deep into the G-protein class, trying to flush them out. But the molecular reconnaissance had turned up nothing. The hidden smell receptors remained tantalizingly elusive.

Then along came a young molecular biologist named Linda Buck. She was at Columbia University, in the lab of Richard Axel. Axel is one of the big guns in molecular biology, brilliant and powerful and brusque. "Richard," says one scientist tightly, "is not known for editing himself." Axel is universally acknowledged to be both blisteringly smart and frighteningly ambitious.

Gambling her career on answering the Sphinx's question of smell, Buck started searching the G-protein class for the smell receptors. After a long, frustrating search, she was sitting at her kitchen table one Saturday night, looking through data results, when she realized she'd found them. Buck and Axel published the smell-receptor paper together in 1991 in *Cell,* which is populated by the great sharks that swim in molecular biology. "In science currency," Luca says, "*Cell* is AmEx platinum. *The New York Times* ran the study on the front page of its Tuesday Science Times the day before it came out in *Cell,* which is of course exactly where we all want to be. It was Huge, Sexy Science, and everyone was in awe. And jealous."

The bottom line was that if a person happened to want to work on smell, that person now had the receptors he needed.

The second thing happened that summer, during a drive home from a trip to the beach near Beaufort, North Carolina. Turin and the Dearborns were in the middle of nowhere east of Raleigh near the intersection of Highway 70 and I-95 when Turin spotted some signs: CIGARETTES, and also LIQUOR, and then one that announced JR PERFUMES. LARGEST DISCOUNT PERFUME STORE IN THE WORLD. He and Anna looked at each other. Mark and his young son sat in the sweltering car with their dripping Tastee-Freez cones, waiting for Turin and Anna. An hour and a half later—"You couldn't print all the names I called them under my breath," says Dearborn—they emerged from the store. Turin was carrying a huge cardboard box he could barely see around, filled with perfume.

They spent the rest of the drive home smelling. Turin explained each fragrance, its creator's oeuvre, its chemical provenance and molecular construction. The Dearborns were astounded at his breadth of knowledge and by how entertaining he made it. "Why don't you just write a damn perfume guide and get it over with," Mark said.

Turin decided he would.

✦   ✦   ✦

AT THIS MOMENT, Turin got word from CNRS that they'd no longer be paying his NIH salary. They wanted him back in France. He packed up and thanked the Dearborns. In Paris, he found that the new lab was unavailable for a few months, so he sat down at his little Mac in his mother's apartment near avenue Wagram, his mother working at her Mac across the room, and started writing perfume reviews. As he finished, he handed them to her. With each one, she was more surprised. She'd only ever seen his writing on biophysics.

For the first three reviews, he didn't even bother to smell the perfumes. He'd smelled them so many times, knew every molecular nook and cranny, each glinting facet as they revealed themselves to him over hours, that he just reached into his memory and pulled out the smells and waved the words into them. *Vetiver* by Guerlain, *Rive Gauche* by Yves Saint Laurent, *Après l'Ondée* by Guerlain.

Rive Gauche (Yves Saint Laurent)

Grâce à Rive Gauche, les mortels connaissent enfin l'odeur du savon de Diane au bain. . . .

Thanks to *Rive Gauche,* mortals can at last know the scent of the goddess Diana's bath soap. A true emblem of the '70s, this sumptuous reinterpretation of the innovative metallic note found in the less fortunate *Calandre* (Paco Rabanne) belongs to the uncrowded category of sculpture-perfumes. Its seamless silvery form, initially hidden by white, powdery notes, soon pierces the clouds and gains height by the hour. Like *Chamade* (Guerlain), *Rive Gauche* enjoys a peculiar relationship with intensity: the more time passes, the stronger its grace becomes, as if fading allowed its inner light to radiate more easily. A masterpiece. A notable example of the perfect agreement between container and content, its atomizer of metal and blue stripes, at once precious and whimsically "industrial," is itself an item of undying chic. The perfume seems slightly superior in quality to the eau de toilette.

Après l'Ondée (Guerlain)

Divinely named ["After the Rainshower"], a prototype of the cold and melancholy fragrance, this stunning creation is the counterpart—the brighter, fresher younger brother—of the mysterious *L'Heure Bleue* (Guerlain). *Après l'Ondée* evolves only slightly with time: its central white note, caressing and slightly venomous, like the odor of a peach stone, imposes itself immediately and retains its mystery forever. Its simplicity, its keen nostalgia, and its unadorned beauty make this an anomaly for Guerlain.

The current eau de toilette seems a bit attenuated, more timid than the marvelous perfume. Choose the latter.

Vetiver (Guerlain)

One of the rare perfumes so named that do not betray the character of this uncompromising raw material, *Vetiver* is a temperament as much as it is a perfume, above all when it is worn by a woman. Stoic and discreet, *Vetiver* scorns all luxury save that of its own proud solitude. At the same time distant and perfectly clear, it must be worn muted and must never allow itself to be sensed except at the instant of a kiss.

His mother edited his reviews. She was, he would say afterward, beaming. So was he. He found it one of the single greatest pleasures of his life. The images came pouring out, and Adela focused her critical energies on paring down the efflorescence. The descriptions took him fifteen minutes or they took five hours, depending, and every day when he had completed his three or four new ones, he felt incredible satisfaction. "I assume it's what a movie director feels when he's got great dailies in the can. When I managed to capture this awesome beauty and greatness in *language,* translating smells into black-and-white words on the page and making this ether tangible and real—that was thrilling."

He pauses, thinks about the words in his head going down to the paper. "You know, perhaps the edge I have in turning smell into language is that for me smell has always had an utterly solid reality that, to my utter astonishment, it doesn't seem to have for other people. Every perfume I've ever smelled has been to me like a movie, sound and vision, which to most people are thoroughly real senses—but not smell, for some reason. To me, *smell is just as real as they are.*"

He called around, took the manuscript to the large French publishers, Hachette and Flammarion and Gallimard and so on, "and most of them told me to sod off." Someone said to him, You know, there's a little outfit that puts out these guides. By the time the third person had said it, he was ready to find the company's offices.

Hermé is actually a huge bookbinding company that, says Turin, "just decided to publish books so they could go to the parties at the book fairs. At the time they'd put in charge a complete scoundrel of a man, very charming and a genuine French cynic. His attitude, delivered with an even smile, was 'It's a nice idea. We'll take it. And you clearly know what you're doing, but frankly if it wasn't you and I'd thought of the idea, I'd have found some jerk in Paris who would have written a completely bullshit guide that would sell just as well.'" He shrugged and reached for the manuscript. Turin shrugged and gave it to him.

The book, called simply *Parfums: Le Guide,* was published in 1992 and became the best-selling perfume guide in France. Perhaps it was the fact that no one had ever done anything quite like it. Perhaps it was the lushness of the critical prose ("Caron's *Alpona* juxtaposes a resinous candied-orange-peel idea with a civilized chypre base"). The FNAC, the French superstore, sold it. It was stacked twelve high at Sephora, the perfume giant (the manager of the big Sephora on the Champs-Elysées told Turin they gave a copy to each new sales associate, which pleased him). That officially it sold eight thousand copies made him figure the publisher had ripped him off—"They've probably sold four times more books than they've told me and just kept all the profits," he says briskly—but so it went. He'd sort of expected it.

What he did not expect was that the guide would change his life in the most wonderful way by cracking open to him the hermetically sealed, well-hidden world of those who create perfumes.

Virtually all the smells in all scented products in the world are manufactured by six huge companies that operate in carefully guarded anonymity: International Flavors & Fragrances (United States), Givaudan Roure (Switzerland), Quest International (Britain), Firmenich (Switzerland), Haarmann & Reimer (Germany), and Takasago (Japan). These are the Big Boys, the industrial giants of the production and sale of a specific, unusual product: molecules. Molecules that trigger the human sense of taste and, above all, the sense of smell. Taste is, actually, a dwarfish, minimally functional sense responding to only six different stimuli: sweet, sour, salt, bitter, umami (richness), and astringent; smell—which in point of fact gives us some 90 percent of what we taste—is thought to respond to ten thousand or so distinguishable molecular smells, but we only say ten thousand because (and this is literally true) we've thus far never touched the limits of smell's power to detect odorant molecules. The Big Boys' molecules generate roughly $20 billion a year in economic activity. They employ hundreds of chemists, molecular jockeys who spend their days welding atoms together to create new molecules with new smells. And, upstairs, they employ an army of perfumers, who spend *their* days mixing these molecules into new scented elixirs.

The Big Boys have two kinds of perfumers. The functional perfumers work with the Johnson & Johnsons, the Procter & Gambles, to scent Tide detergent and Palmolive soap and peach-vanilla candles and the fabric softeners that smell of a million mythical springtimes in distant countries we've never known. These corporate employees create the smell track of our everyday lives, which we barely notice and for which we pay billions of dollars. (A new furniture polish on the market: you open it, sniff—hmm, nice! Buy? Not buy? You sniff again. . . .) The Big Boys won't tell you who they work for. Their names never appear on the toilet-paper label, the shampoo bottle. But where they get positively paranoically secretive is perfume. Because, in fact, all the golden liquid scents sold by the Giorgio Armanis and Vera Wangs, the Ralph Laurens and Jean Paul Gaultiers from their houses of fashion in New York and Paris and London and Milan, these expensive concoctions being sprayed on models and celebrities in the photographs and rip-open ads in the glossies—these scents are not, in fact, created by Mr. Armani or Ms. Wang or Mr. Lauren at all. They are made by professional ghosts working in the locked offices and labs of the Big Boys. These haute perfumers, carefully anonymous and discreetly faceless, are the ones who actually craft the fragrant elixirs in little jeweled five-ounce bottles slipped into boxes that are sold under the names Gaultier and Wang in the department stores' glass cases.

It is the perfumers who transform the confidential briefs from the religious visions and aesthetic hallucinations at the houses of Dior and Calvin Klein and Givenchy—obsessions and poisons and envies and joys; "We want the smell of old melting candles in ballrooms of Italian marble during a Chinese winter," "Give us the fragrance surrendered by a young blue flower crushed under the heated, ivory back of a woman with chocolate eyes," "We must have the scent lightning makes the instant it strikes a platinum rose." The perfumers turn these visions into structures of neutrons and protons and electrons welded together that make our eyes suddenly open, make us sit up, turn and inhale, molecules that blossom and flame, molecules that spin stories.

They never speak to the media. They may quietly attend their chemical offspring's launch parties at Issey Miyake and Donna Karan and Anna Sui (staying out of range of the cameras—to you they'll just look like one more guest), glass bottles lining the walls, or watch from the back as Thierry Mugler and Jean Paul Gaultier are strafed by the flashes. Then they go back to their offices and labs and get back to work transforming more emotion, desire, and smart marketing into actual chemical potions that can be sold and bought. It was the creations of these nameless creators that Turin had dared to transform into language in a book, and to evaluate and judge. And the faceless creators were fascinated.

At first they thought Turin was a spy. That was the rumor. A professional perfumer using a pseudonym? A rogue in the industry? Possibly a thief of some sort. (Son of a bitch.) He wasn't. They thought he was one of them, secretly putting his prose together in the office down the hall. He wasn't. Which made them even more intrigued. A *scientist?* Yes, a chemist, apparently—no, no, a *biologist.* Some kind of *professor,* believe it or not. Suspicious, they checked his curriculum vitae. Well, what did he want? He wanted to meet them was what he wanted. So they obliged. Naturally, they were not uniformly elated. He had not spared anyone's feelings. He was writing in the trade magazines now, in English, and he acted as if he owed nothing to anyone.

57 for Her (Chevignon) ★

Chevignon is a fashion house of such toe-curling vulgarity that one finds oneself hoping that they will never come up with a good fragrance, for one would then have to praise it. Fortunately, that possibility remains as remote as ever. *57 for Her* is a sad little thing, an incongruous dried-prunes note with a metallic edge that manages the rare feat of being at once cloying and harsh.

And this.

Python (Trussardi) ★

The absurdly named *Python* is a poverty-stricken sweet-powdery affair, a very distant relative of the wonderful *Habanita* (Molinard). It belongs in a tree-shaped diffuser dangling from the rearview mirror of a Moscow taxi.

It made their hair stand on end. On the other hand, there was this.

Paradox (Jacomo) ★★★★★

Beauty itself, as with faces, is not simple: perfumes can be handsome (*Mitsouko*), graceful (*Calandre*), gorgeous (*Joy*), comely (*Shalimar*), radiant (*Tommy Girl*), exquisite (*Après l'Ondée*), stunning (*Angel*). Reader beware: *Paradox* is, to paraphrase something once said about Scriabin's music, a perfume of "almost unbearable loveliness." One of the properties of loveliness is that it disarms all attempts to be serious, and turns all critical machinery into a pile of whirring junk. What I find all the more irritating is that *Paradox* isn't even "my type." It is, after all, yet another fruit salad of the type that has kept perfumers gainfully employed since *Deci-Delà*. But this fruit salad does something that it has no right to do: break hearts. If this were music, it would be Bizet's Symphony in C. If it were a car, it would be a Facel-Vega Facellia. If it were an aircraft it would be a 1959 Caravelle in Air France livery. Anyway, go smell it.

And this.

Rush (Gucci) ★★★★★

Gucci hasn't put a foot wrong for some time, both *Envy* perfumes were landmarks, and expectations were high for their latest. The first sniff gave me a shock of recognition, like a long-forgotten but familiar face, and I spent a few busy minutes dredging my memory for the original impression . . . *Dioressence!*

Not all of it, mind you, just a bit I loved, which in the original happened two or three hours into the story and felt like a warm breath whispering crazy things in my ear. That breath is back, now strong, loud, irresistible, a sultry wind fit to keep everyone stark awake and plotting indiscretions. . . . The charm of this perfume is entirely man-made, no mention of Nature, e.g. flowers, etc. This thing smells like a person. To be exact, thanks to the milky lactone note, it smells like an infant's breath mixed with his mother's hair spray. . . . What *Rush* can do, as all great art does, is create a yearning, then fill it with false memories of an invented past . . .

This, words that turned their scents into concreteness, they had never really experienced (except perhaps in the classified briefs they received from Kenzo and Hugo Boss, but those were theoretical marching orders, not synaptic evaluations of the olfactory work they'd wrought). So they began sending out feelers. Turin got messages from legendary names he'd heard, people the public never knows who do the work sold under the names the public does. He got a call from Françoise Caron, née Françoise Cresp, a member of one of the most important perfume families in Grasse and the former wife of the legendary Pierre Bourdon, who did *Cool Water*. Although his guide had said nothing but bad things about her *Gio* for Armani, Caron asked Turin to pay her a visit. She was a top perfumer at one of the biggest Big Boys, Quest International, at their offices in Paris. Turin swallowed hard and knocked on their doors. They let him in, introduced him around; he met all the perfumers and found that most of them had read his guide, that they took it and him seriously. He met the perfumers Christopher Sheldrake, and Gilles Romey, who told Turin he had loved the guide, and Maurice Roucel, the perfumer who had created one of his favorite fragrances, *K* by Krizia, the Milanese couturier.

He was euphoric at being admitted to this closed world. They told him secrets, perfume stories. He met (he could barely believe it) the legendary Guy Robert, and listened with quivering attention to Robert's regal recounting of anecdotes of all the famous scents and their creators. (How did *Chanel No. 5*, one of the greatest perfumes of all time, happen? Well! they said, you see, there are several versions. Some say on the question of the name that the legendary perfumer Ernest Beaux had been messing around with aldehydes and had prepared several samples, and Coco Chanel, called Coco because she threw the most fabulous cocaine parties in Paris, chose the fifth sample. Others say that no, it was actually Beaux's assistant who screwed up the sample Beaux presented to Chanel, put ten times as much aldehyde in the concentration as was specified. Coco loved it, and when Beaux smelled it he realized it was a mistake but didn't dare say anything to her, so *Chanel No. 5* is actually a wildly successful error. Take your pick.) And since Turin had never been in a perfumery lab—Could he see? Please? Certainly he could—they whisked him through halls and halls of glass and metal, thousands of vials of patented, proprietary molecules, plump files stashed in reams of cabinets filled with precious industrial secrets, yard after yard of formulas and structures of molecule upon molecule, the precious corporate data generated by an army of perfume chemists trying to create new smells that would generate billions of dollars for these industrial giants.

As he poked around, they started putting a few questions to him about their creations. What did he think of this one? Was that one beautiful? Surprising? Insouciant? Classic? Reserved? Would this sell? Would that? His ability to describe odors in words mesmerized them. One day he was in Françoise Caron's office, and she asked him what he thought of a new fragrance. It was something she'd created for Escada. He inhaled it, said it was wonderful, that it was like one of those silks that has two colors to it, depending on how the light strikes it. Caron gave him a long look. She reached into her desk and pulled out the brief from the people at Escada and handed it to him. She pointed: Read there. He read, "We want it to smell like the silks that have two colors in them, depending on the light."

Then there was the science of it. The chemistry, specifically. He started meeting the molecule wranglers, including Charles Sell. Sell was a Briton based at Quest's headquarters in Ashford, Kent, an hour southeast of London. Trim and controlled with gray hair and an unflappable professional manner, he ran a team of Quest fragrance chemists. His first lieutenant was Karen Rossiter, an attractive young woman and an up-and-coming chemist at Quest. Sell showed Turin all around. Turin had a great time. The two hit it off—Sell's knowledge of perfume chemistry encyclopedic and Turin's interest inexhaustible. The chemists working away in their white lab coats were doing amazing three-dimensional modeling of the shapes of all sorts of atomic structures that had this or that smell because smell was Shape, and all the secrets of smell were to be found in the shapes of molecules. (Turin leaned closer to the screens.) Sell's responsibility at Quest was the creation of new smells, which meant creating molecules that had never existed before, which by definition meant smells that had never existed before, since no two molecules have ever been known to have the exact same smell. Sell and his team had lately been using computers, the computers' purpose being to predict smells. The prediction of smell determined, after all, the productivity—and profitability—of the industry: how efficiently can I predict what some purely theoretical molecule will smell like without actually going to all the trouble and time and expense of actually building it?

Turin watched molecular shapes flashing rapidly across screens and heard chemists saying, "Well, if it's spherical here and here, it must smell like fresh cedar or burnt sugar." As he took all of this in, seeing what was required for the smell chemists at the Big Boys—Givaudan and IFF and Firmenich and Takasago—to produce a single, marketable smell molecule in their vast, sparkling labs, he was . . . startled. Taken aback, thrown in a way he couldn't put his finger on. It wasn't actually the science that struck him at first. What made him frown initially was the economics.

Consider the way Sell and other chemists made smell molecules. First, Sell essentially took fistfuls of atoms and pieces of molecules he hoped would be interesting (often parts of previous smell best-sellers) and went about putting them together in as many new ways as he could, electrons embracing atoms bonded by other electrons. This created hundreds or thousands of new-shaped molecules. When automated, the process was called, logically, combinatorial chemistry.

It wasn't random. Sell did have some guidelines. Fragrance chemists wanted to make patentable molecules, so they tended toward "theme and variations," took a structure that smelled good and was decently easy to synthesize and started sticking things on it—methyl groups, ethyls, aldehydes. And they only had a certain number of atomic ingredients to play with. They weren't going within a thousand miles of, say, the malevolent fluorophosphonates, which include sarin, a notorious chemical weapon, and which react with absolutely everything, generally in a way that kills it as quickly and painfully as possible. And they would stay away from groups known to smell bad, like isonitriles and sulfides, or to give toxicity problems, like nitros. So it wasn't just anything and everything. But when you got down to it, it was basically a shotgun-blast approach: load, fire, see what comes together, and repeat—random recombination chemistry. In the end Sell would wind up with between five hundred and two thousand (the chemists, forever cagey, would never reveal to Turin exactly how many) different new molecules per year.

Now, having created them, Sell began sorting through the new inventions one by one, smelling and testing each, a ruthless, painstaking process of attrition.

Ninety-five percent didn't smell interesting. So he tossed those out, which meant he had only 5 percent left. Of the interesting ones, many were too weak to use; the customer would have to pour a full pint or so on her body—impractical. So he tossed another 95 percent.

Which meant that after the chemists had painstakingly sorted through a couple thousand molecules (and the company had paid many salaries to the many chemists doing it), maybe twenty molecules remained that were both interesting and sufficiently strong smelling. The smell chemists wrapped these up carefully, said a prayer, and sent them upstairs to the perfumers.

The perfumers sat in their sleek offices in Geneva and Paris and New York, their smelling strips wet with new scents, and stared out their windows trying to think of uses for these things. They'd worked miracles in the past, pulling them out of their bag of tricks, molecules that had launched the megaperfumes, and the megabrands. Tipped pitchers of aldehydes into *Chanel No. 5.* Pumped di-hydromyrcenol, a citrus-lime, into the engine blocks of *Drakkar Noir* and *Cool Water,* run *Escape* by Calvin Klein on Helional. Cast musk R-1 prominently in *Tommy Girl* and powered *Beautiful* for Estée Lauder and Calvin Klein's *Eternity* with Iso E Super. But that was last year. The new briefs with new corporate desires kept land-ing on their desks. Tom Ford was dreaming of a perfume that smelled like fresh cherry wood licked by a green-hot oxygen fire in a Balinese temple, Marc Jacobs absolutely demanding a blossoming daffodil floating on an ocean of smoky Siberian snows—would these molecules work? (The perfumers sifted through their bags.) Was there a smoky metallic here? A wood in green flame? And the answer, statistically, was probably no. In basements beneath the per-fumers, gathering dust, were vast, ever expanding glass-vial grave-yards of molecules the chemists down below had proffered to them and which they had discarded. This maddened the chemists, who had sweated the creation of each one. And the accountants glow-ered over in their paper fiefdoms because with every molecule the chemists created, the company was pouring out money, most of which just flowed into the graveyard. How much money? Turin started asking questions, pointed or oblique depending on where he was and what he thought he could get out of them. This, however, was the perfume industry, everything was opaque and slant, and they never really gave him much concrete information. The best estimate he got arrived during a slightly unguarded moment when Charles Sell named a figure of roughly $4,000 per compound, which in a bad year could have you throwing $8 million down the toilet pretty easily, but as usual this went unconfirmed. The per-fumers, tossing out the molecules they didn't like, culled the few they did for Yohji Yamamoto and Vivienne Westwood. These, they sent back downstairs to the chemists.

And then, on these, came yet *more* triage. First, toxicology test-ing—which was both "Will we be sued for causing cancers if we put this on people's skin?" and "Does this product degrade the ecology, poison streams, and so on?"—a process always done by subcon-tracting firms that charged the Big Boys' accountants around a quarter of a million dollars to test a single molecule. Fixed external costs. It shot the price of each new molecule skyward. If a molecule survived toxicology, the chemists then had to find an economical synthesis process for it, which meant: How can we make this thing cheaply, accurately, and efficiently? Because if it cost millions to make, it was worth nothing. Those they couldn't find a synthesis for were pitched into the graveyard with the rest.

In the end, the very, very rare molecule that smelled strong, was cheap to make, had tested biologically safe and environmentally sound, was patentable, and had a useful odor—that one became a new product in the Big Boys' commercial catalogs. A single decent smell molecule that hit all the right marks could bring money flooding in.

This was why the Big Boys and their stockholders optimally wanted to produce three or so molecules a year. The reality was that each was spending millions every year to create thousands and thousands of molecules, synthesize hundreds, test dozens, and get maybe one onto the shelves. This was what Turin found strange.

The deeper he got into the Big Boys, the more conscious he became that the stockholders were saying to the executives in the boardrooms (and the executives were saying to the chemists in the labs), "Look, to up profits, why can't we come out with ten new molecules a year? How about it?" And he was aware—now it was the science of it that caught him—that the molecular theory that governed these chemists creating these molecules and, thus, the entire massive industry, was Shape. But he didn't really focus. He was busy making friends and having fun. He left for other parts of the building.

Turin is an instinctive egalitarian with an exquisitely refined aesthetic and unabashedly elitist tastes, and so he felt completely comfortable in the perfume world, which is populated by former members of the lower classes who spend their time creating outrageously expensive aesthetically oriented luxury goods for the rich. He met the legendary perfumer Serge Lutens and began frequenting the headquarters of Lutens's Paris empire. Lutens was a working-class kid who started out as a makeup specialist with the estimable French firm Carita and, after successes there, was snapped up by Dior to be their chief colorist, deciding the Dior makeup line each year. In 1980 he left Dior for Shiseido. They wanted him to create their makeup line in Paris, but by this time Lutens had grander aims and worked out a nice deal: he would create their makeup and at the same time open and direct a neck-snappingly chic Shiseido Paris outpost where he would launch a new line of Shiseido perfumery (which he would design), their flag-ship leading-edge offerings. He had no training in perfumery and none in chemistry either, but he knew what he liked, and that, as is ever the case in fashion, was his genius. Lutens chose Christopher Sheldrake of the Big Boy Quest to be his secret engineer, building in chemicals the concepts Lutens would supply. Sheldrake, in Turin's view, is "a really interesting perfumer. He has this minimalist attitude toward perfumery and, under Serge's direction, has been delivering one wonderful fragrance after another."

The first perfume Lutens directed for Shiseido, the infamous *Nombre Noir,* burned a hole into everyone's collective memory. Molecularly blacksmithed by one of Shiseido's in-house Japanese perfumers, it arose from components selected by Lutens (an extremely expensive natural osmanthus straight from the flower and a synthetic, a big-stock damascone molecule of rosy-woody plus prune—"a brilliant juxtaposition of the two," said Turin). The perfume had beautiful packaging, "the most unremittingly, sleekly, maniacally *luxurious* packaging you can imagine: a black octagonal glass Chinese bottle nestled in exquisitely folded black origami of the most sensuous standard." It was a 1982 issue, and Turin had heard the rumors, as had everyone else, that despite its (significant) retail price, *Nombre Noir* lost money because of the packaging (unconfirmable). And then it disappeared. "Just too wonderful for words, one of the five great perfumes of the world, and I have none left, none," Turin said, despondent. "I had no idea they were going to discontinue it."

Lutens's tastes in general coveted extremes, but then, that was arguably what made him a success as a perfumer, and Turin thoroughly applauded its every expression. He would go upstairs to Lutens's shop, where they would talk about perfume, and everywhere he looked were exquisite things, ancient Japanese tables and antiques and works of art. One time, Turin went to the toilet and closed the door and looked down. The toilet seat was dark red. He stared at it, tried to move out of the light, and stared at it some more. What in the world was this stuff, some weird red plastic? And then he got down on his knees to check it out. It wasn't plastic. It was red marble, phenomenally expensive red marble. He'd seen it on ancient Egyptian statues at the British Museum. He did his business, left, went to find Serge, and casually said, "So. Red-marble toilet seat, huh?" Lutens shrugged. *"Bah, oui."* Like why was Turin even bothering to mention it.

It was a blissful time, exciting, full of promise. Turin was here, he was there, information was pouring in. He was beginning to put things together even then, without realizing it. "I was so ignorant," Turin would say later. "I had the confidence of the ignorant, confidence in myself and my abilities and, most of all, in Things Working Out. In good people recognizing good ideas and working together toward the Truth." He paused. "That is truly something only the young could believe. You think everything's going to be just fine."

❖   ❖   ❖

THERE HAVE OVER time been many theories of the sense of vision.

In an age in which people believed we saw objects because they were continuously flinging off copies of themselves ("eidolons" these were called), Isaac Newton proposed a radical new theory of color and light, the fuel for our sense of vision, the food of the eyes. He theorized that vibrations, waves of light, hit the eye and made their colors and forms visible by the way they vibrated.

Thoroughly vested as they were in the reigning eidolon concept of vision, people hated Newton's theory. Goethe—who, it is said, went to his death calling to heaven for "More light!"—emphatically rejected it, going to great lengths to create an elaborate system to counter Newton's new vision theory. Goethe's system was false, of course. His cry of *"Mehr Licht!"* apparently as well; there were new ideas the man simply didn't want to see illuminated.

(Today's quantum-mechanical theory of light makes it both particle and wave, and this is not necessarily easier to accept. "Light's joke on scientists," someone has noted dryly, "is to reveal itself, at last, as something that no one can visualize.")

◆   ◆   ◆

SUDDENLY, TURIN'S PARIS position still in a kind of bureaucratic limbo, a job possibility reached him. He was excited because it came from the Moscow State University Institute of Molecular Biology. He started packing for Moscow. Just before he left, in May 1992, he met someone. Her name was Françoise Le Grand, the curator of a photography collection in Paris, and they hit it off. He felt happy to be, for once, not alone, and she listened when he talked about his science. But then he flew off to Moscow.

He'd had a love affair with Russia and its science since his father's frequent trips there as a U.N. economist. Duccio loved the Russian spirit. He went in 1959, when Luca was six, and brought back a big fur hat for his son, a *shapka*. "For a kid," says Turin, "that's really something. My father was sort of a crypto-Communist, which I never was."

But he was also excited because, in Turin's happy view, Russia has always been a beacon for various scientific weirdos and speculators and wizards. He used to read *Biofizika* in its English-language version, *Soviet Biophysics,* which he found full of astonishing stuff—the "If true, then amazing!" stuff, as he called it. Before the first time he left for Kiev, they called him and asked, "Can you bring a millipore filter holder with you?" So he brought one, no problem, and gave it to them. About four days later he noticed that their lab had had the workshop make a few copies. He picked one up and found it bizarrely light. "And," Turin recalls, "I think, 'Uh-oh . . .' I say, 'What the hell is this made of?' And they say cheerfully, 'Oh, it's titanium.' And I say, '*What?*'" Titanium is bulletproof, one of the strongest metals that exist, and outrageously expensive. They led him down to the lab basement and pointed at a gigantic block of pure titanium, just sitting there. He figured it was a hundred kilos or so. "Russia has the biggest reserves of titanium in the world. When the American military built the SR-71 Lockheed plane to use against the Soviets, they bought all the titanium for the body from Russia through a front company. That block probably cost fifty thousand dollars. Someone in the lab had just *ordered* it. They were carving *soap dishes* out of it."

Turin worked in Moscow five different times, doing research on whatever interested him. Russian biology today, he says mournfully, has been almost completely wiped out. "No funds, no equipment, desperation, lots of emigration. The smartest ones fled to the U.S. or Israel." He shrugs, sighs for an era. What he loved in particular were the science books, which he bought for literally pennies in barren Soviet stores. He would head over to Dom Knigi (Book House), on Prospekt Kalinina, ground floor on the right, and there might be six-foot-tall stacks of these books, books on quantum physics and physiology and electrochemistry and metallurgy. His face lights up. "There was one wonderful one called *Harder Than Diamonds,* about nitrogen-doped gems. I love that—" He laughs with joy, then purses his lips, looks pensive. "All these people with worn-out shoes and poor, shitty polyester shirts who wrote these things. The books I'd accumulate on these visits weighed as much as a small calf. You'd look at it and think, 'I really can't lug this thing home, I'll come back tomorrow,' and you'd come back and they'd be gone. Forever. And there'd be nothing there at all. So when you found them, you'd just lug them to the cash register and have them wrapped in the strangest, most beautiful paper and strange string— everything was strange in the Soviet Union—and then you'd get into a taxi and take them to a post office and have them airlifted out. I bought more books than I could possibly lift, fifty kilos of books, towers of these gigantic, immense, wonderful books.

"And these poor Soviet scientists were just *fucking* brilliant. I remember a pompous English ass gave a talk on a hot summer's day in Moscow. He was wearing a tobacco-colored linen suit and a panama hat, and looked properly colonial. His audience was twenty-five Russian scientists who looked so disheveled, dressed in such bad, worn, pathetic clothing you swore they were begging in the streets. The twit gave them this condescending talk, very English, and then came the question-and-answer, and they roasted him alive. So what if they looked homeless. They were bullshit free. It wasn't a 'career,' it wasn't ball gowns and glamour, it was pure, pure science, it was What's the damn problem? *How do we solve the problem?* God. They inhabited the grim halls of Moscow State University, which was a university exclusively for the sciences, this great fucking building on the top of this hill. The last time I went to work there, they faxed me: 'What academic title would you like?' I faxed them back: 'Would like the title "Grand Duke."' They faxed me back, '"Grand Duke" momentarily unavailable, suggest "Visiting Professor."'

"I loved eating in these crummy Soviet cafeterias where the forks were made of an alloy that doesn't exist in the West—it's like aluminum yet somehow corrodes. Fascinating."

✦　　✦　　✦

EVENTUALLY HE HIMSELF began tiring of the nomadic existence, started wanting to set up a more permanent shop. He went to a Commbelga satellite telephone booth in the lobby of a luxury hotel, the only way you could make daytime direct calls abroad from Moscow in those days, and called his former Ph.D. supervisor at University College London. She was in a chatty mood unfortunately, and the call cost him sixty pounds, but she gave him a tip. There might, she said, be an opening at UCL; he should apply. It was an obvious fit: Turin's father had been a professor there, too, of architecture. Turin applied from Moscow. His old Head of Department (the Department of Anatomy) remembered him. He offered Turin a professor's job for two years.

Turin arrived at UCL in 1993 and set up his lab. Just then the U.S. Navy money came through—$60,000—so he turned his attention to making better diodes that would help the U.S. military smell electrically. He also found some new playmates: Martin Rosendaal, his darkly cheerful neighbor in the office next door; a tall, thin, discreetly impish biologist named Tim Arnett just down the hall; and an attractive, enthusiastic young woman named Jane Brock doing her Ph.D. on tissue repair, who'd set up in the lab opposite his. He met Brock at the No. 24 bus stop. She was reading a copy of *Zen and the Art of Motorcycle Maintenance* and hating it, but due to her good English reserve felt she couldn't just come out and say that, so instead she asked him, "Well, is there something wrong with me?" He looked at her in a friendly, assessing way and said, "Has it occurred to you that it's actually a complete pile of crap?" She felt liberated. On the bus she asked him about him, and he mentioned perfume. She told him she loved Guerlain fragrances for men, and he told her lots about them. They became friends and allies. She was always struck by his openness. "He'd just walk into everyone's lab and start talking to people."

Turin's attempts to measure smell electrically, on the other hand, weren't really going anywhere. And, as usual, he was reading all the wrong things, haunting university libraries, dipping restlessly into this and that, nibbling randomly at weird pieces of biology, chemistry, and physics before returning them, like half-eaten chocolates, to their boxes.

One afternoon, about six months after he'd arrived at UCL and settled into his life in London, he was restless. Not in the mood to experiment. He wandered over to the UCL library and began reading *Aviation Weekly,* "which I'm not supposed to read because it's one of my obsessions." Then he started idly rummaging through recent issues of various journals. He was picking through one he liked with the hyperfunctional title *Review of Scientific Instruments,* and in it he happened on an article about a tool for analyzing molecules and atoms. He'd never heard of this neat gadget, which had been accidentally discovered by some guys at the Ford Motor Company. It was called an electron-tunneling spectroscope. He started reading.

The way the thing worked was just good old spectroscopy, exactly like the machines that shot photons through molecules to tell you what atoms were in them, the machine Dyson had said was somehow contained in the human nose. But *this* spectroscope didn't shoot photons. It shot electrons. *Electron* spectroscopy.

It worked, he saw, basically like a light switch. You flip "on" a light switch, and it just connects a wire, fills in a gap between two sides of an electrical highway, so electrons can flow. The Ford guys had made an observation that was, at least on one level, supremely simple. Electrons are extremely inquisitive creatures, and they want to go everywhere. So they zip along inside conductors until they come to a gap, and then they crowd the edge of this atomic cliff and impatiently try to find a way to jump across to the other side. And you can just insert a bridge into that tiny gap—a single molecule will do, just jam it in there—and the electrons will enthusiastically rush through that molecule (it's called "tunneling" because they actually burrow through the thing like frenetic moles) and across to the other side.

As they tunnel through their molecular bridge, electrons lose some energy and tire (you would, too, running an obstacle course like that). They exit on the other end with slightly lower power. They're just not going as fast when they get off this ride. There was a little old lady who wouldn't pay her electricity bill "because," she argued, "I'm not *keeping* the electricity. It's flowing in and flowing right out again." Which it was, but the power company pointed out that the electrons were flowing more slowly when they left, and they calculated her monthly bill by the amount of energy the electrons had lost burrowing through her refrigerator. The Ford guys had realized that that difference—the electron's Before and After voltages—could identify for you which vibrations the molecule sitting in the gap had. And if you knew its vibrations, well, you knew what molecule it was. You could I.D. it with absolute certainty. Simple.

Now, it is not actually quite this simple. Tunneling happens in everything around you. The very first radios, the old Marconis, for example, used a primitive device based on the tunneling effect, invented by a Frenchman named Branly, whose other claim to fame is that he was the person the French elected to the Académie des Sciences ahead of Madame Curie because he was a man and she was not. Since we're dealing with particles, all this has to do with quantumness, so there's the usual semireligious quantum mechanics mumbo jumbo. Electrons are fuzzy creatures. Because they're fuzzy, even as they're approaching this molecular bridge (or door or lock or tunnel; what it is from their point of view is unclear), part of them is (here we go) *already on the other side*. They literally make a tunnel through a solid door, though it's not really a tunnel or a hole in a strict physical sense. We don't really know what it is. Some physicists say electrons walk through the door without opening it. (This is the basic quantum-mechanical precept that all objects are described by a wave function, and waves have a possibility of passing through all barriers—steel doors, lead walls—unless they're infinitely thick or infinitely high. Which none are, of course. This is also often described as: It is absolutely possible in quantum mechanics for a bus to drive right through Hadrian's Wall.) We do know two things for certain: The electrons *basically* start on one side—and, if the vibrations match, somehow wind up on the other. And (second) the drop in their energy level tells you exactly what molecule they've just tunneled through. And that, for electron spectroscopy, is all that matters.

Turin read the whole article. Because the authors were physics teachers, they actually explained how the machine was built and how it worked. And because Turin had been teaching himself physics in his spare time, he understood this new kind of spectroscopy.

And because of his interest in smell, he knew that we can smell the difference between one kind of atom and another, which only a spectroscope can do.

And . . . wait a minute (he laid the paper on the table) . . . because he had the bad habit of randomly reading everything, he'd read through Dyson's 1938 paper, which proposed that our noses somehow have the spectroscopic power to detect Vibration.

And because he'd been hanging out in the Big Boys' labs (a dividend of his perfume guide), he'd seen that while everyone believed that our noses use a molecule's Shape to get its smell, the fragrance chemists went about making these smellable molecules randomly, which, given the supercomputing artillery thrown at unlocking shapes, made it pretty clear that shape didn't have much to do with smell.

And because he was trying to help the U.S. Navy smell submarines, he happened to be doing electron-transfer work important in smell.

And because he had created a diode out of egg-white protein, he knew that electrons could be transferred by proteins.

And simply because he remembered his high school biology, he knew that proteins are, after all, what make receptors, like the nose's olfactory receptors.

And due to his biology, he'd read the details of the olfactory receptors that Linda Buck had found.

And because he'd been picking up chemistry on his own, he knew that smellable molecules were held together with electron bonds that were identifiable by exactly the sort of electron spectroscopy in this paper.

And in an instant . . .

Sitting in the UCL library, he thought: So electron-tunneling spectroscopy is something you could do biologically. Which means that these spectroscopes, these huge, heavy, expensive machines of metal and glass that sit in laboratories analyzing smell molecules, could literally be constructed of the tiny proteins that sit in your nose, allowing your nose to smell atoms. Tiny spectroscopes made out of living human flesh. Flesh made of proteins that conduct electrons . . .

And suddenly he was hit by a very strange thought: That madman Dyson, the guy who laughably said the nose somehow had a spectroscope inside it, was absolutely right. Turin had perhaps just stumbled across the crucial mechanism that might make this impossible spectroscope work. A thousand irrelevant facts converged in an instant.

At that instant he dropped everything else and started working on a new theory of smell.

III

✦

WRITING

BIOLOGICAL THEORIES ARE created by pretending to be God. Another way of saying this is that you put together a biological theory by reverse engineering the human body. You build a theory by looking at what already is and then trying to think up a good reason why it would be that way, and how it would work.

"OK, so if I were God," Turin thought, "I'd figure, 'Hey, it'd be nice for those poor bastards down there to be able to smell stuff so they can survive.' Because smell is not about sex, contrary to popular belief, it's about food and protection from decaying, poisonous things that can hurt you, to tell you whether whatever's in your hand is good for you. So I'd say, 'They need a system that will determine instantly the chemical composition of a substance, whether it's toxic or not, confirm it's got no nasty nitriles and no sulfides, but esters are OK and also we like small heterocycles, those are good. A system that can in a split second steer us away from big molecules because they're hard to digest (musky, woody smells tend to be large molecules) and away from decay and guide us only toward edible things (most edible smells tend to be have low molecular weights) that fit the limited library of digestive enzymes that I've given them.'

"Now, I, God, have already decided I'm going to build these people out of flesh. Seems like a nice construction material. So then I'd think, 'Well, I want to build a spectroscope because that's a device for telling one of these humans what atoms are in whatever's in front of him.' And I'd have to ask myself, 'Well, can I build a spectroscope out of flesh?' And I'd answer, 'Oh, piece of piss! Here's how I do it. Smells are just molecules that fly through the air. You want to catch them. How do you catch them? You make receptors to catch them. Can you make a receptor out of flesh? In the human body, there are things called proteins hanging around all over the place. So you build your receptor out of a protein with a pocket that the smelly molecules can fall into.' Fine. Then I'd ask myself, 'An electron spectroscope operates by shooting electricity it gets from a power source at the molecules. Can you run this flesh-protein spectroscope on electricity too? No problem: you know that proteins conduct electricity.' But wait! 'If you're going to have an electrical machine, you need a plausible electrical power source made of human flesh, an electron donor. Possible?' No problem: there's *tons* of things in biology that give off electrons, little chemical batteries, and they could be your power source. So—in theory—there are all the biological parts you'd need to make a biological spectroscope."

Now that his mental reverse engineering of smell had produced a theoretic machine that theoretically explained smell, he had to find all these parts for this machine he'd hypothesized. He knew exactly where to look.

✦   ✦   ✦

TURIN PLUNGED INTO the research of his theory through the Big Boys' laboratories, which held riches for him locked away in their vaults and on their disk drives: the data on the thousands and thousands of molecules they'd created. Each Big Boy was at war with the others, each with its jealously guarded cache of gold and its army in their chrome-and-glass vaults, weaving their molecules. He called up Quest and asked to spend a week in their lab. Doing what? they asked. Smelling everything! said Turin. He didn't, he added, want to hang out with the perfumers, who never mixed molecules themselves. He meant with the lab techs. They shrugged and said that was fine.

He went to Paris, got on the subway, and arrived in Neuilly, the relentlessly chic, ruthlessly conformist, breathtakingly expensive Paris suburb between the Étoile with its Arc de Triomphe and the corporate skyscrapers of La Défense. This is where Quest has its Paris headquarters, "a stupid modern-looking building," he says of it, "all very grim. In the entryway there's an old copper still, like at all the perfumeries, to give you a feeling of 'tradition.' Right. And these places all have the same smell, a fruit salad on a color TV with the color turned up way too high."

The lab techs, who were always women, worked at benches in one huge room. It reminded him of a sweatshop. They spent their days mixing the formula orders the perfumers sent down to them. "Give me," an order would say, "jasmine absolute 15 g, rose essence 12 g, alpha-methyl ionone 5 g, Galaxolide 10 g, aldehyde C10 2.5 g. . . ." Barkeeps at a molecular cocktail bar, the lab techs glance over the order, set a little bottle on a scale, which they then reset to zero, and start adding small amounts of chemicals. They have rotating trays. Press a button, and a thousand perfume materials appear at their fingertips, thousands of fascinating molecules to smell. They mix their fragrant molecular cocktails—order up!—and send them upstairs to be smelled.

Every day for a week, Turin arrived, said hello to them (he was getting on with everyone at Quest famously), grabbed a few hundred smelling strips, and pulled on a warm sweater. Then he entered the cold room at the back where the molecules were stored and smelled things. He looked at the perfumes' molecular formulas and thought about them. Some were natural compounds, in which case they were complex and contained hundreds of molecules, and some were synthetics, in which case he would be smelling the odor of a single molecule. He hadn't mentioned to Quest that he was working on a theory, but one day he wound up explaining it enthusiastically to Maurice Roucel, a perfumer (he'd done the female *Envy*) and chemist. Roucel thought about it and said, "I feel like it's right." Turin was having good vibes with everyone at Quest. Roucel said to him, You really should be part of the firm, you're fun to have around. It made Turin feel great to hear this.

Crucially, Turin also now had a collaborator, an intellectual backboard, on the other side of the Atlantic. Turin had met Walter Stewart at a 1983 NATO developmental biology conference in Banyuls-sur-Mer he described as "hilariously boring." Stewart was an organic chemist who had the distinction of having been such a brilliant student at Harvard that his professors considered it a waste of time for him to bother doing a doctoral thesis and sent him directly into research. Stewart was also infamous in a completely different scientific capacity: professional avenging angel and fraud buster. He worked in neurophysiology at the NIH but had made his career investigating science fraud in the two most infamous cases of the late twentieth century, the Darsee case at Harvard and the Baltimore/Imanishi-Kari case (Stewart was the thorn in Baltimore's side). It had made him one of the most feared and loathed scientists in the world; Turin was blissfully unaware of all this and got on with him splendidly. Stewart was a supportive friend and a brilliant colleague, and Turin referred to him as "an archangel thinly disguised as a human."

Stewart knew nothing about smell. What he did know, which Turin did not, or at least not as well, was physics. But smell, Stewart was learning. On Thanksgiving Day 1994, Turin called Stewart at his home outside Washington, D.C., and spilled the whole theory. Stewart's immediate response was that there was a Nobel Prize in it. "This was not pushing the envelope a little further," says Stewart. "This was truly original." At the family's Thanksgiving dinner, Stewart proposed a toast: There was a chance, he told everyone, that Luca had figured out smell.

They began a collaboration on the new theory. Mostly it consisted of Turin in London enthusiastically chucking ideas down the e-mail pipe toward Stewart like some electronic intellectual clay-pigeon machine, with Stewart in Washington calmly blowing them to pieces one by one. This was, certainly, the scientific process, and Turin appreciated Stewart's help, although there was a certain brutal efficiency with which Stewart hit "Reply" and then coolly detailed why this or that brilliant idea of Turin's was crap. Turin would absorb the blow and start generating more ideas. Stewart's attitude was "As a good scientist, of course, you always try to disprove your theory. And this seemed like a good theory to disprove." So he was just helping Turin along in this regard. Sometimes Turin wished he weren't quite so helpful.

◆   ◆   ◆

WHERE TO BEGIN? Well, the striking thing about Turin's theory was that it proposed a code. The code was the secret. He had to begin by breaking it.

A code is basically any word or signal or sign that correlates with another word or meaning. To give a completely simplistic example, if you read "1 2 3" and you knew this was in code, and you knew that 1 = C, 2 = A, and 3 = T, then you'd know that "1 2 3" meant "cat." Two ways of writing the name of the same animal: "1 2 3" and "cat" mean the same thing. They both also mean *neko* (which means cat in Japanese and which is simply yet another code with the same meaning, a small hairy animal with a tail and an attitude). Turin had theorized that each vibration in a molecule, each number from 0 to 4000 on the wave-number scale (a wave number being simply the number of times an electron bounced back and forth as it bonded one atom to another), meant a smell. Every time you had an electron bond vibrating at 840, you would smell, say, ripe papaya. (An 890 vibration might smell of cinnamon.) Read the words "wave numbers of 840" on a page, and you knew—or so the theory predicted—that the molecule containing that vibe would contain the smell of papaya. And so the essential trick here, the very first step, was for Turin to find some specific vibration and prove it coded for a specific smell. Which of course was highly complicated by the fact that you could never get a single vibration alone; molecules, with their numerous singing bonds, always played chords, and it was impossible to get just *one bond* alone by itself (like getting one hand to clap). Instead, he'd have to figure out the smell of a given vibration by finding it in two chords and discerning the difference between them. (This is not so easy even in a field as well worked out as music; in smell, it was completely off the theoretic charts.) But he had to find a smell.

Which smell? He started flipping through molecules randomly, just looking at wave numbers. The bond gluing a Carbon atom to a Bromine atom vibrated, he saw, on the low end, between 500 and 750. The bond welding a Carbon to a Fluorine was at 1000 to 1400. Hmm, here were the Nitrogen-Hydrogen bonds coming in at 3350 to 3500, and Oxygen-Hydrogen at 3100 to 3700. But what interested him most was one bond in particular, the bond holding a Sulfur atom to a Hydrogen atom. It vibrated at a wave number of 2500. What he liked about the S-H bond was that it stood alone, clear as a lighthouse, *and* even better the smell was viscerally distinctive. Sulfur, everyone knows, smells like hard-boiled egg yolk (which contains a lot of Sulfur atoms). The Shapists would say this is because the Sulfur-Hydrogen's shape carries that information (if you only know where to feel for it). Turin was saying no, Sulfur's smell came from the vibration of the electron bonding Sulfur to Hydrogen, that every time you found a wave number of 2500, no matter what molecule it was, you should smell hard-boiled egg: 2500 = hard-boiled egg smell. Or to reverse it, "hard-boiled egg smell" *meant* a wave number of 2500. Now Turin had to prove it. And the way to do that was simply this: find another molecule that vibrated at 2500 like the S-H bond but had no S-H, a molecule that smelled like Sulfur but had no Sulfur in it. He soon began grimly concluding that it was impossible to find.

First, as far as he or anyone he knew understood it, *nothing* except the electrons gluing Sulfur to Hydrogen vibrated at 2500. He spent weeks in the library poring over spectroscopy books and finding nothing. He asked around. No, no one knew any other 2500 bond. Sorry. If you were brave enough to look for one anyway, well, there were hundreds of electron bonds and molecules and vibrations you'd have to pick through, and as many smells. He talked out every possible angle of attack with Walter Stewart, but they came up with nothing.

For Christmas, he reluctantly escaped London for Lisbon with Françoise. She had chosen Lisbon. (She'd tried to get his input, calling him from Paris. Was he in the mood for Lisbon? Well, was he *not*? What he was in the mood for was a damn 2500 non-S-H vibra-tion, and he just replied *Ehhh* . . . into the phone. It wasn't the right response.) He wasn't averse to Lisbon. "It's one of the great cities of Europe, one of the half dozen that prevent God from wiping out the earth. Prague, Paris, maybe Florence, Naples. Seville. Lisbon is a stupendous metropolis on the edge of nowhere because Portugal is this godforsaken place, like Ireland." But he loathed tourism. "I hate looking at monuments. I hate waking up in the morning and think-ing, 'Oh! Today we're gonna visit this *abbey.*' We don't do it at home, why should we do it abroad? The only thing I'm interested in is people, views, restaurants, and a clean, warm place to crap, as What's-his-name said. You never meet real people when you're touristing. I tend to get ravenously hungry when I'm on holiday, like I'm some Holocaust survivor who doesn't know when he's going to eat next."

They walked around the chilly city. Turin froze, since, in his analysis, the coldest one can get is in countries with normally warm climates. Lisbon had gigantic windows with gaps between them. He'd never been cold in Moscow. Also it was raining, and the one thing he hated with a passion was rain. Françoise was still uncom-fortable with his obsessive nature, and she could see him chewing the cud about smell. The food cheered him, a bit. "Astonishing. This wonderful thing called *açorda,* a delicious mixture of bread and sea-food that looks like vomit, and this wonderful liqueur—they have a sherry in which morello cherries have marinated, called *ginginha,* which is heavenly." As usual, he'd forgotten to bring anything to read, and he could read the Portuguese newspapers only with an un-fun amount of effort. It was at this point that they wandered one evening past a lovely old bookstore unchanged since the 1950s. It was a big, dark old place with flat benches, all wooden and somber, run by a family. The elderly owner shuffled about, while his daugh-ter, dressed in black, took care of customers. Françoise went off to search for the photography books.

Turin looked around. On a low shelf on one side he noticed a stack of books. Oh, said the daughter, yes, these are books people had ordered decades before but had never come around to pick up. She stored them there. The books were at their original prices. He started going through them. One of them was a physical chemistry textbook from 1964 written by a Howard University professor. He started flipping pages and found a section on molecular vibration. He bought the book immediately. They went back to the hotel, and Turin lay on the bed reading. He noticed a little table cleanly laying out atom masses and bond stiffnesses. And then, just below, a very nice formula for how you calculate vibrational wave numbers from atomic masses and bond strength.

Then he saw a table with some wave numbers already neatly calculated. He frowned at it. This table listed the C-H bond, the Carbon-Hydrogen bond, with its electron bond vibrating at wave number 3000, and then it showed that the bond linking B to H (Boron, the fifth element, to Hydrogen) had a somewhat lower vibration. Which meant B-H vibed under 3000. Wait a minute, thought Turin. Could it be near 2500? He pulled out his calculator, squinted at the table, plugged in the formula and the numbers. B-H's wave number came in at around 2550, more or less smack on top of the S-H bond's vibration.

It was exactly what he had been searching for. He had a way to test his theory. He'd order some B-H molecules (these are the "boranes" that weren't in your ancestral environment—they are rocket propellants—and that, nevertheless, you can smell), unscrew the cap, and smell. Given that they contained no Sulfur (nor, notably, molecules with Sulfur *shapes* (Boron made bonds with a completely different geometry than Sulfur did), if boranes smelled like Sulfur he would be over the moon, because the only earthly reason they should was that they both had a bond that vibrated at 2500. Turin was making a clear prediction: boranes should smell like Sulfur.

Of course, if the B-H molecule didn't smell like S-H, his theory was garbage.

He went back to London and e-mailed Stewart that the test was smelling boranes. "I must say," Stewart wrote, "the notion of watching a thriller on TV while sipping liqueur and having an occasional snort of stale rocket fuel does define a high level of civilization." But then Turin actually tried to lay his hands on the stuff.

Boranes are, says Turin, "not honest, hardworking molecules. They're complete perverts with bizarre structures." In the vastness of chemistry, they are the only known instance where Hydrogen atoms form stable bridges between other atoms. (He heard, to his delight, that boranes smelled satanic, which usually referred to brimstone, which was loaded with Sulfur atoms.) Their structure was so hard to work out that a Nobel was given to Lipscomb at Harvard for doing so. They are viciously poisonous to human beings, and all other carbon-based life-forms for that matter, and tend to spontaneously ignite on contact with air. Turin keeps in his lab a copy of an old book he loves, *Ignition!* by John D. Clark, an irreverent, whimsical personal history by a crusty old inorganic chemist recounting the search during the 1940s and '50s for rocket fuels. His copy of the book is suffused with the odor of his lab, a thick, incredibly complex, darkish musk—Turin says he can no longer describe it because he can no longer smell it—from the bottles of perfumes, the perfume chemists' molecules, and all the vials with black-on-orange skull-and-crossbones strewn everywhere. His papers, his computer, and his clothes have stewed for years in this smell like the subtle, constant background radiation that prompts the *click click click* of the Geiger counter.

In Clark's day, he and his team had a great time playing with compounds like dicyanoacetylene, which has no hydrogen atoms at all and has three triple bonds, and which they burned in their lab with ozone, getting a Steady-State temperature of 6,000 degrees Kelvin. This is the temperature on the surface of the sun. There were molecules they loved—Clark has a lovely little sequence about producing a very nice one called hydrazine, which was so civilized, it even decomposed (the problem for the U.S. Navy was that the stuff froze at -1.5 degrees Celsius, which basically limited its usefulness to the tropics and the ground)—and molecules they loathed.

Some they loathed because of the smell. "Mike Pino," Clark wrote of his colleague, "in 1949 made a discovery that can fairly be described as revolting." Butyl mercaptan spontaneously ignited when mixed with acid. This was great for Standard Oil of California, since they had to strip tons of butyl mercaptans from their crudes to make their gasoline socially acceptable to the noses of

California's residents and had drums and drums of the stuff left to deal with. "If they could only sell it for rocket fuel life would indeed be beautiful.

"Well," wrote Clark,

it had two virtues, or maybe three. It was hypergolic [highly explosive] and had a rather high density. And it wasn't corrosive. But its performance was below that of a straight hydrocarbon, and its odor—! Well, its odor was something to consider. Intense, pervasive and penetrating, and resembling the stink of an enraged skunk, but surpassing, by far, the best efforts of the most vigorous specimen of *Mephitis mephitis.* It also clings to the clothes and the skin. It was rumored that certain rocket mechanics were excluded from their car pools and had to run behind. Ten years after it was fired at the Naval Air Rocket Test Station, the odor was still noticeable around the test areas.

Clark adds that when Pino started working with mercaptans, he and his crew were banished from his lab's posh headquarters near San Francisco to a wood shack two hundred yards away. He had begun playing with new compounds, ethyl mercaptans of acetone and acetaldehyde, which were garlicky, but then, tragically, got heavily into a certain dimethylamino group that he hooked to a vile mercaptan sulfur "whose odor can't, with all the resources of the English language, even be described. It also drew flies. This was too much, even for Pino and his unregenerate crew, and they banished it to a hole in the ground in the tule marshes. Some months later, in the dead of night, they surreptitiously consigned it to the bottom of San Francisco Bay."

Then there were molecules they loathed simply because they were diabolical. Red fuming nitric acid (RFNA), which Clark experimented with in 1945, was "hated by everybody who had anything to do with it, with a pure and abiding hatred." It was fantastically corrosive. It sat in its aluminum drums and produced a slimy, gelatinous, white sludge that screwed up the rocket engines. No one knew what the sludge was, "but," said Clark, "the aversion with which it was regarded was equaled only by the difficulty of analyzing it." Put it in stainless steel, and the stuff turned a ghastly green color as it chewed through its steel cage. It attacked human flesh like a school of piranhas, and when poured it gave off dense clouds of nitrogen dioxide gas, which had the odd habit of causing a person to cough for a few minutes, then insist there was no problem—and then the next day, while walking around, suddenly drop dead. (The alternative to RFNA was WFNA, which had its own personality; Clark used to test the mettle of job seekers to his lab by having his assistant drop a bit of old rubber glove in some WFNA. The rubber would squirm and swell for a moment like some satanic worm and then erupt in a magnificent, shrieking jet of flame. "I could," wrote Clark, "usually tell from the candidate's demeanor whether he had the sort of nervous system desirable in a propellant chemist.")

But boranes were particularly malevolent. Alfred Stock discovered most of the better-known ones between 1912 and 1933. When rocket-fuel chemists began working on boranes, there were only forty pounds of diborane existing on earth, and the rocket chemists called fuels that used boranes "exotics." Clark described some of the problems they presented:

> Boranes are compounds of boron and hydrogen, the best known being diborane B_2H_6; pentaborane, B_5H_9; and decaborane, $B_{10}H_{14}$. At room temperature the first is a gas, the second a liquid, the third a solid. Diborane and pentaborane ignite spontaneously in the atmosphere, and the fires are remarkably difficult to extinguish. . . . When the stuff spilled, it burst into a pool of flame and made the area it covered look like the floor of hell. It seemed to laugh at the water thrown in hopes of extinguishing it. If the burning pool eventually did go out, the unburned molecule would immediately shroud itself in a solid crust of boric acid. When you tried to clean it up, you would inevitably break the crust. When the crust broke, the pool once again erupted into a highly poisonous inferno. They not only are possessed of a peculiarly repulsive odor; they are extremely poisonous by just about any route. They are also very expensive since their synthesis is neither easy nor simple.

There were other difficulties, not least of which was that diborane boils at 92.5 degrees below zero Celsius. Even as rocket fuels, they are satanic: burning with a flame of lurid green, they have a fiendishly hot combustion, about 50 percent higher than jet fuel, and when unchained tend to melt the engines that dare burn them.

These were the molecules Turin was trying to find. They were not available over the counter.

He went down to Piccadilly, to the Royal Society of Chemistry library and took out a book on chemical suppliers. Listed in it was a company in Pennsylvania "in some place with a low-density population. You understand why they're not in Orange County. Might be a good idea if they were, but they're not." He called their chief chemist and said he was a scientist in London and would like to purchase some boranes, please.

What, the chief chemist asked, did he want to do with them?

He wanted to smell them.

A long pause. You wanna *what?*

In any case, the voice from Pennsylvania informed him decisively, the minimum order was a ton.

A *ton.* Well, could they provide him with a sample?

No, they could not provide him with a sample.

Huh. OK, well, could he just ask a question then.

A suspicious instant on the line. Go ahead.

What did the things smell like?

There was a distinct pause. Sir, said the chemist with deep sincerity, we do our best not to smell them, and hung up.

In desperation, Turin went out and got the fattest chemicals catalog on his shelf, from a company called Sigma that supplied biologists. He was sure they wouldn't have boranes, "because there's no reason for a biologist to get within a mile of them." But he thought he'd just confirm that they didn't have decaborane, which, though toxic, doesn't explode. They had it. Why, he had no earthly idea. He ordered one gram. When it rolled in the next morning, he took it up to his lab, holding it as if it were an armed land mine. Open it? His hands were almost shaking. Open it? He was just tightening his fingers around the container when Tibor Krenacs, a Hungarian cell biologist with a lab down the hall, walked in. You've come at the right time, said Turin, and in a single motion opened the vial and shoved it under Krenacs's nose. There was a heavy pause. Krenacs took a cautious sniff. Then, slowly, in a thick Hungarian accent, he remarked thoughtfully, "It smells like boiled onion, Luca." Turin almost jumped in the air. Onions and garlic contain Sulfur-Hydrogens. Look at the label, he said, and explained in a rush. Krenacs looked, saw the word *decaborane,* and realized there was no Sulfur in it. The two of them stood in the lab with a small tin of onion-smelling poison, looking at each other.

Turin finally managed to track down some borane chemists, and they replied that, oh, sure, *all* boranes smell like Sulfur, everyone knew that. And yet they contain no Sulfur at all. None.

He had found the first piece of code for deciphering smell, and it was a number, a wavelength, an electron vibration: wave number 2500. The number linked two code equivalents (an S-H and a B-H borane), two completely different molecules, to one meaning: the smell of rotten eggs. And they were shaped completely differently. As far as Turin could see, there was only one possibility: they both contained a 2500 vibration. And that vibration had a smell.

✦   ✦   ✦

TURIN WOULD WRITE a paper. He decided to submit it to the prestigious science journal *Nature*. Edited in London and reigning over the scientific field, *Nature* is (along with the Washington, D.C.–based *Science*) one of the world's two most prestigious publications of record. Appearance in its pages guarantees a serious and thorough hearing for important new discoveries. It is membership in an exclusive club.

✦   ✦   ✦

THE TIMING WAS what made it feel particularly odd. In the labs of the Big Boys, Turin had just learned the dominant Shape theory, and here he was trooping back to check the fine print. But Shape had never really added up to him, and the closer he looked, the more he stumbled over clauses with one too many footnotes, tiny irregularities in the theory, convenient little loopholes. When you really looked, Shape, bit by bit, started to come apart at its neatly sewn seams.

Shape's basic thesis is extremely simple: as in immunology, neurology, virology, and on and on, so in olfaction, molecules with similar shapes should carry similar information and behavior. Just as a cop identifies a perp by his unique fingerprints, the immune system identifies a virus by its unique shape. You find a molecule smelling of rose, Shapists said, the olfactory system must be reading, somewhere on that molecule's complex, bulbous, molded surface, shapes that say, "Rose smell here." (Incidentally, although every single species of rose has an identifiable "rose smell," no two species of rose have the same rose smell. Next time you're in a flower shop, smell each rose variety. You'll see.) If you're a perfume chemist, your task is clear—to track down the shape of rose smell, the shape of burnt-wood odor, the shape of the scent of ocean water, in order to sell these smells.

So the smell chemists at the Big Boys would take all the molecules that smelled of, say, sandalwood and morph them on their powerful computers into a thousand slightly different versions—Turin, curious, watched as they did this—and look for the shapes they had in common. And sure enough, Turin found out, going through their published literature and chatting with them in the white, fluorescent-lit hallways, they came up with shape-smell correlations. "Mostly" or "typically," they would write in the papers they proudly published in the prestigious scientific journals (carefully verifying the spelling of their names and the names of the institutions they worked for), "sandalwoods have certain shape similarities, and to get a molecule that smells like sandalwood you stick a methyl group here and a hydroxyl group here, this distance apart and pointing in this direction." These were shape-smell rules, empirically derived, and they showed these rules off lovingly; they'd talk to him about them with confidence. Look at a lovely little molecule called beta-santalol, they said to him, it smells deliciously of sandalwood. It behaves according to all the rules, they said with satisfaction.

There was just one small problem. He ran across it pretty quickly. One evening a few decades earlier, an Indian smell chemist named Rahman Ansari had been working in his lab at Bush Boake Allen in Walthamstow, in North London. He was trying to find a new way to synthesize levo-citronellol, a molecule that occurs naturally in geraniums and has a warm, sweet, slightly green rosy scent (roses synthesize it naturally). Levo-citronellol cost a hundred dollars a kilo, and everyone was hoping to make a synthetic version costing ten times less; people estimated that such a molecule would be worth $2 to $3 million a year in sales. Ansari was cleaning up the lab for the evening. A younger chemist had just done the reaction for purifying levo-citronellol in a pot full of boiling liquid (he had been working it up into a vapor, then condensing it), so Ansari dumped the condensed vapor into a flask, carried the flask over to a bottle, poured it in, and capped the bottle. Then he went to the sink to wash the flask. He turned on the hot water, and suddenly the room blossomed into an astonishing, mesmerizing sandalwood smell.

Alone in the lab, the chemist shouted out loud. He dashed to the bottle, but the purified levo-citronellol didn't contain this marvelous smell. So he ran with the flask to have a friend in the next lab smell it. They analyzed it, realized the sandalwood smell was coming from a completely new molecule no one had ever smelled before, which had somehow been created in the reaction. With some time and effort, they worked out a synthesis process for it. Ansari named it Osyrol because, he said, well, they had to name it something, and he liked the name. Osyrol had a rich, full range from bottom notes to top, was extracted from a natural, renewable resource (turpentine), and performed beautifully on the skin—it radiated when put on a warm body (the bloom of odor had come from the hot water, which had volatilized the oil). Plus, it was completely nontoxic. The problem with Osyrol was that it smells almost exactly like beta-santalol, a sandalwood fragrance, and all the power of the smell chemists' computers together could find no correlation in shape between them at all. None. Zip.

But the problem only started there. When you looked at the literature, you then found at least six other ways of getting sandalwood smell that didn't fit the shapist rule, didn't even *remotely* share beta-santalol's shape. (Osyrol drove them particularly mad—small where other sandalwoods were large, simple where they were complex, noncyclic where they were cyclic.) Worse, the amount of heavy computer firepower turned on the problem contradicted Shape only that much more.

The more Turin looked, the more counterexamples he found. There were—now, here was something—some seventy-five molecules that basically smelled of bitter almonds, and the fragrance chemists had dumped them in their computers, pressed a button, and out had popped the bitter-almond shape they all had in common. Then along came hydrogen cyanide. "HCN?" says Turin. "What most people call cyanide, you know, the classic Victorian-novel poison where you smell bitter almonds on her breath? It's a truly tiny molecule, three atoms. H, C, and N in a row, and—please—you can't get a simpler footprint. It's the most famous bitter almond in the world." It refused to fit into any of these other bitter-almond shapes.

Turin started turning his attention to the scientists, but he found that when he asked them uncomfortable questions their reaction, as far as he could tell, was that you had to keep the faith. The faith that Shape worked. That bigger, more powerful computers and imaging would, someday, somehow, get them out of this tight corner. Turin went and burrowed into learned reviews of shape-odor relations, and he had the sensation of imbibing religious texts. "You sit there reading these things," says Turin, "and the sandalwood chapters inevitably start out with complete assurance, 'We have great understanding of what makes sandalwood smell like blah blah,' and then they say, 'And here are the rules,' and then at the end there's a sentence tucked away that says, 'Oh, well, someone found a molecule that smells of sandalwood—Osyrol—that's shaped nothing like any of the reference sandalwoods and doesn't follow any of these rules.' Or they simply don't mention HCN. Which, you have to admit, is the easiest way."

He read a major 1995 *Scientific American* article, "The Molecular Logic of Smell" by Richard Axel, "the god of olfactory genetics," as Turin describes him, "and leading Shapist." Axel dismissed the entire mystery in two sentences: "Scientists believe that various receptors respond to discrete parts of an odor's [shape]. . . . [T]he scents of jasmine and freshly baked bread are . . . different structural groups, and each group activates a distinct set of receptors [by shape]." As far as Turin could tell, you'd read this stuff, and if you didn't know, you'd have no idea you'd just fallen down a chasm.

Shapists also had another problem, which was that we can smell ten times the number of smells that, according to Shape, we should be able to. Linda Buck only found maybe a thousand different receptors in our nose. But we can distinguish by smell ten thousand different molecules (and counting; we have yet to touch any ceiling here). If each receptor was measuring one shape, and if each shape equaled one smell, the math didn't work.

Turin could see for himself that if there *was* a coherent theory, it wasn't jumping out and biting anyone. And—this was galling—he could see glaring mistakes just in the way scientists (who, from Turin's instinctively rigorous point of view on this matter, apparently didn't give a damn) were mischaracterizing smells, writing that molecule X smelled woody (because it happened inconveniently to have what was supposed to be a woody shape) when it was clear to him that it smelled of *musk*. But to Turin, "the ultimate proof that Shape was bullshit was this: I went down to Kent and gave a talk on my growing ideas on Vibration at Quest International, to their chemists. These are guys who invest millions in time and equipment based on Shape, who publish on Shape, who spend hours looking for molecules based on Shape, who are completely vested in Shape. Their findings they keep secret. 'Confidential corporate research by perfume companies.' What you see published in journals is the tiniest tip of the iceberg, because if they found the algorithm that predicted smell, believe me, you'd never hear about it because it would be worth billions and it would be supersecret. So what is a theory? If you're a business guy with stockholders breathing down your neck, a theory, followed by the algorithm you derive from it, is a labor- and money-saving device. It allows you not to screw around wildly at random for years. I was standing there in the room talking to all these Quest chemists about a Vibrational theory, and some guy piped up and objected, 'But we already have a perfectly good theory of smell. Shape.' And I said, 'With all due respect, if you had a theory there wouldn't be thirty-seven Quest research chemists in this room. There'd be three; the others would have been fired, and the three wouldn't be here—they'd be churning out new molecules on a regular basis so Quest could make millions.' If you're a chemist and the number of people who work for you and your status and your power in the company hierarchy all depend on your R & D budget, you don't want a laborsaving device. Unless you're actually inherently interested in efficiency and productivity and not in feeding and clothing yourself and having a powerful position. This is kitchen sociology.

"So the reason I believe Shape is garbage is because they were sitting there listening to me talk about Vibration."

Shapists, playing a little defense (Turin was not the first to notice the cracks in the foundation), had countered quickly in the 1970s and '80s with a nuanced version of Shape, what might be called Shape 2.0 or the Weak-Shape Theory (it's formally known as the Odotope Theory). Weak Shape was a kind of smellable molecular Braille: why (Weak Shape argued) couldn't Buck's one thousand smell receptors be binding to the shape of *parts* of smell molecules? One receptor would feel a certain shaped knob on the molecule, another a rounded hump, another a groove, and you'd then just add "knob" and "hump" and "groove" together and get the smell of asphalt. Or popcorn. Or whatever. Moreover, that, they said, is the answer to the Mystery. It's combinatorial. That's how we smelled boranes, instantly, even though they never existed in our ancestral environment. We just recognize a bunch of curves and nooks, add them up, and get borane's hideous sulfury smell. Mystery solved.

So Turin took a good look at Weak Shape. Yes, it solved the Mystery (theoretically). And he duly noted that Weak Shape—"Each receptor just adds its little piece of info to the others' to get the whole picture"—got Shapists around the ten-thousand-smells-but-only-one-thousand-receptors problematic math. But it immediately occurred to him that Weak Shape had created its own problem, which was that since the receptors were now feeling much less of the molecule, they must by definition be getting less information. And *that* meant, axiomatically, that it was now both more difficult for the receptor to tell two molecules apart and easier for it to mistake many now much-more-similar forms. Like Sulfur and Oxygen, for example. The reason one is right above the other in the periodic table is because they have very similar shapes and very similar chemistry. But humans never, ever mistake Sulfur (SH) for Oxygen (OH) when we smell them. (Otherwise vodka would sometimes smell of rotten eggs.)

But the final case against Weak Shape came back to the exact same problem facing Strong Shape: they still couldn't predict smell. Weak Shape hadn't managed to change the functional Shapist question, which (now) was simply OK, so then which *part* of a molecule's shape carries its smell information? Turin's ruthless analysis was that for Believers in Shape, Weak Shape merely delayed the day of doom when their story would be shown to be worthless. The Shapists could always argue they still hadn't figured out exactly which piece of the ambergris molecule's shape with exactly which other pieces produced "ambergris smell," and they'd figure it out any second now, please hold, your call is important to us. But he observed, uncharitably, that they had been putting these shapes through their computer grinders for years, throwing the greatest calculatory power that human beings possessed at them. And their theory *still* had zero predictive power. Otherwise they wouldn't be tossing atoms together doing combinatorial chemistry. They'd be designing each one. The test of a theory is simple, he noted: how much predictive power does it have? And when you asked how much predictive power Shape had, Strong or Weak, you were forced, reluctantly and warily (if you were the sort to be wary about rocking the foundations of a multibillion-dollar global industry, not to mention a bedrock rule of biology), or quite straightforwardly and cheerfully (if you were Luca Turin) to come up with an answer:

Zero.

✦   ✦   ✦

TURIN STARTED WRITING a draft. He opened the paper with the observation that we can, bizarrely, actually smell atoms, reintroduced Dyson's absurd and fantastical explanation of this, that we must have a biological spectroscope inside us, and then explained why this fantastic machine could, in fact, exist, in the nose, made out of meat: electron tunneling by human cells, since, as he himself had proved with the egg-white diode, proteins conduct electrons and can play wave numbers. At which point he dropped his discovery of a wave number of 2500 for both Sulfur and borane squarely in place as the first piece of proof in the puzzle.

Then he drummed his fingers on his desk and squared his shoulders and tackled the dreaded Enantiomer Problem, the bugaboo that had killed Dyson's theory.

The Enantiomer Problem was that two mirror-image molecules called carvones, which came in an R (*rectus,* or right-handed) version and an S (*sinister,* or left-handed) version, had the same vibrations—yet (frustratingly for Turin) different smells. R smelled of garden mint, S smelled of caraway seeds. But the same vibrations should give the same smell.

The best offense is data. Turin invaded the UCL library's chem texts and marched his computer into the Internet and retrieved bits and pieces from his memory. He wound up with one fact that particularly interested him: R. H. Wright, the big promoter of Dyson's Vibration theory, had, Turin discovered, bizarrely enough never been particularly fazed by this problem. In the 1950s Wright had pointed out that if enantiomers are right- and left-handed, so are the receptors in your nose (and they are; all receptors are, a quirk of biology). To say that a receptor is "right-handed" is just a metaphor for saying "it has one of two orientations." When "right-handed" receptors hold things in their (metaphorical) hands, they hold them differently than left-handed receptors do, and the shape of the object they hold matters. Anyone who's ever cut anything is familiar with this: pick up a pair of left-handed scissors in your right hand and see what they feel like. (Now try cutting a piece of paper with them.) Wright figured that the reason the two carvones smelled different might be simply that holding them in different receptor hands was somehow giving different vibrational readings. But none of the Shapist critics ever got far enough to pay any attention to this because Wright never established the most fundamental thing his theory needed: a plausible mechanism by which a spectroscope could exist in a human nose. For that matter, even if there *was* a spectroscope in the human nose, actual spectroscopes made of metal and glass can't distinguish any vibrational difference between enantiomers. Which brought everything back to the start of the problem. So they ignored him. Next, please.

Except that now, sitting in his office at UCL, Turin set aside for a moment the problem of how to build a spectroscope in the nose (he'd get to that) and focused on his enantiomer difficulty. OK, so: To spectroscopes, enantiomers had identical vibrations, yet they had different smells. Hm. Except . . . (argued Turin, thinking his way forward), except that, come to think of it, everybody's been conceiving of a nasal "spectroscope" as being a spectroscope that uses the standard technique: dumping the molecules you wanted to analyze in liquid and beaming light at them as they tumbled about like clothes in a washer. It was a nice technique, because that way your beam would soon hit every possible side of the molecule, which was showing you all its faces. You saw every bit of it, and you heard every one of its bonds sing.

But there was another way of doing spectroscopy. Not used much, not as well known, but another way: instead of dumping it in liquid, you could fix the molecule still (you stuck it firmly into un-moving crystals) and then aim a laser at it. Since your light beam hit only one side of the molecule, it was like being able to shine a flash-light at only one side of a used car at midnight; the driver's side might look great, but you had no idea what the passenger side looked like because your light beam wasn't reaching it. The beam would hit only one side of the unmoving molecule, strike only some of its bonds, and thus you'd hear only some of its bonds singing. The (few) people who did "crystal spectroscopy" knew this perfectly well. Everyone else was sort of generally aware of this, too, but— here was where doing a little thinking mattered—astonishingly, given that the Shapists had used enantiomers to destroy Dyson's Vibration theory, no one had ever bothered to actually apply this fact to enantiomers.

And Turin realized something pretty simple: when molecules got stuck in receptors, they were essentially sitting still, unmoving. Just like in crystal spectroscopy. If your nose was doing "receptor spectroscopy" (now, that was a new term) as he was saying it was, the molecules were sitting stuck in a receptor, not tumbling around in some wash. So if there was a tiny nasal spectroscope beaming light at them, it was shining its flashlight at only one side and getting only some of the bonds to sing. And some, not.

That was his realization. He now turned his attention to the mint and caraway enantiomers, peering into their guts to figure out exactly which of their vibrations *weren't* getting played.

How about a carbonyl?

Carbonyls are a Carbon atom soldered by a double bond—two electrons—to an Oxygen atom. $C=O$. Read that "C double bond O." They have a stretchy vibration with a wave number of 1800. And both the R and the L, the mint and the caraway, had one implanted under the hood. (Point number one.) If these two mirror molecules were giving different vibrations, the nose's light beam must not be reading one of these carbonyls. But which one? The one in the mint or the one in the caraway? Well, since he'd spent his life looking over structures of smell molecules just for fun, he'd noticed a while ago that (point number two) many mint molecules didn't have carbonyls, but all caraway molecules did. The L carvone smelled of mint, the R of caraway. So he figured that in the L carvone, the mint one, the electrons must not be hitting the carbonyl, and just because the thing was facing the wrong way you weren't smelling the vibration of that double bond in $C=O$. So he deduced that in the left carvone, you got mint. That was the difference.

Nice.

Did it work experimentally? He quickly did some mathematical estimates. Sure enough: it appeared the receptor was gripping the left molecule so that the electron beam couldn't hit the carbonyl. The carbonyl was right there, but the spectroscope just wasn't seeing it.

Very nice.

(This also meant, he realized, that a molecule's shape did matter at least in one basic way: its shape determined the way the receptor would hold it in front of the electron beam. But its smell—his theory said—came from the vibrations that the beam then read.)

Then he suddenly got an idea of how to prove this experimentally. He'd get some molecules with a mint smell. He'd then take pure carbonyl vibrations and pour them in. Like a cook pouring buttermilk into the flour and sugar to transform it all into pancake mix, he'd essentially be pouring in pure 1800, the numbers combining rapidly, wave numbers meshing and recalculating in the velvet liquid. And, he hoped, at the right mix, suddenly, magically, you'd get the smell of caraway. The formula was Mint + Cabonyl = Caraway. That was the bet, anyway. To use vision as analogy, you'd pour yellow into blue until, suddenly: green. Part of this was his own instinct. Turin had smelled the mint carvone, and he'd smelled its caraway version, and effortlessly, without giving it any thought, it had come to him that the difference in smell between the two, the shade that was missing, was the smell of . . . nail-polish remover. Which, when you buy it in those little glass bottles, is basically a molecule called acetone. And acetone happens to be nothing but carbonyl.

Thus (and he had now not only theoretically solved the deadly enantiomer problem; he had set up another experiment) the molecular recipe for the odor we call "caraway" should be something like a cup of mint vibration plus a half cup of nail-polish remover vibration.

Like some molecular chef, Turin went to his lab, poured out some left carvone, and then started pouring carbonyls into it in the form of acetone.

Immediately he ran into a problem. Acetone is such a small molecule, and it evaporates so quickly (in seconds), that he couldn't smell the result before it vanished into the air. He literally couldn't get the stuff into the carvone quick enough. The damn mixture's ratio of acetone to carvone was changing constantly because it was so volatile. In frustration, he glanced around the lab. How about butanone, which has a carbonyl like acetone's but doesn't vanish as fast in air? He grabbed it, grimly started again with his mixtures: 90

percent mint carvone with 10 percent butanone? Nope. 80 percent mint, 20 percent butanone? Still no. When he got to 40 percent mint, 60 percent butanone, he leaned over to sniff, and suddenly there was an unmistakeable caraway smell.

Turin had discovered—it certainly seemed—that when we smell caraway seeds, we are smelling the vibrations that we read as mint plus the vibration that smells to us like nail-polish remover.

He inhaled the smell he'd created.

Then he wrote it up and put it in the paper.

◆   ◆   ◆

TURIN'S NEW THEORY of smell proposed an incredibly sophisticated machine, these thousands of tiny flesh spectroscopes embedded in the nose's mucus, shooting electrons at smelly molecules. How in the world would that machine work? *Nature,* and the rest of the scientific world, would demand that he locate each part—the electrical power supply, the wiring—in the cell's machinery. Time to build the machine.

The first thing to do was learn a lot more about everything. The biology, the chemistry, and the physics, with which he'd started and which meant, most immediately, electron tunneling. He got on a train to Cambridge University, the physics department. Came back exhausted. E-mailed Stewart: "Was in Cambridge all day (great place!!). Visit to C. J. Adkins, inelastic electron-tunneling-spectroscopy specialist, head of the low-temperature physics lab at the Cavendish [the main Cambridge physics laboratory], fellow of Jesus College. Great lunch in the Tudor dining room (curious how all Tudor looks fake, even the real stuff), then long discussion about electron tunneling." Adkins had reeled off information, suggested this and that. Turin had sat and absorbed, had been surprised that "*probably* the best way of doing it is with a cheap STM," which was nice, "just put a droplet of the stuff between substrate and point and get spectra at room temperature." Very simple. "Adkins a very nice man, took a lot of time over it, all afternoon in fact. Showed me a nifty piece of work they'd done where they look at the C-H stretch vibration at high resolution. . . . Cambridge itself too small as a town for comfort, but still impressive. Much better to be lost in London when you leave work." But he drooled over the lab. "The Cavendish great place, full of wonderful-looking hardware carved out of solid stainless steel."

From the day the theory was conceived, when he'd found out about electron tunneling and had experienced the emotional jolt as the pieces fell into place, everything had started moving forward, edging first, then rushing together in a flood—or at least that's what it felt like to Turin. Sometimes he quaked before the idea he'd set himself to birthing. Other times he simply plunged ahead. Several times in his life he'd gone through periods of extremely, almost painfully intense creativity. He loved the monastic, obsessional feel of it, a spiritual agony in intellectual form, the interior emotional buzz of the thing. It was a rhythm that worked for him, spending most of his conscious hours in the dusty crystal silence of the library stacks.

And then it started getting less silent library and more chemical party. He had to find smells now, match them to molecules, match molecules to vibrations. He had to start creating, and he began mixing chemicals, whipping up electron vibrations, wholeheartedly in his mode as mad cook. He was running into Jane Brock's lab, down the hall into Tim Arnett's office, tracking down Martin Rosendaal and hunting Tibor Krenacs, armed with smells, dragging molecules around the old department building on Gower Street and shoving things under their noses several times a day, ordering, "Smell this!" They always did. He'd demand, "What does this smell like?" He'd wait till they'd smelled it and tried to identify it before he'd propose his own ideas. And they'd say whatever came into their minds, "rusted iron" or "hot cotton cloth" or "hand cream and plastic," and he'd nod or frown or say, "Well, does it smell like *this?*" and then, effortlessly, he'd give the words that *exactly, precisely* described the way that the molecule smelled, exactly the description they were groping for. Or he wouldn't bother waiting and would simply demand, "This smells like Styrofoam and fresh basil, doesn't it?"

They watched him. It was having an effect on them, too. Very subtly, without her noticing it happening, Jane Brock realized he had completely changed the way she perceived the space she lived in. It was, she said, as if he'd added a texture to everything, a dimension she'd never perceived. Everywhere she went now, she was conscious of smells.

As Turin's guinea pigs, they all reacted differently. Brock was always interested, supplying him the choice descriptors as best she could, though she was sometimes apologetic about her lack of "expertise." ("Oh, hell, 'expertise'!" Turin said. "Doesn't exist! Everyone can smell as well as everyone else!") Arnett was attentive and utterly sincere and completely petrified of the beasts shoved toward his nose. He produced adjectives warily. Rosendaal, just next door, was more cynical, though game enough, offering sardonic olfactory definitions that Turin then took away to think about. Tibor Krenacs, the Hungarian cell biologist, a darker presence parsimonious with his reactions and wary of facile description, enjoyed growing renown on the floor for purist adjectival obstinacy. If he didn't think something smelled like something else, he absolutely wouldn't supply the descriptive, no matter what Turin threw at him. But, Turin would say, it had this or that vibration! Krenacs the purist refused to be foxed. He approached the molecules and their smells with an admirable seriousness of purpose, determinedly impartial as a referee, analytical as a sommelier, sober as a judge.

When something finally worked, they celebrated. They'd go to Tim Arnett's office and open a bottle of the really good wine, since Turin insisted, and drink it in honor of whatever molecule had graciously agreed to smell the way Turin thought its tiny vibrations should make it smell.

Turin was monomaniac. "I don't *have* a social life," Turin said to them. "I don't give a toss about a social life. I'm only interested in either extremely intimate personal relationships or productive professional relationships." He was living in London and Françoise was, as always, in Paris, so in London it was all concentration. He would come home and fix dinner by himself and sit in front of five hours of TV, thinking about the theory the whole time. He passed weekends in which he uttered not a word to any human being. His flat was an absolute mess. He wouldn't touch it for two weeks at a time, and so he lived, said Brock, who actually witnessed the phenomenon, "in a total pigsty. Filthy, unwashed plates from days before, rubbish overflowing from the trash can onto the floor. It was great." Bare white walls, nothing at the windows, plain blue carpet, the cheapest possible blue sofa you could buy, his stereo system and a piece of wood sitting on top of a trunk, which was the table on which all his papers and everything else got piled. Hundreds of classical CDs strewn across the floor. The bathroom hadn't been cleaned for months. On the rare occasions when Françoise came to London, he'd make an effort to clean. The trash was emptied, the papers were arranged in neater piles. Then she'd leave, and it would go to hell again. It bothered him (but not enough to do anything about it) that if he died and people came to find his body they'd see the apartment and think, "My God, he was living like an *animal!*"

But he just didn't have time—or, more precisely, interest. The thing was *moving*. Turin would come bouncing into their offices at the most inappropriate moments and rip the lid off something extremely evil-looking and shove it forward and say, "Smell this!" They would get nothing more than a glance at the lid, S-Cs and S-O-Hs forming dimers. Turin would say cheerfully, "Don't worry, not toxic, perfectly harmless," which is what he said about everything, including the deadly poisons. Brock and Rosendaal and Krenacs would brace themselves and lean forward, but Arnett was—and he was quite insistent about it—"a coward with a natural instinct to caution," and because Turin worked with S-H groups a fair amount, even if it wasn't extremely toxic, it was fair odds the thing would smell horrific. If you passed by in the hall you'd hear Arnett saying for the fifth time, No! I won't smell that, and Turin saying, Oh, *smell it!* and in the end Arnett would brace himself and grimace and have a little sniff. (Oh, good *Christ,* Luca, what the *hell* is that?! Turin [very interested]: So how would you describe that?)

Arnett was walking the linoleum halls with an increasingly guarded, uneasy look. Rosendaal and Brock came to expect Turin's exploding through the door, recounting astonishing things about smells. At the same time, Turin's attention span was short, and they'd often find him on the Internet reading about some American air force base or how to land a plane. When he was bored, he went and played.

To Arnett's dismay, Turin had little conception of the niceties of fume cupboards, "where," Arnett reminded him, "you're supposed to store these things so you don't shorten everyone's life to thirty-five years." Turin grumbled. Arnett was the safety officer, conduct-ing inspections: no toxins left out, no eating, no smoking. Turin did all of those. When one day an absolutely asphyxiating rotten-egg smell came rolling into his office, Arnett ran down the hall (it was getting stronger as he approached Turin's lab) and burst in, and Turin, wearing a look of glee, shoved some compound at him and said, "Smell this, *it smells really bad, doesn't it!*" Arnett roared that he should put the damn things in the fume cupboard, to which Turin hotly retorted something about "bureaucracy," to which Arnett replied, objectively if not calmly, that Turin might hate boring things like safety and loathe the idea that anyone would control him, but he was poisoning them all and being antisocial. So they had a huge row and didn't speak for a fortnight. Geoff Burnstock, the department head, got them to be friends again. For goodness sake, Luca, sniffed Arnett, can't you work on something that doesn't in-volve S-H groups?

"The thing about Luca," says Arnett, "is that he has this reality-distortion field. Which he freely admits." ("Bullshit," says Turin, half the time, and the other half "Yes, that's true.")

There were a million knickknacks he had to track down and buy, pieces of software, measuring tools, smell molecules. Turin waited for what seemed like forever for them to arrive in his postbox so he could inhale their atomic fragrance, meanwhile setting things up, looking things up, downloading bits and pieces. Brock was saying to him, "I know you'll figure this out," and everyone on the Depart-ment of Anatomy's second floor was pushing him on, "Go, go, go!" He was a bit awed by it, the enthusiasm from others, the support, but he generated it by laying each new piece of Vibration's puzzle before them, and they responded. "I was devoting complete con-centration to making this work," he explained later. "I was manic. I didn't have a life."

But he did have a life. He had a creative life.

✦　　✦　　✦

ON A TRAIN from somewhere in silvery-gray, rainy England, rushing toward London, and Turin muses: "Remind me to tell you why
only manic-depressives can do science properly."

Are you manic-depressive?

He says promptly, "Not in the clinical sense," and then goes back
to staring out the window at the English countryside flashing past
the train.

When he gets around to discussing it, he says, "If you look at Darwinian evolution, Nature is just generating tons and tons of mutations and then, because most of them are duds, ruthlessly cutting
them all down. Not very nice for the mutations. That's what you do
as a scientist: generate tons and tons of ideas and then shoot them
down. To generate them you have to suspend disbelief. You have to
believe that everything you come up with is 'Wonderful! Brilliant!
Plausible!' That's manic. Then you have to shoot 'em all down, one
by one, 'This won't work, this one's crap.' That's depression. But——"
Thinking about it, he starts laughing. "——But since just about everyone else is depressive, you can just be manic all the time, and they'll
shoot the ideas down for you. So it helps to have manic-depressive
disease, and to have it in a particularly acute, aggressive form." This
gets him started on the state of professional science. "The rewards
system is equally hilarious. You slave your whole life in some
Formica-covered lab, you have a couple of double bypasses, your
wife leaves you, your kids don't talk to you because all you've done
is generate The Humungous Idea. Then they fly you to Stockholm
first-class and they give you some *medal* made out of *chocolate,* and
the thing is, it isn't intended to make *you* feel good at all, it's intended to inspire envy among all the little ones still churning out
product in the labs. It doesn't even have a good evolutionary benefit
in the Darwinian sense—in terms of spreading your genes by
screwing all your pretty graduate students impressed by the dominant silverback in the gorilla troop. Because, see, by the time you're
a silverback, the problem is you're a silverfront." He sighs happily,
exhausted with laughter. "I get such a kick out of making these sinister statements."

✦　　✦　　✦

EVERYONE IN UCL's Department of Anatomy was wondering, not necessarily with any charity, what he was up to. The department, per academia's usual eternal politicking, had its doubts, and it had its concerns, and it had its questions about funding and research and *what,* if you please, was the Turin lab really turning out? Certainly not papers; he wasn't publishing a damn thing. And his two-year contract was expiring. Wasn't it. (It was.) And so the question of Luca Turin's professional future at University College London arose.

He had his camp. Geoff Burnstock, the department head who had given Turin a job when he was fleeing France, was supportive, tensed to spring at the right moment for a meeting with the Provost of UCL, Sir Derek Roberts, about Turin's future. But Turin wasn't exactly helping his cause. His experiments were inciting Paris Commune–style riots in the corridors. "The funniest thing in the world just happened," he e-mailed Stewart. Some chemist had mentioned to him, offhand, that some SH molecules didn't smell like his decaborane ("Boiled onion, Luca!" Krenacs had proclaimed). *Huh?* said Turin, alarmed. If this was true, he was in deep trouble, so he nervously ordered a dozen different sulfurs from Aldrich, the chemical-supply company, and prayed for foul odors. "So I'm busy unpacking them and notice they smell pretty bad even when sealed, the packing material itself has taken on the smell, etc. I decide to collect all the packing and go to the main trash can. When I get back, the *entire floor* is in an uproar, with the safety officer accusing me of dangerous (wrong) and antisocial (not his remit) behaviour. When I point out to him (nice guy, by the way) that instead of listening to him, I would prefer to be dealing with the origin of the stench and put the things in a fume cupboard, he nearly bursts into tears with rage and fear and calls me names." Turin heaved a sigh through his keyboard. "Anyway, it's all over."

"Btw," Turin added (needlessly, given the floor's reaction), "boranes *do* smell like sulfurs. Fun, what?"

He cut a figure in the anemic fluorescent academic light.

Rosendaal didn't mind that Turin was a sharp dresser and quite vain about his appearance, but Turin's lab manners drove him up a wall. He'd quite flagrantly pilfer Rosendaal's equipment or his calculator, or the right color of rubbish bag that the department insisted you use (medical waste in yellow bags and so on). Rosendaal, a self-described bit of a tight-ass, got into terrific fights with Turin that mostly consisted of Rosendaal yelling, "What the fuck have you done with my things!"

The anti-Turin camp armed themselves with the fact that, as Rosendaal reluctantly but quickly concluded, if you were one of the uninspired or slightly slower students, Turin was an absolute disaster as a teacher. Either he pitched way over their heads or he simply didn't turn up. On the other hand, for the students who could keep up he was a marvel, a wizard; they gave him top grades across the board, and he loved teaching them. He was also great, his colleagues duly noted, at selecting good-looking women for his courses, which he made no bones about. He was enormously flip and entertaining in the classroom and made them gasp (when he showed up), but when he didn't show up he was incensed that people were cross. Turin decided to go on vacation in Corsica at one beginning of term and couldn't understand why everyone was furious. Arnett and Rosendaal took turns explaining that when the students came back to school, the teachers were supposed to be there to help them out and point them in the right direction and wipe their noses as necessary. Arnett explained patiently that Turin had accepted a position as a lecturer, he'd taken the king's shilling, and now he had to be there. Turin thought they were being boring, small-minded people. Arnett said, Luca, if there's *one* time of the year you're supposed to be here, it's now. Turin said, furiously, Tim, you're moralizing. He'd thought Arnett of all people would understand. He didn't have many responsibilities anyway, he said, and Arnett replied that he didn't have many responsibilities because everyone knew he was completely irresponsible, that one would see six students sitting forlornly outside Turin's office because he'd forgotten and was in Paris or being flown in a private plane to the south of France or wherever. That he always did the most interesting thing that day, said Arnett, and the hell with everything else. Turin shrugged. Off he went to Corsica.

People whispered about Turin's research methodology, which was, at moments, the opposite of double-blinds with controls. He'd barge in excitedly and say, "This smells like shit, doesn't it!" On those rare moments when Arnett did not, in fact, think it smelled like shit, he would dig in his heels and say *no,* it *didn't.* ("I'm from Lincolnshire," says Arnett. "We aren't to be convinced when we don't agree.") So Turin would blast into Brock's office and do the same, and she'd dig in her heels ("From Yorkshire—even worse than Lincolnshire"), and Turin would try to convince them in an openly partisan manner. It was not, to put it mildly, the standard scientific approach. Every once in a while Turin would write a grant request for some bizarre grant. In five years in the department, he published one paper and, in Rosendaal's estimation, thought that generous of himself. Of course, he managed to publish it in the most obscure journal humanly possible to find. Geoff Burnstock was producing twenty-five papers a year, and Arnett pointed out to Turin that all he, Turin, had to do was write one paper, just one—it would take him two afternoons! But Turin couldn't bring himself to do it. He simply wasn't interested. It made him enemies in the department. At least one professor was doing what he could to get Turin, whom he considered a disgrace and a scandal, fired.

If Turin was not publishing, he was at least leading a high-profile lecture series on Thursday nights, very popular with students, on the philosophy of science. The problem here was that as speakers he invited, by his own happy description, "mavericks, iconoclasts, odd-balls, and weirdos." One had just finished building the Babbage computing engine, which was a purely theoretical computer that had been proposed in the mid-nineteenth century and that, to everyone's amazement, when built actually worked. That was fine, but another lecturer, a scientific journalist working for the London *Times,* explained why there was actually no AIDS in Africa, which wasn't fine at all, and which aroused a certain reaction in the faculty lounge and prompted one UCL colleague to wonder aloud why Turin didn't just invite a goddamn psychic and have done with it. Who knew how much of this had reached the Provost.

And then there was the question of what kind of creature Luca Turin was, exactly. He'd been trained as a biologist. Fine. But he was metamorphosing in his intellectual chrysalis by reading all these books, voluntarily transforming himself through his curiosity into . . . a biophysicist, an in-betweener, a disciple of a newish (faddish, in the strong view of some) neither-fish-nor-fowl science. The cult was quietly tolerated among the mainline academic sects but not, certainly, embraced. And not understood.

Even the name is wrong. "Biophysics" leaves out chemistry. This is anomalous, given that chemistry is the universal mediator between biology and physics and a crucial link every biophysicist must know as well as the other two. As for any orthodox Christian, God in biophysics is a trinity. But perhaps "biophysistry" just sounded too strange. Still, biophysics is about the interaction, the fusing, of the three temples that had always in the traditional university stood clearly separate. It is biology—genes with the infrastructure of cells and receptors and proteins and the complex systems they produce—meeting chemistry—the frenetic microscopic commerce between the fancy molecular products these systems churn out—meeting physics—the behavioral psychology of the forces and particles that are the mechanics of that commerce.

It is said that both chemists and physicists study the atom, but chemists mess around with the electrons and physicists pass their time on the nucleus. Biology (which at its birth could conceive of nothing smaller than the entire human body, slowly perceived the system, suddenly caught startled sight of the organ, swooped down from there to the cell, and only recently zeroed in on the tiny molecule) has now metamorphosed into the study of the gene, a string of molecules that blueprint the construction of other molecules, which build cells, which assemble into organs, which organize as systems, which make up the body. This is the historical reason people still say "*molecular* biology," which is actually a name without meaning. As if there were any other kind of biology anymore. And if people believe there is another kind, it is in part because the very idea of biophysics is, for various ideological and religious and political and emotional reasons, anathema to many. Are we great and noble animals, possessed of creative genius and free will, the sum greater than the parts? Or are we compilations of buzzing pieces of molecules, our hearts cells, our cells atoms, human beings just big physics projects made of flesh? Is there no immortal soul? There is only one biology that matters anymore, and it is molecular.

What this means is that the three separate kingdoms—biology, physics, chemistry—which have always seen themselves as their own fiercely independent city-states, are now, for biophysicists, unifying. The coming scientific One-World Government is particle science, and biophysicists are its soldiers. We are atoms, moving about restlessly. They are us. The borders are meaningless, although the schools and universities have not yet caught up with this reality. They still turn out biologists, chemists, and physicists, the nations and their peoples divided, each speaking its own language. There are a few interpreters here and there, a few cross-cultural forays, but from the three traditional tribes, very few choose to live abroad for long. Turin experienced this as a sort of constant surprise. He didn't throw the three together out of conscious intent, necessarily, but just because he was *interested,* because one thing always led him, beckoning, to another, and that one inevitably and insistently to a third. And he was too impatient to bother with the boundaries. So he crossed borders, no passport, no visa, didn't ask anyone's permission or stop at the consulates. He called it being "a true four-wheel-drive creature that could go anywhere." This basically meant reading everything he could get his hands on, regardless of which principality claimed it. He wheeled into a cell that was under Biology's traditional control, looked it over, jumped down from the cell to a neutron in territory claimed by Physics because it seemed the obvious place to go, caught sight of the buzzing electron cloud overhead and flew upward into what was supposed to be Chemistry's exclusive terrain. It was intellectual federalism. He would find that those who ran the three ancient fiefdoms did not appreciate it. They favored unification, but strictly on the margins, and strictly in theory. They were nineteenth-century nationalists: "Stay inside your boundaries, keep to your own kind." Which he simply hated. He thought it stupid. He was no diplomat. He slagged them off. It was instinct. They said, "Passport, please." He had no time for it. He pissed off their envoys, the diploma granters and the department heads and so forth, and they refused to stamp his papers. He continued anyway, not really noticing. He had the books he needed heaped in stacks at his bedside.

Turin would panic about his contract, and then he would pop back. "Forgot to mention in the last msg," he wrote Stewart. "Burnstock informed me this morning that my job was practically 'in the bag.' It turns out some guy who was supposed to come did not, and his position can apparently be recycled into mine w.out having to create a new one. That means a 5-yr contract!! Good, no?" Françoise, for one, didn't think it was so good. The job was in London. But that, he could work out later.

He needed to do something proactive, so he screwed up his courage and went to Burnstock and proposed something he had never done before: give a talk about his budding theory of smell. To the entire department? OK, replied Turin, wondering what he was getting into. Burnstock said yes.

Turin approached the lecture with dread. The dread deepened when so many people showed up—over a hundred—that the audience had to abandon the normal seminar room en masse and re-assemble itself in an ampitheater. He gulped and gave the talk. Afterward, after Vibration's slightly shaky baby steps into the world of science, and the world of science's first wary peek at Vibration, he reported to Stewart with relief, "Talk went very well, much appreciated it seems, I think I made it reasonably entertaining. Chemists in the audience v. impressed, rather a good sign since they've actually had more experience of smells. Glad it's over, tonight champagne."

Then he heard the gossip and wrote a bit more: "Talk: *tremendous success*, as it turns out, people have been coming to see me to compliment me, a good feeling. One colleague, Candy Hassall, said that several people had come to the talk anticipating that I would screw up, and I bitterly disappointed them . . . what nice people academics are! Geoff Burnstock actually *signed* my job appointment when he returned to his office, apparently! I asked him today whether my job description could be Lecturer in Biophysics (not usually done at this level). It may seem like nothing much, but it means a lot to me that biophysics should exist as a subject without apologies to all the cell and molecular people. He said he'd try for that. All in all, at a local level, I pulled it off OK. Phew!!"

Stewart replied: " 'Lecturer in Biophysics,' God knows you deserve it."

Turin: "Thanks!!!!!!! fingers crossed. . . ."

Perhaps the fingers worked. The next day Turin typed: "I got the *JOB*!!!!!!!!!!! Geoff Burnstock went to see the Provost this morning and had my appointment approved." He was awestruck: "Five years of thinking time ahead."

"That's really great news!!" Stewart e-mailed and then prompted "What about the Vibration paper for *Nature*??"

Turin replied cheerfully: "It's half-written, just working up to finishing it."

This was a lie; Turin was gearing up for more experiments.

To his surprise—and, to a degree, disbelief; it seemed rather too good to be true—his fledgling theory was turning some heads.

Date: Fri, 3 Mar 1995
To: stewartw@helix.nih.gov
From: l.turin@ucl.ac.uk
Subject: at the prince's request . . .

At 3PM, I get a phone call from the Provost: Could he come to my lab to get a firsthand account of what I'm up to. Naturally, I offered to go to his office instead. We had a very pleasant conversation about science, first mine then his, for an *hour*. He then said he'd set up an informal group to explore the future of biophysics @ UCL, consisting of a few people in chemistry, physics, and biotechnology. Did I want to be part of this and would I mind explaining what my smell work was about as a basis for discussion. I said yes please. . . .

Stewart: "God Almighty!! This is the Kingdom Come to Earth!!! Good news, I presume."

Turin: "Yes, excellent news if you like that sort of thing." He meant the politics of academia.

❖   ❖   ❖

MARTIN ROSENDAAL LATER said of Turin's lecture, "This was when I first realized there was something special about him. In the embryology lecture theater. I realized half of UCL was there, all the big shots, and so on. And I thought, 'He's the first person to apply quantum mechanics to a physiological problem.' One of the reasons why we're not going to live on in memory is because we're using nineteenth-century physics to tackle our problems in biology. I said to Tibor, 'What an extraordinary piece of luck that we should be next to a man who will get a Nobel.' Of course, I'm sure he won't get a Nobel. There's a fatal flaw in Luca's personality: he isn't a terrier. He doesn't take a subject and sink his jaws into it and shake it and worry it obsessively. He's impatient."

❖   ❖   ❖

TURIN AND STEWART were playing with gadgets. They bought Net Phone software, and Turin bought a really fast modem (28K! very exciting) (it was 1995), and soon he was sitting at his computer doing midnight crawls through molecular biology databases and airplane-design websites. One night he stumbled into the home of a rather amazing computer in Heidelberg, Germany. The computer's name was Blitz (an acronym, nicely Germanic). He e-mailed Stewart about Blitz: "Check this out: highly parallel computer compares a sequence to *entire* protein database in less than 30 seconds !!!! holy cow !!!" He was excited because he loathed all the gruntwork of molecular biology, digging out data in this field that was, as Jane Brock put it, "simply following recipes." So Blitz was a pleasant little oddity, his own friendly German molecular biology supercomputer. Purely for fun, he sent Stewart Blitz's address: www.ebi.ac.uk/searches/blitz_input.html.

❖   ❖   ❖

"GRASSE," SAYS TURIN, "is twenty-five kilometers from Nice, fifteen kilometers inland, just behind Cannes. The story I heard is this: Grasse was a big leather town in the early nineteenth century, particularly gloves. Gloves used to be scented because people believed disease was carried by bad odors. They used to strew castle floors with thyme and stuff because they thought it would fight off typhoid. So a guy named Antoine Chiris, originally Italian, set up a natural raw-smell-materials distillery—the climate's ideal for growing flowers—to make scents to scent the gloves. He had a patent on steam distillation, Antoine Chiris et Compagnie, he was the first, and his method was so powerful that more and more fragrances started to be made there, and suddenly Grasse was the perfume capital of the world, the origin of virtually every high-priced perfume molecule you could want. This lasted for years.

"Then in the 1960s, of course, the bomb exploded. Synthetic raw materials, which people had started to make in the 1880s, arrived in full force—synthetic heliotropes, synthetic rose molecules. Suddenly anyone with a basic chemistry set could start welding atoms to each other and exporting them. And then French labor costs shot up, and today almost all the naturals, the roses and jasmines and greens, come from the Third World, where they're cheaper to make, and the synthetics come from labs everywhere you can imagine. Some naturals do still come from Grasse, and these ingredients are the most expensive in the world today, and the highest quality. Laboratoire Monique Remy makes a pure distillation of fresh hay that is . . . *unpronounceably* wonderful. Distilled hay is the smell of liquid summer sunlight.

"The French perfumers," says Turin, intently. "There were people of great class among them, but the industry basically was just a bunch of kids from Grasse, which means typical Côte d'Azur, which means a bunch of criminals. I was talking to a perfumer raised in Grasse once, she said, 'Either you became a perfumer or you stole motorcycles.'

"They're quite familiar with sensuality. One of them, a man, once gave me a guide to Rome that he'd written. It was twenty pages, typed, and it was a shopping guide. It consisted of nothing but expensive shoes and ladies' lingerie. He'd obviously known Rome entirely as a place for fucking. This guy once described Henri Alméras, who did *Joy* for Jean Patou, to me as '*Vous savez, Alméras . . .*'" Turin makes a lecherous expression, puts out his hands, and flexes his fingers. " *'Il était toujours les mains en avant.'* " Groping.

"I got to know Guy Robert particularly well. He's a professional-level jazz pianist, writes fiction, is a terrific cook. You should hear him talking about olive oil. He knows the only place to get it. He took me to one of the best restaurants I've ever been to, Le Bistro le Paradou, west of Aix. He's in his seventies now. He's been in the business a long time, has bad relations with Jean Amic, the old head of Givaudan. It's a small world, Grasse. Everyone's screwed everyone else at some point, literally and figuratively. There are some real scam artists. A *very,* I mean *very* small world. Often the scam is buying natural raw materials from India and passing them off as real Grasse products, and I swear to God I think it's not the money; it's to see if they can outfox the damn gas chromatograph. Everyone gets swindled." He mentions the filthy-rich head of a private perfume house. "She's gotten taken for millions. She's battening down the hatches a bit. They sell you the best stuff the first time, and then they resupply you with some Chinese shit. Or Madagascar, or the Comoros. So you have to keep incredible quality control.

"These perfume people—their obsession is what's so terrific. They get a flight to Rome, connection to Palermo, and the supplier, who basically greets them on bended knee, says, Here's our new citrus for this year, and they smell it, and it's the best, the best in the entire world, and they snap it up. At Chanel, when they have to dilute the perfume with ethanol—Jesus, ethanol! It costs nothing, and it *smells* of nothing!—Chanel still gets ten competitors from Europe to bid for it, they put all the samples in wineglasses, everyone is standing around smelling this stuff, and then they decide OK, this Spanish guy is going to supply us with ethanol for *Chanel No. 19.* This is the kind of obsessional *mania* that makes great perfume. You *have* to be this obsessed. Then they go to Tunisia and lock up *one* guy's total jasmine supply for a full decade. He's got guaranteed sales, at Chanel rates—imagine those—he gives them a jasmine that is absolutely drop-dead stupendous (and on his life he doesn't dare do less), and no one else in the world for any price can get their claws on that jasmine.

"The best Guy Robert story is this. The House of Dior started making perfumes in the 1940s. Very small scale. The first two were *Diorama* and *Miss Dior*. The former was made by Edmond Roudnitska, a Ukrainian émigré who'd studied with Ernest Beaux in Saint Petersburg because Beaux was the perfumer to the czars. The second by Paul Vacher. So Dior approached Guy Robert—they invite him to dinner, they're talking over the cheese course, no sterile meeting rooms, this is a brief among gentlemen—and they said, 'We're doing a new perfume we want to call *Dioressence,* for women, but we want it very animalic. The slogan will be *le parfum barbare,* so—propose something to us.' Oh boy. Guy can hardly wait. Of course he wants a Dior commission. And the challenge of mixing the florals of the traditional Dior fragrances into an animal scent (because this isn't just any animalic, this is a *Dior* animalic, if you can imagine such a bizarre thing) is just a bewitching challenge, who else would have the guts to attempt joining those two. So he gets right to work, plunges in, and he tries all sorts of things. And he's getting nowhere. Nothing's working. He's frustrated, he doesn't like anything he's doing.

"In the middle of this, someone in the industry calls him, and they say, 'There's a guy with a huge lump of ambergris for sale in London—get up here and check it out for us.' Ambergris is the whale equivalent of a fur ball, all the undigested crap they have in their stomachs. The whale eats indigestible stuff, and every once in a while it belches a pack of it back up. It's mostly oily stuff, so it floats, and ambergris isn't considered any good unless it's floated around on the ocean for ten years or so. It starts out white and the sun creates the odorant properties by photochemistry, which means that it's become rancid, the molecules are breaking up, and you get an incredibly complex olfactory result. So Guy gets on a plane and flies up to see the dealer, and they bring out the chunk of ambergris. It looks like black butter. This chunk was about two feet square, thirty kilos or something. Huge. A brick like that can power Chanel's ambergris needs for twenty years. This chunk is worth a half million pounds.

"The way you test ambergris is to rub it with both hands and then rub your hands together and smell them. It's a very peculiar smell, marine, sealike, slightly sweet, and ultrasmooth. So there he is, he rubs his hands in this black oily mess and smells them, and it's terrific ambergris. He says, Great, sold. He goes to the bathroom to wash his hands 'cause he's got to get on an airplane. He picks up some little sliver of dirty soap that's lying around there and washes his hands. He leaves. He gets on the plane, and he's sitting there, and that's when he happens to smell his hands. The combination of the soap and ambergris has somehow created exactly the animalic Dior he's been desperately looking for. But what the hell does that *soap* smell like? He's got to have that goddamn piece of soap. The second he lands in France, he sprints to a phone, his heart pounding, and calls the dealer in England and says, 'Do *exactly* as I say: go to your bathroom, take the piece of soap that's in there, put it in an envelope, and mail it to me.' And the guy says, 'No problem.' And then he adds, 'By the way, that soap? You know, it was perfumed with some *Miss Dior* knockoff.'

"So Guy put them together, and got the commission, and made, literally, an animalic Dior. *Dioressence* was created from a cheap *Miss Dior* soap knockoff base, chypric, fruity aldehydic, plus a giant cube of rancid whale vomit. And it is one of the greatest perfumes ever made."

Something passes over Turin's face. He says "*Dioressence* is still being manufactured, and sold everywhere, and everyone buys it, and it's now a total lie, a total lie to the original, to what it was. *Miss Dior* is also still around, and it's only half a lie. Dior have continuously cheapened their fragrances and substituted less expensive materials till the gods departed and all that's left is a gorgeous, empty, lamented name."

◆   ◆   ◆

AROUND THIS TIME, Turin got a phone call from a young woman named Alison Baum. Turin had tutored Baum when she took her master's in neuroscience, after which she chose, instead of looking out from the laboratory, to look into it as producer of a BBC science series called *Horizon*. One day when she'd stopped by his UCL office for a visit, he told her about his theory. Baum went away, thought about it, then called him and asked more questions. She rang off, wrote a two-page proposal, and sent it on June 23, 1995, to John

Lynch, the series' executive producer. Then she called Turin: *Horizon* wanted to make Turin the main subject of a substantial BBC documentary.

He was elated. Someone was paying attention to Vibration. This could be a phenomenal opportunity to get the theory out there. The problem was that playing the BBC card could be dangerous, or fatal, to the bet he'd placed on *Nature*. The bitter jealousy of peer-review journals is legendary, *Nature* being perhaps the premier example. If you get more press than they do, "they have your guts for garters" is the way Turin put it. "The peer-review process is the best we've got and it's corrupt, inefficient, and wrongheaded, not least because it is run by human beings, who happen to be competitive, territorial, and jealous." If the documentary ran first, *Nature* might decide the BBC had stolen their thunder. But he decided to do it, because what the hell, and besides, television takes forever, right? By the time the BBC broadcast the program (Isabel Rosin, the producer, told him they were aiming for the fall of 1995), *Nature* would have already safely published the paper, right? So everything would be fine.

❖   ❖   ❖

"I WENT TO a primary school in Paris, then my parents moved to Switzerland and I went to school for four years in Geneva. At the Paris school I did very well. I was in love with my teacher, who seemed very tall to me and apparently was a short young lady. At the school in Switzerland I did appallingly badly. I had no idea what people wanted from me, and my life had a nightmarish quality that I've never since quite managed to dispel whenever I'm in contact with institutions. And then fortunately my parents divorced and I went back to France, because within weeks I was top of my class and stayed at the top of the class for years. Got every prize and everything, and then when I got to high school, I didn't work hard enough. You know the slogan the Situationists painted on the wall: '*Ne travaillez jamais.*' [Never work.] And I agreed. I couldn't see the point.

"I have an abiding hatred for the Swiss educational system. Actually, I don't know anything about the Swiss themselves and I don't give a shit. What I know about is their educational system, which was"—Turin suddenly articulates every syllable with envenomed precision, the words popping like water droplets falling into hot fat—"*designed* to destroy human beings and turn them into Swiss citizens. Switzerland is Germany without the random noise. As Noël Coward said of a really bad twentieth-century musical, 'It was like Wagner's *Parsifal* but without the jokes.' They try to take kids with hearts and heads and imaginations and turn them into Swiss taxpayers, gelatinous beings with a fanatical belief in nothingness. I occasionally dream of flying over Geneva and bombing my old school. A simple example that still sticks with me vividly. Those fucking assholes—and I choose my words carefully—conceived of having children sell postage stamps for charity. So you're six years old, and you're supposed to go and ring doorbells in your apartment block. You got the stamps, and a book in which you had to record how much everyone paid. So I rang the doorbells, and I sold every damn stamp. I brought all the money back. But because I'd been too busy running around, ringing doorbells, asking, 'Lady, would you like to buy some stamps?' I hadn't done the proper bookkeeping, 'Six stamps to Frau Schroeder' and 'Twelve stamps to Madame Dupont' and 'Ten stamps to Signora Nonino' and all this horseshit. And I was told off. In front of everyone. Humiliated. I was a complete failure because, no bookkeeping. That is Switzerland for you. People like that destroy human beings.

"I think my libertarian streak started then. Also my view of institutions as abnormal and insane. Nobody is more ambivalent about institutions than I am. I mean, I'm capable of getting tears in my eyes at the thought of the Academy of Sciences. Or the Royal Society, this group of scientists. I'm a great believer in symbols and totally convinced that symbolic acts carry a tremendous force, and that honor and recognition are really what we strive for, the notion of someone who does it simply for the heck of it being utter bollocks. I really love these institutions. What I find totally incomprehensible is the everyday madness that everyone in institutions seems to live in. You'd think the ninety-nine percent would tolerate the one percent of us who are different, the weirdos, the fanatics, you'd think they wouldn't resent us so *goddamn much*. I'm prepared to live with those bastards! I don't want everyone to be like me! But they want everyone *to be like them!* Second-rate! I shouldn't be blamed for not contributing what everyone else is. And you know my old head of department at UCL, Geoff Burnstock, God bless him in eternity, was that kind of guy, he said to me, 'Look, Luca, we have two hundred people in the department. We can afford half a percent of weirdness. Stick around.'

"Then Burnstock left and I got fired by his replacement, Nigel Holder."

◆　　◆　　◆

WHAT THE BIG papers are built on, what gets you publication in *Nature* and the front page of the *New York Times* Science Times section, what hooks the grants and hauls in the big prizes, is the airtight, foolproof experiment. That was what Turin needed for *Nature*. Since everyone measures everyone else's theory by predictive power, the obvious way to prove that Vibration was smell was to predict a smell based on vibrations. The question was how. It wasn't simple.

He pushed the problem around. OK, here was a possibility: what if you took two different electron bonds whose smells were, clear as day, different (one was ripe tangerines, say, the other kerosene). If you glued those two vibrations together, added their wave numbers, you'd get a new vibrational chord—and according to Turinism, you should get a new smell. So the experiment was simply this: could he, purely from his theory, predict what that smell should be? He'd try and see and hope to God his crystal ball got it right.

OK. Which smell to predict and then build? He decided on the smell of bitter almonds. First of all, there was a little molecule he knew of, HCN, that smelled of bitter almonds, and conveniently enough HCN only had three vibrations, two prominent ones—a carbonyl (same as the acetone), which vibrated at around wave number 700, and a nitrile (close to the carbonyl of acetone) that vibrated around 2000 and had a bending mode around 800—which simplified things. And there was another molecule he knew, benzaldehyde, which also smelled of bitter almonds, and which (again conveniently) had the carbonyl and a stong 800 ring bending mode. His theory's prediction was that if you grabbed any off-the-shelf 700 vibe and any 2000 vibe you had lying around the shop and glued them together, that two-note molecular chord should also play bitter-almond smell; but since this molecular arts-and-crafts was impractical, he'd just find a third molecule that had the 700-2000 chord and confirm that it, too, played bitter-almond smell. Which would be neat enough. The clincher, however, would be that this new molecule's *shape* would be different from benzaldehyde's and HCN's. Yet its vibrations and smell would be the same.

So much for hypothesis generation. Now to find this molecule. Turin carries in his head a compendium of chemical knowledge from having essentially memorized Cotton and Wilkinson's *Advanced Inorganic Chemistry.* His copy is filthy and dog-eared from years of being read in bed, in cars, on subways. His mind thumbed it, looking for molecules as in a hardware-store catalog.

Ah. Now here were some that might do the trick. They had the 1800-2000 carbonyl and 800 benzene ring, hooked together in a totally different structural way (which meant they were shaped nothing like the others). The benzene and carbonyl were glued up with a metal ion sitting in the middle of their guts. They were possessed of, first, a rather gruesome name (cyclopentadienyl-metal tricarbonyls, nicknamed "metal carbonyls"), second, an odor ("One of them," he e-mailed Stewart offhandedly, "is reported to have a camphor smell!"), and third, a strange structure: they were basically molecular hamburgers, the two five-Carbon rings like buns with burgers of the various metal atoms—Iron, Cobalt, Nickel, and Manganese—slapped in between. But he didn't pay this any mind.

When they arrived by Royal Mail, he was trotting down a corridor at UCL with them when he passed the famous synthetic-organic chemist William Motherwell. The dry Scotsman frowned suspiciously at him. "What airr ya doin'?"

Turin said cheerfully that oh, he was just going through a bunch of metal carbonyls.

"Going through 'em *how?*"

Well, he was smelling them.

Motherwell went white as a sheet. "Ehhhh," he glowered, "aire ye tairred of livin'?" Metal carbonyls, he informed Turin, are extremely poisonous, ate at your fingers, gave you diseases.

Huh, said Turin (he knew this), and trotted off down the corridor carrying his booty.

(Turin's attitude is: Who can worry about this sort of thing. "A sniff here and there isn't going to kill you," he says. Motherwell says that a sniff here and there of violently toxic molecules is exactly what kills you. Turin shrugs. "I'm still here." And so far, he is.)

He did attenuate his organometallic-sniffing habit ("I'm trying to cut down"), but mostly because, disappointingly, none of them smelled of bitter almonds. The nickel burger (nickelocene) had a nasty chemical-oily smell. The iron burger (ferrocene) did indeed smell of camphor, and the cobalt-flavored one smelled like— well, it turned out that it exploded into flames on contact with air, which made it impossible to smell. So he counted this experiment a failure.

On March 9, 1995, he seized on a new, improved angle. Plan B. "You know about these cryptate molecules," he e-mailed Stewart with enthusiasm, "a cage molecule that encloses another, smaller one?" His new idea was to prove that the nose functions like a metal detector.

Take a thick rubber foam ball. Slit a very thin opening deep into it with a razor, slide a dime down into its center, and allow the rubber foam to reseal itself so it looks exactly the same as before. Then give it to someone and ask him to tell you what is in the ball. If all he can do is feel the outside shape of the ball, he has no idea. The dime is invisible. But if he has a metal detector, he can detect the dime inside. Turin looked around for a molecule he could open, tuck a vibrational dime in, and then zip up again, encasing the vibration. Then he'd loose on it the biological metal detector that, his theory said, the nose was, inhale this dime-filled molecule, and see if the detector worked.

What vibrational dime should he try to smell? And which molecular foam ball to hide it in?

The electron ropes that hold all atoms together can be single strands (one electron circling two atoms like a lasso), double (two electrons), triple (these are rare), or (almost never) quadruple bonds. Each molecule has a name that, at a single glance, will tell chemists which of these bonds the molecule has inside it: if its name ends in *ane* you know there's a single bond; *ene* means a double, *yne* is a triple.

Dime and ball. For his hidden dime, he had an idea, something rather strange. It seems we can, Turin had noticed, actually smell the difference between a single and a double electron bond. All perfume chemists know that the molecule hexANal (single bond) smells harsh and like swimming pool bleach, but hexENal, the exact same molecule but with a double bond, smells very different, more like bitter almonds and much sweeter. So Turin figured a double bond must smell sweet. That would be his dime: he'd test his theory by taking a double bond—all by itself, two electrons holding two atoms—sticking it inside the foam ball, and seeing if he could smell the sweet odor of its rapid shimmer.

Now the foam ball. He already had one in his sights. "Ever heard of 'betweenanenes' (I kid you not, my friend)?" Turin e-mailed Stewart. "Fascinating compounds, synthesized in the early '80s. Found them in a book about weird molecules." These rare creatures had a highly unusual structure in that they were made of two interlocking rings of Carbons and, joining the rings, a double electron bond like two tiny diamonds hidden in a velvet box. Like having them served on a silver platter. Feel the thing from the outside, and you'd have no idea there was a double bond in there. But if the nose worked by vibration, its receptors should blast the betweenanenes with a buckshot of electrons, the electrons should tunnel through, hit the double-bond dime in one of them, and report its presence "by an unmistakable sweetness," Turin enthused. "If you can smell the double bond, my case rests."

He dove into it. And was brought to a dead halt by a simple problem: he couldn't find any betweenanenes. He couldn't make them himself—they are horribly difficult to manufacture, and he wasn't a chemist, didn't have the facilities—so he tried hunting down Alex

Nickon, the guy who had created betweenanenes. Nickon had just retired. Turin tried a colleague of Nickon's, James Marshall. On May 4, 1995, Marshall e-mailed:

To: l.turin@ucl.ac.uk
From: prynne@psc.psc.edu
Organization: USC College of Science and Math

Dear Dr. Turin,

I regret that it has been nearly ten years since we engaged in be-tweenallene and related chemistry. I have been unable to locate any of our previous samples. If our program in that area were still active, we would be willing to prepare additional samples, but under the present circumstances it is not possible.

With sincere regrets.

Turin went to Plan C: "Another line of inquiry," he wrote Stewart, "things called carceplexes." The name meant, basically, "cage," and essentially they were big rings of benzenes. If you dangled a small molecule next to a carceplex (a double-bond dime, for example) and then chopped off part of its rings, the rings would snap shut, swallowing and imprisoning the small molecule inside, a version of molecular S & M (hence the molecule's bondage-redolent name).

"Good news," Turin e-mailed Stewart. "Potential imprisoned molecules are potent odorants: H_2S,"—a very strong rotten-egg smell—"thiophene, pyrazine, pyridine"—a distinctive harsh inky odor—"etc."

And then: "Bad news: damned things"—he meant the carceplexes—"are probably too large to smell at all." (Generally we cannot smell molecules over ten angstroms wide.)

Plan A, dead. Plans B and C too. Turin thrashed around a bit and hit on Plan D. Plan D was a molecule called a fullerene.

Fullerenes are very weird and extremely beautiful molecules, platonic solids called polyhedrons, and they do amazing things, not least of which is superconducting. Harry Kroto, the man who created fullerenes, got the 1996 Nobel Prize in Chemistry for it. What interested Turin was that they have a trunk into which you could pack other molecules. He decided on a fullerene called C_{60}— simply sixty carbons linked together. There are only three forms of pure carbon: graphite, diamond, and C_{60}. And—the point— loading a dime into C_{60}'s trunk didn't change its outer shape at all.

For his dime, he decided on the evil-smelling little molecule H_2S, which stank of classic Sulfur. If pure Carbon fullerene with H_2S in it smelled sulfurous, then the nose must be a metal detector, because the Sulfur atom sure as hell wasn't showing up in the shape.

At the same time, Turin was doing reconnaissance on *Nature*. Casing the joint. In April he phoned John Maddox, *Nature*'s editor in chief, to tell Maddox he'd be submitting a paper on olfaction and that he'd like to illustrate it for *Nature*'s reviewers by sending them real smell molecules along with the paper "because they wouldn't believe me otherwise." Maddox said that sounded unusual but rather fun and Turin should absolutely tell Nick Short, the articles editor, that he'd said so. A very good sign, Turin thought.

As for wrestling an H_2S into a fullerene, he was thinking of heating it in a glass tube with charcoal. "Heat the hell out of it," he wrote Stewart, "(wear glasses, stand back, etc). *Liquefaction* of H_2S was actually achieved like this in 1873!!!"

But the more he looked at it, the more the low-tech approach seemed futile. Turin had no way of blasting his H_2S dime into the fullerene cage. The betweenanenes had imploded on him. The carceplexes and betweenanenes were intransigent, and Turin was left with a terrific experimental idea and his floor littered with failures at implementing it.

Suddenly he figured it out. The answer had been there all along, literally in his hand. He'd simply been asking the wrong question.

Go back to the throwaway comment he'd made to Stewart almost a year earlier. He'd been trying to make a bitter-almond smell, and when he'd smelled the metallocenes, the burger molecules, he'd e-mailed Stewart offhandedly, "One of them is reported to have a camphor smell!" (What a funny thing . . .) Yep, a sniff of the nickel burger (nickelocene) confirmed that it had a nasty chemical-oily smell, and the iron burger (ferrocene) "a definite camphor smell!!!" But he'd been stalking a bitter almond, and they had two other smells, and so he had simply walked past them.

Until now. Because he suddenly realized that . . . *that was the point.* The metallocene burgers had strikingly different vibrations because of the different metals sitting in their guts, the iron versus the nickel—but virtually identical shapes and very different smells. Which meant—"To hell with bitter almonds!" said Turin—that they did exactly what the betweenanenes, carceplexes, and fuller-enes had failed to: they constituted same-shaped molecular balls encasing different vibrational dimes inside them. And they smelled *different.* You were—you had to be—using the metal detector in your nose.

It was exactly what he'd been looking for.

He wrote it up, added a graphic that looked like this:

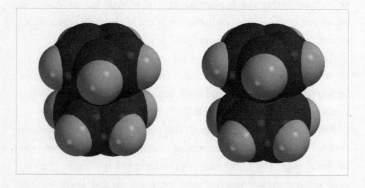

Space-filling models of ferrocene (left) and nickelocene (right) showing that the two molecules have virtually identical shapes (and very different odors). They also differ in the frequency of their strongest vibrational mode, involving an internal motion of the metal ion between the two rings.

And stuck it in his paper.

✦   ✦   ✦

THERE IS, IN various philosophy departments, and also in the cheese section of Bon Marché department store's lavish, expensive food hall (where foreigners in Paris eyeing the Bries and the Camemberts come nose to nose with the literally breathtaking Reblochon for the first time and unamused Parisians observe their sometimes violent reactions), this question: How much of what we consider good and bad smells is instinctual and how much do we learn? Nature or nurture.

Turin starts here with two views, the first being "Relativism is utter bullshit." He means the Leftist notion that everything is nurture and everything is subjective (except of course the Leftist belief that everything is subjective, which is itself objective). "I'm not a relativist at all. Let me put it this way: it's apparent in fashion. Yes, Yves Saint Laurent was influenced by what was going on around him"—nurture—"but nevertheless, his clothes, particularly the 1978 collection, are beautiful." (Objective.) "The extreme relativist view is due to sociologists having physics envy. All the nonsciences, the 'social sciences,'" (he barely bothers to roll his eyes to dismiss them) "are simply jealous of the hard sciences. They'd dearly love to reduce real science to their pathetic level because it would make them feel more comfortable about their useless lives. So they say to us, 'Since you guys at one point said the sun went around the earth and now you say the opposite, why should we believe you?' Which means they are completely missing the entire point of science— which is, itself, news to no one. As a friend of mine says, in philosophy there's no new data. In science there is. This is the point: with new data, one changes one's mind."

His second view on the nature versus nurture of smell, firmly held, is that one should seek the full spectrum of smells in one's life. "France," he says, "is a country that understands that, much as in music an orchestra is not just violins, the range of smells that makes life interesting includes some rather severe ones." So what determines what we like to smell? "Your taste in smell is part biology and part culture. Everyone who smells rotten cheese the first time— take Époisses, where you smell it about three rooms away, and one that is even more rare and heavenly and makes the Époisses positively spartan by comparison: Soumaintrain, from Bourgogne, specifically from Saint-Florentin, near Auxerre. When they smell that, Americans think, 'Good *God!*' The Japanese think, 'I must now commit suicide.' The French think, 'Where's the bread?' Why? The quality of decomposition: amines, short-chain aliphatic volatile fatty acids, the typical products of the decomposition of organic material. Oh, incidentally," he says, frowning, "the worst natural smell I've ever encountered in my life is rotting octopus. Octopuses are brilliant, at least as smart as dogs, and can be used to study neural function, and in Naples I worked as an assistant to the great John Zachary Young. I used to train them to do things like distinguish colors, play Rachmaninoff, and stuff. And then Young would remove half their brains to see if they could still do the left-hand part and thus figure out what the neural wiring for playing Rachmaninoff was. But sometimes they'd not survive the operation and would be found floating belly up—which was hard for a species that has no belly—in their furnished tanks, decaying, and the smell simply made you retch your guts out. Once you smell dead octopus, you never forget it. The only thing that approaches that is isonitriles." He grimaces.

"That was Naples during the cholera epidemic of 1974." He brightens. "Our lab got vaccinated with vaccine from London, and you could walk into the best restaurants in Amalfi and get a terrace-side table. But back to the question of culture's role in our taste in smell. Look at beer, which is a very interesting cultural product. Beer smells like a burp. Gases from someone's stomach. Lovely. Again, a product of fermentation, which is to say decay. Decay enhances smells and flavors, yet we have a sharp ability to I.D. decay, because decaying things will kill you. Bacterial and yeast decomposition. Which can give you 'I wouldn't touch that in a million years' and, at the same time and in the same culture, mind you, 'I will pay great sums to consume Rodenbach,' which is a miracle of a beer from Belgium. A miraculous powdery apple flavor. Those Rodenbach yeast have an I.Q. of *at least* two hundred. Fucking genius yeast.

He thinks about it for a moment. "My father used to go completely crazy about a cheese called Carré de l'Est. Hugely powerful. He'd say 'It's like the entire Grande Armée taking off its boots after a thirty-mile march in August.' To me as a kid, that he loved all this vile stuff was fascinating. He bought the worst cheeses and gave me the pieces he didn't eat. I ate them. But look, fecal smells are different. We produce shit, we don't produce cheese, and I would imagine the reaction to feces is hardwired. That's a guess. But finding *rules* for what we like and don't like? Aesthetics? Look, aesthetics is parochial ideas professing a spurious generality. In music that's been shown a thousand times. We hear harmonics that strike us as absolutely wrong, and then we get used to them. Having said that, there may well be things we never get used to: feces in smell, and Schoenberg in music. As Charles Rosen pointed out, Schoenberg took extreme chromaticism, where you no longer have a key, to its logical extreme—no harmonic center at all. And it simply doesn't work. It's not beautiful, ever. It's music for Ph.D. theses.

"There's a vibrational fifth in esters, you know. I've always thought that esters, fruity, are Mozart. The melon notes—helional, for example—strike me as the watery Debussy harmonies, the fourths. Beethoven in his angrier moments is quinolines, which you get in green peppers. Thus *Bandit,* a dark, angular Beethoven string quartet. There's a lot of perfumery that smells like Philip Glass's minimalism, a deceptive simplicity. *Mitsouko* I think is pure Brahms, the string sextets, extremely intricate but rather monochrome. *Tommy Girl* gives you Prokofiev's First Symphony.

"But the rotten cheeses. Put it this way: Sauternes, this incredible thing, is a wine that is the direct result of rotting grapes being eaten by a mold. I mean, in an American hospital they'd hand out antibiotics to exterminate half the food in France. In 1982 at Villefranche, a colleague of mine had a brother who was a wine dealer in Bordeaux, and he did a little wine tasting for us at the marine station. We all got into a room, and he had brought the first good Sauternes I'd ever tasted, Château Lamothe Despujols 1981. It must have been a blessed year for the Lamothe Despujols. I bought a case of this stuff, and every time I had a glass it was a religious experience. The guy showed us a photo of the fungus attacking the grape. That, of course, got me seriously into Sauternes, which is, believe me, an expensive habit to acquire. They're no good until you spend real money, and there's no competition from the rest of the world to lower the price. So there we are.

"When I sold my flat I bought a 1959 Rieussec, a Barsac, a sweet white, one hundred and ten pounds. Tim Arnett loves them, so he, Marty Rosendaal, and I wolfed it down. We drank it in the lab. *Utterly* sensational. Fresh as a trout. Sauternes are very saturnine, a honeyed summery exterior covering a late November liquid. There are three elements—a beeswax, a woody, and a floral banana—with a perfect balance between extreme acidity and huge, heavy, oily sweetness, like a blend of jasmine and musk. A great Sauternes is a perfectly proportioned thing. Rieussec makes big-boned, stocky affairs. The '59, in a bottle for forty years, comes out the way James Bond emerges from a wet suit in a perfect tuxedo. It looks at you and murmurs, 'What kept you?'

"Of course a '76 Rieussec would have been even greater. The most definitive statement of the Sauternes one can imagine. Unless, of course, you're going to buy the equivalent Yquem, '75 or '76, which will blow every fuse in your body."

Turin actually never really gives an answer on the culture versus biology question, probably because it's not scientifically answerable at this point. Also because it doesn't particularly interest him per se, not next to the smell of rotting lipids.

◆   ◆   ◆

TURIN WAS VERY nervous about the paper for *Nature*. As an elitist publication, *Nature* rejects a huge number of manuscripts. *Nature*'s articles editor was a man named Nicholas Short, a man with a rather mysterious personality. Short, a biologist himself, was one of the most guarded, uncommunicative, opaque people Turin had ever spoken to (they never met, and, through all that followed, never would). It was Short who would be shepherding the paper up the *Nature* chain of command and through the refereeing, and he seemed competent—as well as guarded, uncommunicative, and opaque. Which was to say, the polar opposite of Turin. But Turin didn't spend too much time thinking about it. Stewart tried to temper Turin's *Nature* monomania: "Keep in mind," he advised in an e-mail, "that *PNAS* [the journal *Proceedings of the National Academy of Sciences*] is a perfect fallback from *Nature*."

Turin (not believing it): "Absolutely right."

Since at the time *PNAS* considered only items nominated by fellows of the exclusive National Academy of Sciences, Stewart began searching for a white knight, and found one in the form of biophysicist William Hagins. Turin venerated Hagins, a sorcerer of photoreceptor research, and he was somewhat in awe that William Hagins might be going to bat for his theory. "I'll make sure the manuscript blows his socks off!" Turin assured Stewart.

The paper had the sulfur = 2500 = boranes section. It had the enantiomers, it had the metallocenes. But it needed more, and experiments are not easy things to think up. Stewart was still hedging bets, talking about *PNAS,* getting Hagins on board, but what could hook Hagins's interest? Turin mulled it over, glowering at his computer screen by day and staring at the ceiling at night. And then he had it: he would present Hagins with the solution to a perfume mystery. It was the next piece in the puzzle.

His pursuit of the puzzle began on a chilly mid-March day, when he'd gotten yet another mysterious feeler from the perfume industry. He e-mailed Stewart:

Date: Wed, 15 Mar 1995
To: stewartw@helix.nih.gov
From: l.turin@ucl.ac.uk

Interesting phone call an hour ago: a guy who does the marketing and pr for 6 of the biggest perfume firms in France (that's what he said, no idea which . . .) wants to organize a lunch with me and their respective directors to "discuss my book, which they all loved . . . in parts." The fellows in question are sufficiently busy that this won't happen for weeks yet, but I'm dying to know whether they want to bribe me, intimidate me, hire my services, or all of the above, and if so how they will actually get round to broaching the subject. Interesting, no? I *think* what they're worried about is not so much that my book will influence buyers (it would have to sell a whole lot more than it is doing before it made even the smallest dent in their sales), but that it would start a fashion for disparaging perfumes in the popular press and negate their byzantine marketing strategies. Alternatively, they may think that I know what the *next* fashion is, and they'd be entirely wrong.

The phone call put him in a Paris mindset, and rather abruptly he decided on a weekend with Françoise. It included catching up with perfumer Serge Lutens. Turin e-mailed Stewart the debriefing ("Subject: weekend"):

Supper with Serge Lutens of Shiseido perfumes in one of the best restaurants in town, called Le Grand Véfour. Food actually indifferent, particularly when the price ($200 ea.) is taken into account. Honest, I can cook better stuff at home, and the wine was far from great. *But* . . . the waiter came round with a basketful of black truffles and Lutens asked me to select one, since I reputedly had the best nose. I picked a good-size, egg-shaped one and it was promptly sliced with a small microtome-like object and put on warm toast dampened with olive oil: heavenly stuff, truffle aroma is like nothing on earth (dimethyl sulfide actually).

Lutens actually wanted a) to have my opinion on his two new perfumes (rather good, really, I'll bring some samples) and to offer me a job, but he promptly relented on the latter when he found out I already had one. Four of us at the table: Lutens's partner and business associate, a withdrawn character exact opposite of his flamboyance, and his assistant, a sweet lady named Liliane Menard. Lutens looked tired. Drove me home in his chauffeur-driven 1962 RR Silver Cloud, quite a car.

("P.S.," Stewart e-mailed him back, "what's one of those truffles cost, for my own edification??" Turin: "Literally more than its weight in gold. I estimate the one we ate @ around $200." "Sad about the food," wrote Stewart, "but I'm sure you expected that." Turin: "I didn't, as a matter of fact: my only previous experience of stupendous French haute cuisine was in one of Michel Guerard's restaurants in SW France where the food was *so* good that I felt euphoric for 24 hours afterward.")

He and Françoise traveled a bit. "Weekend in Ghent and Bruges, lovely places in Belgium, the cheapest restaurant we went to better than the Grand Véfour!!" And he was really trying to make things work romantically. "Good vibes with Françoise, discussions still simmering but sorting things out it seems."

Back in Paris, Turin decided to go talk to the Grasse perfumer

Guy Robert at the flat Robert maintained there. He was groping for a new angle (he wasn't sure what), more ammunition for his theory, good experiments. He was somewhat directionlessly pumping Robert for information: Had he ever come across any weird relationships between similar smells of molecules of different shapes? *Non,* said Robert, *désolé.* Hmm. "Have you ever noticed any chemicals that had unexpected smells or strange behavior?"

Robert thought about it and smiled and, with typical regal grace, said, "*Au fait,* there's one thing . . ." The thing, he said, was a mystery, which became an abiding obsession for years among perfumers, surrounding the molecular structure of one of the world's greatest perfumes, *Chanel No. 5.*

Chanel No. 5 was created in 1921 by the legendary perfumer Ernest Beaux, and it was the first runaway success to use a molecule called an aldehyde. Aldehydes are basically just snakes of Carbon atoms—four Carbons, five Carbons, six Carbons, and so on. You write them C_4, C_5, C_6, etc., with an aldehyde group, a Carbon atom double-bonded to an Oxygen atom, stuck on the head.

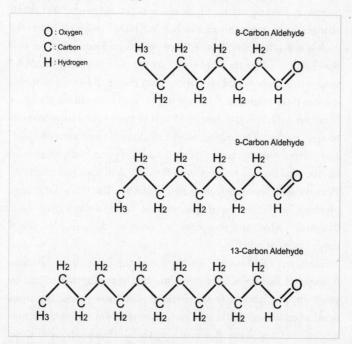

Below seven or eight Carbons, they all smelled pretty bad and couldn't be used in perfumery, but above eight, aldehydes start smelling good and make good perfume ingredients. But the gnomes of Grasse, spinning their olfactory spells, had noticed that these molecules behaved in one odd way: all the aldehydes that had an even number of Carbons (ten Carbons, twelve Carbons) smelled like mandarin orange. But all the odd ones (seven, nine, eleven) smelled like smoky candles.

Now, the aldehydic secret to *Chanel No. 5* was that Beaux had used almost entirely the even aldehydes, with just a touch of the odd. When people figured it out they started copying it right and left. ("Actually," says Turin, "*Chanel No. 22* is the ultimate aldehydic. *White Linen* is Estée Lauder's attempt to do a modern construction of it, and it succeeds. It's fantastic. I, in fact, sort of prefer *White Linen* to *22*, which has always struck me as a tad sweet.") But, said Robert, what was strange was the bimodal, almost digital fluctuation. Why were the odds (C_7, C_9, C_{11}) waxy and the evens (C_8, C_{10}, C_{12}) citrus? Why, when the shapes of C_8 through C_{12} changed progressively (and significantly), would you get not progressive smell changes from one point to another but rather this weird bimodal back-and-forth? If smell were Shape, you would expect one of two possibilities. Either there'd be no pattern and the smells would be random, or there would be a pattern but the smells would be incremental: nine would smell closest to ten, which would smell closest to eleven, which would then be closest to twelve, and so on. In fact, you got neither. The pattern wasn't random. It wasn't incremental. The pattern was alternating. Why would you get citrus with an even number and then go to waxy with the odd? And then *back* to citrus? Why would a receptor feeling Shape give you that? "It's the strangest thing," said Robert quite pointedly at Turin (it was a challenge), "because—what? the receptors are *counting* the atoms to see if they're even or odd?"

Turin left for the Gare du Nord and the Eurostar to London. It sounded like the smells were due to alternating vibrations. To prove this, he needed to watch these molecules dance. Electron-bond vibrations move very differently. Some go in and out, some go side to side, and some (for instance, the aldehyde groups in these molecules) go in a *rotating* vibration as they dance around the Carbon-Carbon bond. Turin was suspecting (hoping) that the vibration might differ in the odds and the evens. To watch this molecular dance he'd have to get his hands on one of the new, superadvanced molecular-modeling programs that did the calculations showing you the molecules as they rotated and bounced on their springy electron bonds. Those programs, until recently the preserve of experts, had now been "ported" to desktop PCs and given interfaces a human could understand without five years of study. It would bring him one step nearer to actually *seeing* a molecule's smell.

The problem was that these calculations were fiendishly difficult. In fact, his theory was asking questions of molecular behavior and the human ability to measure it that sat on the outer horizon of scientific knowledge. And the technology that *was* available was hard to use. Back in his lab, he started auditioning modeling software he could run on his desktop Mac, programs with names like "MOPAC" and "Ab Initio" that were completely new to him, and he spent months figuring out what they could and couldn't do. Some of them used quantum physics, some classical physics. A program might tell you how much force you'd need to bend an electron bond .01 of an angstrom, then .02 angstroms, .03, and so on, which was wonderfully informative if you were trying to figure out how molecules bobbed around on their electron springs when you whacked them (which was exactly what Turin was trying to figure out). But the program still had some serious limits, and he was having trouble understanding exactly how those limits were obscuring his attempts to peer into the complex heart of molecular space. Moreover, because the molecules' vibrations were so computationally intensive, MOPAC (he discovered) could give him only simplified quantum physics; if Turin wanted a proper quantum analysis, he'd have to use Ab Initio, which would then take days to calculate the simplest molecule. If he wanted to calculate the vibrations of a musk, MOPAC would take five minutes, and the simple version of Ab Initio, even on the fastest Mac, would take about two weeks. But, he reminded himself, fiddling with them, he shouldn't complain—just two years ago, these calculations could only have been done on $10 million

Cray supercomputers, and he would have had a much harder time working on his theory.

Turin toyed with Ab Initio ($500), briefly considered a program that ran on Unix before dumping that ("Life is too short for Unix," he declared to Stewart), and then came across a program named CAChe—Computer Assisted Chemistry—from a company in Portland, Oregon. He contacted one of the Oregonians—actually a transplanted Englishman—a nice guy named Dave Gallagher, who found his project interesting. "Smell, huh! *Cool.*" Then Turin looked at the program's price. $29,000. Hair-raising. But one thing led to another, CAChe gave him a 90 percent academic discount, he sent $2,900 to Oregon, and soon he was booting up CAChe.

He fed in the *Chanel No. 5* molecules and unleashed CAChe on them, telling the program to calculate and display all the different vibrations. And lo and behold . . . "the aldehyde rotates much more freely in the evens (8, 10, and 12)," he excitedly wrote Stewart, "but remains confined in the odds. Wow!! Another mystery explained." CAChe was reporting that the different rotations meant the waxies' vibrations alternated with those of the citruses. (Their shapes, meanwhile, thank you very much, did *not*.) "By the way," Turin added, "I phoned up Olivia Giacobetti, young perfumer genius, and she said the systematically different odd/even smells were self-evident to anyone who smelled them. I'm really glad about this one."

Stewart, never an easy scientific lay, was as skeptical as ever. "Quite hard to credit the story about the odd and even chain lengths," he wrote from Washington. (In London, Turin read it and grimaced.) "What *exactly* is the source of this info? I'm real curious!"

Turin: "Which info? Smells or dynamics? Dynamics utterly reliable, *clear* difference in the short simulations so far, I'm running longer ones as we speak. Put it this way: the program does not 'know' to count carbons."

No, no, Stewart meant the smells: "Did Olivia describe the difference in smells to you???"

Turin: "Yes. She said that it was citrus vs wax respectively for even and odd, just like Guy Robert had."

Stewart frowned, thought about it. "OK, here's my question: *what* exactly does the modeling program spit out?? Are you doing this by eyeballing a simulation, or does it print out some sort of values?? Extremely curious about this."

"So far, eyeballing," Turin replied carefully. "Using standard parameters in augmented MM_2, a piece of software inside CAChe, takes into account everything except the moons of Saturn."

Stewart relented: "Roger on citrus vs wax, that sounds consistent. Aldrich Chemical sell these guys????" Stewart meant C_6, C_7, C_8, C_9, C_{10}, C_{11}, and C_{12}.

"Yup," Turin wrote. "I'm ordering them today." He added, "Guy Robert warned me about two things: first of all, the things age ungracefully, and secondly the perfume suppliers actually supply impure ingredients *on purpose* to personalise their supply and make it smell better!! (Aldrich does not, to my knowledge)."

(Stewart, convinced, now wondered if he was too tough a critic. "Tell me if I'm missing the boat here . . ." he e-mailed doubtfully.

"No, no!!" Turin replied quickly, if exhaustedly. "All good and useful comments.")

The aldehyde finding was only getting stronger. MOPAC and CAChe were whispering encouragingly to him. These were all preliminary results, but they looked great. Now he had to do the final, most exacting calculations.

Before he could start on them, he got an offer from a Paris radio station to discuss perfume and promote his perfume guide. It happened to coincide with yet more feelers from the perfume companies, asking, Would Dr. Turin have time for a lunch? Maybe two? Back again to France on the train. He stayed with Françoise and her teenage daughter, Sabine, and debriefed afterward to Stewart.

Date: Thu, 20 Apr 1995
 To: stewartw@helix.nih.gov
From: l.turin@ucl.ac.uk

Hi Walter (this written on the train back this morning),
Fascinating week in Paris, couldn't report on it before because of crappy Compuserve link, forever interrupted by incoming calls for Sabine (desperate young men by the dozen).

First the radio program: presenter, sixty years old, total phoney, astrologer sexologist radio host and "expert" on literature. [Jean Paul] Guerlain was supposed to be there but did not come, apparently his brother had been taken very ill. Went there with Jean Laporte, smart guy, former chemist and owner of a small and very successful firm manufacturing relatively cheap feel-good perfumes. Interesting conversation on the way there and back, all sorts of tiny tidbits about the perfume world. On air, we gas on for two full hours about strictly nothing.

Next day, go to my appointment with the two perfume ladies, one in charge of creating a perfume for Celine, an upmarket clothes manufacturer, the other a perfume composer for Quest, the multinational which resulted from the fusion of Unilever and Naarden. I get there bang on time, maître d'hôtel informs me that no table is reserved in the name of the Celine lady, frequent customer (works opposite). Phone her, turns out that the two had waited for me for two hours exactly one week earlier!! This due to the Quest lady being asleep at the wheel when I told her my timetable. Anyway, the woman from Celine comes down from her office and we have an interesting lunch. Alarmingly well groomed, steeped in chic and totally optimized. She did a good (?) job at Kenzo perfumes and has been put in charge of starting up the next fragrance.

On which she is proceeding *very* cautiously: no fewer than five perfumers are submitting tenders for the job, one of them has already gone through one *hundred* changes since it started. She sort of knows what she wants (same as everyone else): a classy job, nice and old but really new, same only different, etc. ad nauseam. LVMH is forever doing "clinics," asking a bunch of morons what they think, a sure recipe for disaster. Anyway, far from clear what she wants from *me*, save perhaps to figure out how much money I got paid for writing good things about certain firms in my perfume guide (she tells me this quite candidly). I assure her that if I was going to get paid, I would have said good things about the big firms, whereas I praised to the skies those that will be out of business before the year is out. We part on good terms, she wants me to smell the darned thing when it's nearly ready.

I make a separate appointment to see the second lady at Quest. Though possessed of a disconcertingly bluff telephone manner, she turns out to be an absolutely charming person about 45, typical Côte d'Azur product, all chains, bangles and suntan, 20 years' experience but totally and sincerely modest, says she is not all that pleased with any of her work. Anyway, after a few pleasantries we start talking smells, she lets me smell her uncompleted submission for Celine, half a suspension bridge going nowhere, she *writes down* everything I say, then she starts calling the lab (on the same floor, 60 by 40 ft, a few thousand ingredients, two assistants preparing strips and weighing things) to bring in interesting ingredients she is working with and asks me what I think of them. One of them, which Quest appears to be obsessed with at the moment (through the glass, I can see one of her colleagues, one of 8 noses in all on the floor, smelling the same stuff) comes up. It's called gingerbread and smells stunning, of liquorice and biscuits, not ginger. I suggest using it against the grain in an animal-like context à la *Bandit,* she writes it all down (!), etc. etc. for one and a half hours.

I score a major hit at one point when discussing an evil piece of work by Cartier called *Pasha:* I say that the only other perfume which, though different, gives me the same impression of dimly lit confusion is another piece of junk by Gaultier. She looks at me as if I'd just moved the ashtray by telekinesis: how did I know that they were composed by the same person? (Didn't, just blind luck.) At this point she has decided that I have supernatural powers, and is asking aloud how Quest can use me (something not unlike psychics called by the FBI when really bereft with ideas, I guess). I am beginning to understand what it is that they find puzzling: I gave *Tocade,* a perfume uniformly disliked by the professionals (why? no idea) a "heart" in my perfume guide two weeks after it came out. To everyone's surprise (but not mine), the thing is a runaway success despite a relatively low-key advertising campaign. By now I think I know what these guys are thinking about me: "This weirdo can smell *money*."

Tocade was, in fact, more or less a complete mystery to the professionals. Turin had a detailed theory of why they disliked it, which he expressed with anger masked, typically, as scornful succinctness: "Too simple, too legible, no new raw materials, seemingly straightforward." He loathed snobbery. In his perfume guide, he had written:

Tocade (Rochas)

Studies have, it appears, shown that the decision to buy a perfume is made in the ten seconds that follow the first contact with the molecules that attach themselves to the nasal velcro. Does that mean adieu to deep perfumes, to those who believe in making one's acquaintance before launching into their life story?

This would be forgetting that for some, conciseness is not a constraint. Just when we had given up hope of smelling anything but superficial slogans, *Tocade* produces a poem, a perfume as immediate, abstract, and evocative as a flag. Ten seconds suffices amply, and one immediately feels marvelously well in the golden light that suffuses a summer evening.

Indispensable.

People often forget to consider this fundamental factor when buying a perfume: time. Yet it is a crucial component in a fragrance's structure. Turin's perfume guide had assessed the immortal *Chamade,* the best exemplar of a brilliant manipulation of time in perfume, this way:

Chamade (Guerlain)

Une note de départ verte et anodine donne le coup d'envoi à un miracle qui se produit sur plusieurs heures, voire plusieurs jours. A green and somewhat nondescript top note launches a miracle that happens over several hours, even several days. As soon as the initial fog dissipates, a splendid form appears, all of one piece, smooth and seamless, a strong white note, powdery and sculptural, that strengthens without losing complexity until complete evaporation. Typically Guerlain in its flattering and tender character, *Chamade* is nevertheless a haughty perfume, pure and distant and miles away from the slightly catty chic of *Jicky* and *Shalimar.* Its tenacity is prodigious, and one would believe it conceived to be smelled two days later. Put it on at least two hours before asking it to have its effect.

A masterpiece of elegance and poetry. One of the greatest perfumes of all time.

What he had feared would become extinct in their modern versions was the time dimension of older French perfumery, and *Tocade* entranced him by showing he needn't worry. It didn't matter that it revealed its depth swiftly. What mattered was that it was deep in whatever time it chose to work its magic. And if *Tocade* made the professionals look like idiots while the public snatched it off the shelves, so much the better. ("Making a good fragrance has very little to do with making money in the short term," Turin observed later, "but in the long run, the reason Guerlain still sells *Jicky*— created in 1889—by the trainload is not because of hype but because it is great.")

Anyway [Turin's e-mail to Stewart continued], she wants to talk the firm into using me as a consultant. In the meantime, she says if I want to come back and spend a week in their lab smelling everything (and sharing my impressions), I'm most welcome. Naturally, this would be for me like dying and going to heaven without the attendant disadvantages, so I accept enthusiastically. This lady thanks me profusely when I leave, saying how much she learned from me, I feel stupid saying the same thing to her (should have said it first). I leave, struck by the dearth of collective intelligence in perfume composition owing to the lack of words: they can't really discuss things with each other, tremendous waste of intelligence. Amazing that the rate-limiting step in a field should be mere words, never thought of it, though I guess in science we're minting them all the time as we go along.

Back to London, and the lab, and confirming the aldehyde data. Fingers crossed. He was creating "histograms" (bar graphs), into which he was dumping his data. The process was nerve-racking, feeding data into his impassive electronic twins, CAChe and MOPAC, which were graphing it out, letting them work their hushed magic comparing C_9 with C_{10} and then C_{11}, implacably spitting out their scores. He would pounce on the mathematical runes the twins spit back, praying the histograms would say what he wanted them to.

And then he hit it big. He sent an outwardly nonchalant e-mail to Stewart. "Your eagle eye will notice a change in the histogram for

C_{11}." He was e-mailing his bar graphs across the Atlantic. "Btw," he added casually, "the [alternating] pattern ceases at C_{12}."

Stewart: "Pattern? Pattern?? What pattern??"

The pattern was the whole point. Turin's heart almost stopped: "The PATTERN, silly!!!!!!!!" (Stewart was an ogre on statistics. Christ, had he screwed these stats up?) He spent a nervous night, opened his e-mail the next morning to see from Stewart: "OK, looked again, now I see the pattern!!"

Turin: "Phew!!! That's a relief!" (Jesus Christ! . . .)

The key to the *Chanel No. 5* mystery was clearly that the alde-hyde's smells alternated according to their alternating vibrations, and not to their shapes.

Hello, William Hagins! This would get them their white knight. *Send* him this, Turin said to Stewart. Stewart agreed—time to bait the hook. Stewart packed Turin's data into an electronic package, and it vanished into the wall. Silence. Turin waited. He checked his e-mail to find a message from Stewart. It was dismaying: "Ran this amazing discovery by Hagins," wrote Stewart. "He is taking para-noid position [that it is the result of] impurities." The molecules weren't pure, Hagins conjectured; they had junk with other vibra-tions floating in them, which was confusing the electronic twins, MOPAC and CAChe, and Turin's nose as well. Stewart said Turin might do well to be paranoid too and contact Aldrich about how the stuff was purified.

Turin set his jaw and replied, as calmly as he could, that Aldrich's record for purity was exquisite. Furthermore, he, Turin, had smelled each of the molecules, and to his nose what the computers said checked out. He sent over some more data. Stewart hurried off to deliver it to Hagins in another part of NIH. In a little while, Stewart returned to his computer to file his reconnaissance. Turin frowned at it on his screen. This was getting weird: Hagins was now suggesting a way to purify the molecules. Huh? Turin queried, "Don't Aldrich do this already anyway?" He was a bit bewildered by Hagins's excruciating details. "I'd rather not have to learn chemistry in the next few weeks," he e-mailed, desperately cheerful, "if it can be avoided. Be happy to in the following decade, though." His mind was racing. What was going on? He shot some more data to Stewart, then waited. Nothing from Hagins. Nothing from Stewart. "WHAT NEWS!?!?" Turin e-mailed.

Then something from Hagins. The phone rang, which was odd right there. Turin picked it up, and it was Stewart. Stewart cleared his throat and started explaining something. Turin was frowning, sitting in his lab before the huge window over his desk, trying to grasp this. Hagins had a problem, Stewart said, clearing his throat.

With what?

With the calculations.

What about the calculations?

Well—some of the calculations Turin had sent? There'd been one piece of surprising results, Turin's finding that two isomers happened to rotate very differently from each other.

So? said Turin.

So Stewart had said to Hagins: Wasn't it amazing that these two molecules with slightly different shapes should behave vastly differently! Hagins apparently thought it was, indeed, amazing. In fact Hagins thought it was so amazing that he had taken Turin's work and done a completely different sort of calculation and gotten completely different results.

Yeah? said Turin. Holding the receiver. So?

So he's claiming, said Stewart very quietly, that you made up the results.

The London traffic was flowing by on Gower Street outside, the gear-grinding sound of the double-decker buses, a hotshot roaring by on a motorcycle. Perhaps he had misheard. He frowned into the phone. Hagins thinks I *committed scientific fraud?*

Turin took a breath. He told Stewart that he knew these calculations gave that result because he'd already done the calculations that way—just to see what would happen—and, like Hagins, had gotten different results too.

Oh, said Stewart quickly, listen, I believe you.

I mean, how stupid would you have to be, continued Turin, when anyone can replicate these figures with the CAChe molecular-dynamics program, to try to fake something like this? Jesus, at least you'd do it with software not everyone in the world owned.

Stewart agreed. Stewart was himself rather furious.

William Hagins is saying I committed *scientific fraud?* said Turin.

Turin hung up. Stewart went off to repair the damage, and Turin went off to wait for it to be over.

Hagins didn't pursue it (although he didn't recant), and Turin, with an emotional itch he couldn't scratch, tried to let it drop. That Hagins had been a hero of his didn't help, nor did getting what felt like an unpleasant, condescending phone call from Shuko Yoshikami, Hagins's collaborator, telling him he'd lied. Hagins, Turin explained (again, gripping the phone), was doing *a different calculation,* getting a different result. Whatever, said Yoshikami.

It gnawed at Turin like a toothache.

✦   ✦   ✦

IF YOU THEORIZE a highly unlikely machine that does an amazing thing—say, a spectroscope made of human flesh that grabs molecules and shoots them full of electrons, measuring the ways they vibrate and sending that information to the brain as a smell—eventually you have to produce that machine. Or your theory disintegrates.

The moment was approaching when Turin would have to produce the machine, point out its gears and wires and the power it ran on, and he had to find the pieces of this machine—or, rather, machines, a thousand tiny spectroscopes in a thousand tiny human receptor cells. The thing was, the smell receptors had a history in biology almost as weird as the machines he had to show they were, and the weirdness was a wild card.

After Linda Buck had found the smell receptors, Mark Dearborn had handed the *New York Times* Science Times section to Turin over the breakfast table with an apologetic look. The look came because these receptors were part of a large, well-known class called G-protein receptors. *All* known G-protein receptors operated by Shape, so it seemed axiomatic that smell thus had to too. *Quod erat demonstrandum.* Turin had gripped the *Times* and thought desperately, "Oh shit. It is Shape."

G-protein receptors are long snaking threads of amino acids, each acid like a pearl on a necklace, but a better image is worms, or perhaps threads, because the necklaces are always threaded like embroidery through the cell's skin, its membrane, seven times. No one has ever figured out their exact structure, which is phenomenally complex, but we think they look something like this:

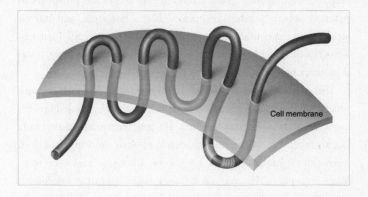

Cell membrane

But after Buck's paper came out something very interesting happened, which was that as months and years passed, nothing happened. The standard process is that someone discovers receptors for something, and someone else does the experiments confirming that they are, in fact, the receptors for this thing, and everyone in the field accepts it, and then ninth graders learn it in their textbooks. People were trying, but no one was confirming that the smell receptors were in fact the smell receptors for the simple reason that no one could get these receptors to react to any smells—which was "primary reception," what happens when the smell hits the receptor. After a while, people sat up and noticed, and frowned at what wasn't being found and what wasn't being published in the journals, and the silence became deafening. It was bizarre. Everyone agreed that these were the smell receptors. But they didn't work. Then Richard Axel pushed the entire question into the shade. Through some truly wizardly biology, Axel published a paper showing that the receptor neurons were continually shooting new axons—neural connecting wires—up to the olfactory bulb, and that where they ended up in the bulb depended on which exact smell receptor they carried. The olfactory bulb is smell's neural control center in the brain (which happens to be the only part of the entire human nervous system that is constantly dying and regenerating; we don't know why). This demonstrated that these receptors had a role in wiring the olfactory system, at which point everyone stopped wasting their grant money trying to get the receptors to react, dropped "primary reception" like a hot rock, and started working on the neural wiring of olfaction. ("In America," Turin observes of this, "the herd instinct in science is incredibly strong. It's as if primary reception never existed.")

This was excellent for Turin. His theory was all about primary reception, and he needed some breathing space. He needed breathing space because he was terrified. He was terrified because Linda Buck's receptors, which he had been studiously ignoring, had been a near-death experience for his theory. Everyone said they were Shape receptors. He was saying they were Vibration receptors, working in a spectrograph machine. He'd now been given a window of time to *prove* this with some evidence. He waded into the receptor's guts to find the machine's parts.

OK, thought Turin, you want to build a machine inside this receptor that reads the vibrations of electrons. A spectroscope. Let's start logically, with the machine's basic design. This machine is probably going to function like a light switch. When you switch a light switch "off," you're just putting a gap in the wire from the electricity to the light bulb, creating a chasm in the electrons' highway. A stream of electrons flows out of the power company till they screech to a halt before this gap in the wire in your front hallway, at which point the electrons wait impatiently on the edge of the gap for someone to turn the switch on. When you flick the light switch on, you're laying a metal bridge across that gap, and the electrons rush over the bridge to the other side and pour into the light bulb, lighting it up. Until you turn it off, which removes the bridge again and re-creates the gap.

So, OK, let's get down the basic design here, Turin figured that the smell receptor would have a gap in it. On one side of that gap, electrons would enter, and on the other side, they'd flow out. Like this:

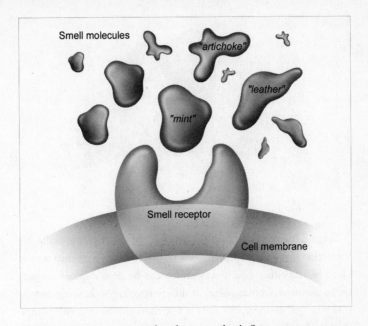

But! In a spectroscope, the electrons don't flow across a temporary bridge of wire between other wires. First, the bridge they flow across—through, actually, since they burrow through it—is the complex structure of a molecule. As they rush through, they jangle all the electron-bond strings inside the molecule. The electrons are waiting impatiently on one side. A person inhales a smell—peach flowers or whiskey or asphalt—and a molecule of peach or asphalt is sucked into the nose and tumbles into the gap. The gap nicely accommodates all molecules (at least those up to ten angstroms wide), and as the molecule slots into it, suddenly the electrons have before them a bridge reaching from the "in" side to the "out" side, and they hurl themselves across this bridge:

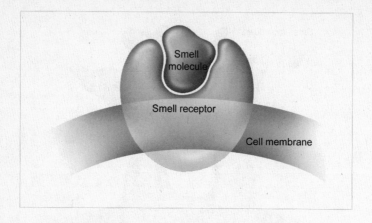

Second, there's an important catch, a catch that provides the information that makes spectroscopy possible: the two connectors for electrons on either side of a receptor can be *set at different energies,* or, to use electrical language, at different voltages. In some receptors, the "in" connector is only a few thousandths of a volt higher than the "out" connector; in others the difference might be as much as half a volt. Receptors come in different classes, each class with its own, specific voltage drop from in to out. This is handy because the electron is somehow going to have to be lowered by just that drop as it rushes through the molecular bridge. (The bridge, it turns out, is actually more of an escalator, both crossing a distance and descending from one level to another.) The electron needs to lose some energy (some height) before it can rush on. So get a complete set of receptors of every height class and fill each one with the same molecule (inhale, perhaps some molecule naturally created in orange blossoms). Then set loose at these receptors the pack of pushy electrons waiting on one side of the gap. Once inside a receptor, each of the electrons, just like each person in a crowd, has its own individual energy. Every single electron will try to get through the molecular escalators. The trick, however, is that they will come out the other side only when they can lose just the right amount of energy to gently deposit them at the low end of the escalator. What do they give their excess energy to? A molecular vibration! In other words, if you observe this process, you will see that only when the height of the escalator matches a particular molecular vibration does the current flow. Look at all the escalators, count how many electrons come through each, and you will know which vibrations the molecule has.

It won't be perfectly accurate, because thermal agitation—your body temperature, which is constantly stirring molecules around at a very low internal simmer—will blur things. It won't be as precise as a human-made spectroscope of calibrated glass and polished aluminum and fine-tuned lasers. But it will work. It will be able to tell you within a few tens of wavenumbers what vibrations some molecule of shoe leather or tea rose or shrimp shell has. It will be able to tell you whether you have a Sulfur-Hydrogen or a Carbon-Oxygen. You will be able to smell.

That was, Turin figured, the basic design of the human spectroscope. Now he had to find all these components inside the human nose.

First he needed a power source, a source of electrons to run this machine. In first-year biochem they teach you that there are millions of little biological batteries inside us, tiny things that pack electrons in their guts and cruise around inside cells, regurgitating electricity to processes that need it. It's called bioenergetics, a way of carrying energy around in a cell electrochemically, and these little floating, flesh CopperTops are needed to power lots of well-known chemical reactions. They come in many kinds. Phosphate groups, for example, power various electronic processes in the body. And so do things called NADPHs (nicotinamide adenine dinucleotide phosphates), which are actually a kind of vitamin and which dutifully lug electrons all over the place (every living cell is full of NADPH).

Turin figured he'd assume that NADPHs were powering the cellular spectroscopes in the nose. He had a neat method of finding out. Like the plugs on Compaq computer power cords that *only* fit Compaq sockets and no other computers', NADPHs only plugged into specific sockets fitted just to them, a unique sequence of amino acids that said to the NADPH, "OK, plug in right here." (The various biological batteries in your cells will plug in only where they see their own sockets, say, the specific combination of the acids AAGHT or GPTAG or whatever.) If he could find NADPH's specific socket on the smell receptor, *Nature*'s peer reviewers would have to admit that NADPHs could be powering his machine.

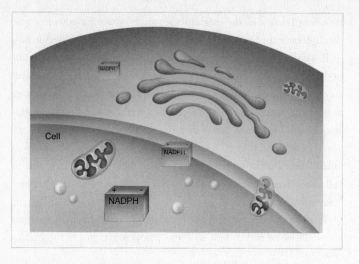

The first thing he had to know was NADPH's socket sequence. He happened to be in North Carolina visiting Mark Dearborn, and he popped down the hall to see Dearborn's professional neighbor, Dick Philpot. Philpot was a big, handsome, manly guy, an outdoorsman, mostly monosyllabic, and an expert in electrically powered enzymes. "So listen, Dick," Turin began explaining, "I'm trying to track down the sequence for the NADPH binding site, and I—"

"GXGXXA," said Philpot, "or GXGXXG. Either one."

Turin blinked. "Ah. Uh, thanks, Dick." He got up and left.

G is Glycine, A is Alanine, and X can be any neutral (uncharged) amino acid at all.

So the socket would have to be these six acids, in one of these specific orders. But now Turin had to figure out how to search through all of these letters—the thousands of amino acids strung together to make a smell receptor—and find the six that exactly matched Dick's sequence. It was the ancient era of 1995, and sequence search engines weren't yet everywhere on the Web, so not knowing quite what else to do, he came up with a low-tech solution. He turned on his laptop, went to the Web, and downloaded the sequence of amino acids in the receptors, Serines, Lysines, Glutamates, Tryptophans, long strings of letters.

When the complete protein was coiled inside his Mac, he called

up his word processor (a program called Nisus) and clicked the
"Word Search" function. He typed "GXGXXA," clicked on "Search"
and sat back, watching the Mac's screen.

The program clicked and whirred and, almost immediately, out
popped one of the sequences: GSGLLA. He thought: "Jesus.
There's the socket." It was sitting right on the sixth of the receptor's
seven coils.

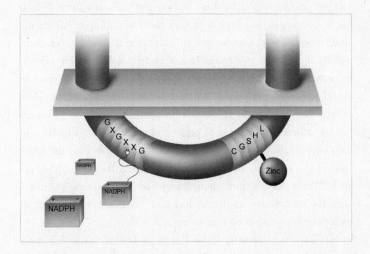

So he had a place to plug in his battery.

Wait. Damn it. He'd forgotten to check: Did these NADPH batteries deliver enough of a current to power his machine? He looked
up their voltage, and found, to his great relief, that his little batteries would give each microscopic spectroscope up to about half an
electron volt, which happened to be just enough to power detection
up to about 4000 wave numbers, the upper reaches of the spectrum, where O-H and N-H sat. The power source just fit the
amount of power the machine needed.

He now had evidence that there was a battery to power this spectroscope and a power socket to plug the battery into. He needed
one last part of the machine: a metal ion. If you're going to do electron transfer in biology, you'll need a metal ion for the job because
that's your wiring, where electrons are stored. The metal has to

coat the spot on the receptor where the spectroscope sits (the spectroscope is only going to be a part of the receptor, not the whole thing), the place where the smell molecule gets gripped in the receptor's hands to be shot through with electrons. The question now was, Which metal was this wiring made of?

The body needs any number of metals: molybdenum, calcium, selenium, copper, nickel, which all do various things. (We can carry oxygen in our blood because hemoglobin contains iron, which binds to oxygen and lugs it around the body.) Turin was having lunch one day with Charles Sell at Quest, and Sell told him a story. Sell had been frustrated by the lack of understanding of why certain odorants smelled very, very strong and others very weak. No one could figure out odor *strength*. Not what they smelled of. How strong they smelled of it. So Sell had drawn twenty or so super-strong odorants on a sheet of paper and taken them up to UCL in London and shown them to Turin's chemist neighbor on the other side of the campus, William Motherwell. Sell had asked Motherwell, "What do you think these things have in common?" Motherwell (Sell recounted to Turin) had said, "Oh, simple. They're all exceptionally good at binding to metal."

So Turin was thinking about this as he started his search for a metal. He also had to find another binding site, a place on the receptor where the metal could glom on to. To further complicate things, the site where the metal was attaching and the site where the electrons were flowing in from the NADPH battery had to sit right next to each other on the receptor's snaky body, no more than ten angstroms apart, because tunneling only works at tiny distances. (Electrons hate to travel far.)

Turin thought and read and talked to people. He found a clue, tracked it down, and decided to place his bet on it. One common piece of medical trivia that mystified doctors concerned Captopril, a drug for high blood pressure. More or less every doctor who regularly prescribed Captopril had noticed that a common side effect was that some of their patients lost their sense of smell. When people looked at what exactly the drug was doing down on the molecular level, they saw that it was binding like crazy to a metal: zinc. It was also known that people who became deficient in zinc lost their sense of smell, which was circumstantial evidence that zinc was somehow essential to smell, though no one had any idea how.

No one except possibly Turin. On a spring evening in May 1995, he went down to his UCL lab on Gower Street, sat down at his computer. Each metal—iron, copper, and the others—has its own unique binding site on any receptor, a code of amino acids that only it can bind to. He wanted to find the chain of amino acids that locked onto zinc.

He started by crawling through the Web, searching enzyme databases for amino acid sequences that acted as zinc binding sites. The databases spit out twenty-five different combinations of amino acids that could bind zinc. Twenty-five codes. Now he just had to match one of the codes to the smell receptor, and he was golden. He took his twenty-five zinc-binding site candidates and fed them through the computer to the database, which then set off to see if they were integrated into the smell receptor he'd found.

Not a single one was in the smell receptor. The machine was missing this piece. Turin sat back, deflated and baffled. He took a deep breath—it was 3:00 A.M. now, nothing on Gower Street outside except an occasional car, the streetlights, the Department of Anatomy completely quiet—and tried feeding various sequences, ten amino acids long, into the computer. No matches. Nothing.

OK. Alternate strategy. He Telnetted into an enzyme-database computer and started feeding in parts of the receptors themselves, hoping the database would snag a match to any zinc-powered enzymes. It handed him various things, but nothing that made sense. Christ. He suddenly remembered Blitz, the friendly German supercomputer living in Heidelberg that was expert in protein database searches, so he jammed the computer into reverse, Telnetted into Germany—Blitz was free to anyone with e-mail, no registration, no passwords, and, more or less like Turin, open twenty-four hours a day—and started throwing in bits of the receptors. Blitz was so powerful that in twenty-six seconds it could match your sequence with one of 150,000 known sequences. But it snapped up the sequences, spun them around at light speed, and shot back its report: zero matches. Blitz went off to attend to other business.

For several weeks Turin tried feeding things to Blitz. He got nothing. And then late one night, at home, he was trying, yet again, a piece of the receptor sequence. It was only five amino acids long, CGSHL, and it sat on the receptor just a few short acids away from the NADPH socket. He sighed exhaustedly, selected it, hit a key, and the sequence zoomed off from London to Heidelberg. Blitz thought about it for a half minute, spit something back at Turin, then slipped away again, leaving Turin before a screenful of names and numbers in neon green. He frowned, leaning toward the laptop's gently glowing square in the dark in his Clapham Common apartment.

Subject: Results for: CGSHL
Date: Sat, 27 May 1995
From: Blitz@EMBL-Heidelberg.DE
Organization: European Molecular Biology Laboratory, Heidelberg

Sequence: CGSHL

No.	% Match	Length	ID	Description
1	100.0	84	INS_PIG	PROINSULIN
2	100.0	51	INS_RABIT	INSULIN
3	100.0	81	INS_SHEEP	PROINSULIN
4	100.0	70	INS_TORMA	PROINSULIN (FRAGMENT)
5	100.0	54	INS_SQUAC	INSULIN
6	100.0	51	INS_ZAODH	INSULIN
7	100.0	110	INS_PANTR	INSULIN PRECURSOR
8	100.0	57	INS_PETMA	INSULIN
9	100.0	105	INS_ONCKE	INSULIN PRECURSOR
10	100.0	50	INS_KATPE	INSULIN
11	100.0	116	INS_LOPPI	INSULIN PRECURSOR
12	100.0	110	INS_MACFA	INSULIN PRECURSOR
13	100.0	52	INS_CALMI	INSULIN
14	100.0	110	INS_CANFA	INSULIN PRECURSOR
15	100.0	51	INS_CAPHI	INSULIN
16	100.0	52	INS_LEPSP	INSULIN
17	100.0	50	INS_MYOSC	INSULIN
18	100.0	86	INS_HORSE	PROINSULIN
19	100.0	59	INS_HYDCO	INSULIN

No.	% Match	Length	ID	Description
20	100.0	51	INS_HYSCR	INSULIN
21	100.0	51	INS_ELEMA	INSULIN
22	100.0	51	INS_FELCA	INSULIN
23	100.0	108	INS_GEOCY	INSULIN PRECURSOR
24	100.0	51	INS_GADCA	INSULIN
25	100.0	107	INS_CHICK	INSULIN PRECURSOR
26	100.0	51	INS_CHIBR	INSULIN
27	100.0	51	INS_CROAT	INSULIN
28	100.0	106	INS1_XENLA	INSULIN 1 PRECURSOR
29	100.0	106	INS2_XENLA	INSULIN 2 PRECURSOR
30	100.0	110	INS2_RAT	INSULIN 2 PRECURSOR
31	100.0	51	INS2_THUTH	INSULIN 2
32	100.0	52	INS_AMICA	INSULIN
33	100.0	51	INS_ALLMI	INSULIN
34	100.0	81	INS_ANAPL	PROINSULIN
35	100.0	51	INS_ANSAN	INSULIN
36	100.0	51	INS1_BATSP	INSULIN 1
37	100.0	234	GU38_RAT	POSSIBLE GUSTATORY RECEPTO
38	100.0	234	GU33_RAT	POSSIBLE GUSTATORY RECEPTO
39	100.0	312	GU27_RAT	GUSTATORY RECEPTOR GUST27
40	100.0	51	INS_PSESC	INSULIN
41	100.0	50	INS_ONCGO	INSULIN
42	100.0	51	INS_BALPH	INSULIN
43	100.0	105	INS_BOVIN	INSULIN PRECURSOR
44	100.0	110	INS_CERAE	INSULIN PRECURSOR
45	100.0	51	INS_DIDMA	INSULIN
46	100.0	108	INS_CYPCA	INSULIN PRECURSOR
47	100.0	110	INS_CRILO	INSULIN PRECURSOR
48	100.0	110	INS_HUMAN	INSULIN PRECURSOR
49	100.0	464	L2AM_DROME	ALPHA-METHYLDOPA HYPERS
50	100.0	88	BXB8_BOMMO	BOMBYXIN B-8 PRECURSOR
51	100.0	314	OLF9_RAT	OLFACTORY RECEPTOR-LIKE PR
52	100.0	314	OLFI_HUMAN	OLFACTORY RECEPTOR-LIKE PR
53	100.0	310	OLF0_RAT	OLFACTORY RECEPTOR-LIKE PR
54	100.0	314	OLF1_RAT	OLFACTORY RECEPTOR-LIKE PR
55	100.0	312	OLF4_RAT	OLFACTORY RECEPTOR-LIKE PR
56	100.0	51	INS_BALBO	INSULIN

No.	% Match	Length	ID	Description
57	100.0	51	INS_CAMDR	INSULIN
58	100.0	50	INS2_BATSP	INSULIN 2
59	100.0	110	INS2_MOUSE	INSULIN 2 PRECURSOR
60	100.0	51	INS_ACOCA	INSULIN
61	100.0	313	OLF5_RAT	OLFACTORY RECEPTOR-LIKE PR
62	100.0	820	CHIA_ALTSO	CHITINASE A PRECURSOR
63	100.0	312	OLF8_RAT	OLFACTORY RECEPTOR-LIKE PR
64	100.0	313	OLFD_CANFA	OLFACTORY RECEPTOR-LIKE PR

He sat staring at his screen. Blitz was saying that CGSHL was found on two and only two receptors, the receptors for smell (that, he was sure of, since that's where it came from) and the hormone . . . *insulin?* Well, there were also No. 49 and No. 50, some weird enzymes, and No. 62 (chitinase, which makes soft-shelled crabs soft), but those aberrations aside, it was smell and insulin, straight down the line. (The taste receptors—"gustatory"—were probably smell receptors that happened to be on the tongue, which in the scheme of things was not the most unusual place for them; they'd found a genetic sequence for smell receptors in human sperm, who the hell knew why.) So essentially he had smell receptors and insulin. That was it. The key was, it seemed, the connection between the two. But they had absolutely nothing, as far as Turin could tell, in common. Was it merely coincidence that both insulin and olfactory receptors happened to have those amino acids on them? Possibly. But that made little sense. He glared at the screen. Where the hell was the connection? (And—wait a minute, why hadn't the first computer given him this?) Maybe his brain had shut down. He pressed the off switch on his laptop, and it popped and died, a bubble of strangled energy. It would be dawn soon. He stared blearily at the delicate luminescence creeping over the edge of London's skyline, rubbed his eyes. His mind felt grainy. He went to sleep as the luminous edge turned into day.

Perhaps he'd got something wrong. The next day, at his lab at UCL, he fed in the same sequence: CGSHL. Blitz patiently threw back at him the same results. He stared at them. *What* did olfactory receptors have to do with insulin? He spent the entire day on it, winding up furious and having got strictly nowhere. When evening came again, he closed up shop, jammed his hands in his coat pockets, trudged down to the Gower Street tube station. He got on the Northern Line and sat there as the train hurtled forward. He was walking across Clapham Common past a church when, from some deep, dark, dusty place in the back of his mind, from some ancient undergraduate course the singular fact surfaced: "insulin," as he put it, "binds to zinc like shit to a blanket." Which fit exactly with the side effect of Captopril. He had turned up, on the insulin receptor, a binding spot for a metal, and the metal was zinc.

Wait. Could this be right? He seemed to remember that the Sigma catalog sold insulin in two forms—with zinc, and zinc-free. He went home and grabbed his Sigma catalog. Sure enough: insulin came in two grades: zinc and zinc-free, which meant zinc must bind like hell to insulin, or Sigma wouldn't bother charging for stripping it away. He jumped to the computer, and downloaded the crystal structure of insulin with zinc bound to it. There was the zinc atom, and then the sequence that was binding it. Yep, the zinc binding sequence was CGSHL. Which was exactly the same on the olfactory receptor.

That was it. The insulin receptors strongly implied that olfactory receptors were binding zinc too—that, in other words, they had a metal to conduct electrons at exactly the place they'd need metal. The machine was wired. He dashed off an exhilarated e-mail to Stewart: "I think I've *cracked it*!!!!!! Found the link between the 'known' receptors and electrons! Explains everything neatly, paper now ready for completion."

Turin spent the following day cobbling the data together into coherent form. It was still bugging him why the first computer, the one before Blitz, had neglected to show the insulins. And then he realized: Insulin is a *hormone.* He'd only asked the first computer for *enzymes;* Blitz had looked at everything.

He was really progressing on the paper now, working on it every minute. To Stewart: "Today is a national holiday, wonderful weather, city completely empty, back at work (Françoise took off this morning, more abt that later)." Every detail counted. He inserted a credit to Motherwell for the zinc part in the paper. He mentioned this to Motherwell. Why me? said Motherwell. Turin was surprised: Charles Sell said it was your idea, he said. Actually, replied Motherwell, Charles was the one who suggested that. Turin rolled his eyes and credited them both.

"I think," he wrote Stewart, "this is the baby!!!!!!!!!!"

+   +   +

HIS LONDON-PARIS relationship had always been stormy, and it was becoming stormier. His conversations with Françoise were strained. He wanted children, she didn't; he was attached to London, she (deeply) to Paris. Stewart had suggested that Turin make a list of all of Françoise's good qualities, and Turin had readily agreed—then kept putting it off. "How goes the list?" Stewart queried delicately. "Are you reluctant to tackle it? (Would be completely understandable. . . .)"

Turin tapped out a reply: "Working on it." (He wasn't.) "Françoise back this weekend!" he noted, then immediately added, "Enclosed the phenylacetaldehyde-phenylacetonitrile picture." Which, whatever that was, had absolutely nothing to do with Françoise and her qualities.

Good idea, Stewart replied the next day about the phenylacetaldehyde, and then asked, "What about the list??"

Oh. Right. "Coming up . . ."

It never came. What came instead was, finally—finally—the actual paper for *Nature*. June 8, 1995: "Here it is!!!!!" The first complete draft.

And then a revision of the draft, and a revision of the revision. Turin was getting punchy. He was trying not to feel sick to his stomach with nerves, triple-checking his numbers, making corrections, trying to ensure it would be perfect when the *Nature* referees looked at it. He was fairly flinging drafts at Stewart and others for criticism. He was bouncing absurdities back and forth. He finally cracked. He e-mailed Stewart, "Hi Walter, *if* you received the latest draft, don't bother because I took it to Nature yesterday." On July 25, 1995, Turin submitted "A Spectroscopic Mechanism for Primary Olfactory Reception" to Nick Short, the articles editor at *Nature* magazine. It was off.

He did feel a little sick to his stomach.

IV

✦

NATURE

$\mathcal{N}$OW TURIN WAITED.

Nature represents itself as a "rapid-review" publication. The claim seemed true. Already, by August 7, Turin was e-mailing Stewart nervously: "Just spoke to *Nature:* it *was* sent to referees, one has already answered (no clue as to content), they're waiting for the second one . . . fingers crossed."

He and Françoise left for Argentina on vacation. They'd always wanted to go to South America together, but they chose to go in winter, which turned out to be less than great, and they found Buenos Aires expensive, so they went to Chile. They were in La Serena when he couldn't stand it anymore. He found a public international telephone booth and, heart pounding, dialed UCL in London.

He reached the department secretary. She knew exactly why he was calling. It's come, she said. *And?* She paused. It's been rejected, she said.

He held the receiver for a moment. Can you fax it to me?

When the fax came through, he found a bar, planted himself, and read through what the reviewers thought of his new theory of smell. The referees were, in their tight, precise, scientific way, hysterical. They hated it. They loathed it. By the time he finished, Turin was furious. He went back to the phone, called Walter Stewart in Washington, and faxed the reports to him. Then, ignoring the bill he was running up, he called Nick Short. "Nick, listen, I can counter every damn point in here. I want to resubmit." Ah, yes, said Short in London, mildly, with no enthusiasm but no aversion to the idea, either.

I'll rebutt the criticisms point by point, said Turin.

Ah, yes, murmured Short over the phone to Chile. Turin got off the line as fast as he could.

Back in London. Turin went over the referees' comments and prepared to launch into his reply. Stewart helped him, in Stewart's way, which meant simultaneously noting "what shit" the comments were—which hardly stanched Turin's already volcanic sense of injustice—and hectoring Turin to be polite: "They're like muggers, Luca. You don't like them, but they've got the knife."

So Turin gritted his teeth, plastered a smile on his face, and started with exquisitely good form: "I am very grateful to the referees for taking the time and trouble to write a detailed and penetrating review."

After that sentence, he ran into trouble. He turned initially to Referee 3 because, as he put it, 3 had got on his tits first thing by sniffing, "[Turin] contends his [Vibration] theory explains all observations"—an imprecise and provocative statement. Stranger, though, was that if he or she dismissed Vibration's explanatory power, 3 then immediately turned around and dismissed Shape, a theory, 3 sniffed, "proposed when little was known about the biology of the olfactory system." Turin, not sure where this was going, replied that he happily agreed that Shape should be discarded because it didn't account for the facts. (Oh, and he *didn't* claim his theory could explain "all observations"; it was just better than Shape.)

Then 3 made a rather astounding comment: "[Shape] is no longer argued." Turin: *Really!* Then what *was* argued, exactly? (3 didn't bother to say.) Or, rather, on the very next page, 3 did say: "The current view is that the identity of an odor is encoded by a combination of different receptors that recognize structural features of an odorant." Which—since "structural features" referred to and had in olfaction science always referred to the shape of a molecule—meant that 3 was arguing Shape, which directly contradicted 3's statement "[Shape] is no longer argued."

Turin tried out various responses like a diplomat rehearsing possible tones of voice for hostile governments. He showed off his knowledge, forecast smells, elucidated his theory: "Where my approach differs [from Shape is] in being predictive. Boranes should smell like Sulfur . . . benzaldehyde and ecyclooctatetraene should smell like cinnamon." He gently corrected gross errors. (Referee 3 in his confusion had thought that the alternating smells of C_7–C_{13} aldehydes were "in direct conflict" with Vibration; actually, Turin noted with acid words dipped in sugar, they directly *supported* it: "The referee misunderstands my point . . ." he purred). He got a bit snooty at times—"As is well known," he tossed out, "catecholamines are redox reagents"—but ultimately (Stewart was riding herd) responded in a more or less gentlemanly fashion.

With Referee 2, however, he started to let his impatience show. Referee 2, he wrote, "makes three points which, if correct, would certainly invalidate . . . the paper." Pause for a frosty breath. "Fortunately, the referee is incorrect on all three."

Referee 2 complained that Turin's "argument" for a zinc-binding site on the receptor "seems a bit thin." *Really,* retorted Turin. Sixty-four proteins that *just happen* to exactly match CGSHL, which *just happens* to be the zinc-binding site on insulin, is thin? Seemed rather clearly diagnostic of olfactory receptors. And as for 2's protesting that the smell molecules would have to punch through the cell membrane to get to the receptor, Turin pointed out that 2 "appeared to forget that odorants are small hydrophobic molecules"—which meant (as any chemist could tell you) that "a membrane, far from being an obstacle, is actually where an odorant would most likely be found!"

Referee 2 ended with the snide jab that an "equally fanciful" part of the proposal took "no account whatsoever" of G-protein structure and docking difficulties. And so Turin calmly downloaded X-ray structures of G-proteins, threw them in, and shot back: "No docking difficulties arise."

Then there was referee 1, who began, rather breathtakingly, by casually questioning whether any of "the authors" had actually done any original work at all. (Turin cleared his throat: "First, a minor point: there is only one author.") In Referee 1's view, Turin was claiming credit both for 1) originating Dyson's theory and 2) pointing out the difficulty of building in the nose a spectroscope of metal gratings and glass mirrors. Simmering, Turin replied that, first, he was, thank you very much, well aware of Dyson, "to whom full credit is given in the paper." And second, he observed acidly, "I take no great credit for pointing out the 'difficulty' of putting a spectroscope in the nose, given the conspicuous absence of gratings and mirrors in the nasal cavity." But what was truly breathtaking was a comment that 1 seemed to toss off absentmindedly: Instead of using shape to recognize smell, he said, Turin instead just "uses electron tunneling." ("Like, 'Great,' " said Turin, incredulous, " 'you invented the wheel, so what else is new?' ") To *Nature* he wrote: "For Referee 1 to sum up the central and novel idea of the paper merely as 'instead uses inelastic electron tunneling,' as if that were the most obvious thing in the world, is, I believe, unfair to the subject and to the theory being advanced. The referee's comment implies that this is in some sense an obvious idea, but," he drove home the point, "the extensive literature contains not a single reference to electron tunneling."

Referee 1 complained that "the authors at no point provide a clear, plausible display of the *nature* of the currents." "I am not sure," replied Turin, thin-lipped, "what the referee means by 'plausible display of the nature of the currents.' They are electron currents, as suggested by the fact that the word 'electron' appears 22 times in the manuscript."

Then Referee 1 wrote: "The important part of the paper is nonexistent."

Now, what the fuck, Turin asked Mark Dearborn, do you say to that? Stewart had had the same reaction. He'd e-mailed Turin, "How do you refute 'The important part of the paper is nonexistent.' What the hell is he talking about??"

Referee 1: "The major body of the paper is an extremely rambling case-by-case discussion of specific molecules and their shapes. I find this quite unconvincing and virtually irrelevant."

If, Turin responded, you think that a discussion of specific molecules and their shapes is irrelevant to a paper on molecules and shape, then you are quite out of your mind. (He phrased it on the page as: "I do not share his view . . .")

Referee 1: "I doubt if this paper could be adequately revised, thus I find it not too convincing."

"[T]here is," Turin wrote silkenly, "no specific list of points that the referee thinks should be changed or added. In this sense I agree it would be difficult to revise the paper to meet his objections, but that is the fault of the referee, not the paper."

So much for the referees.

Turin launched himself into the rewrite, calling in debts, searching for information. He beamed stuff to distant sources, they sent back hints and references, and he wrote and rewrote and sweated every line. He put the rebuttal in an envelope and mailed it to Nick Short. There was a carefully polite letter ("Dear Dr. Short, enclosed you will find . . ."), but on the referees' competence to comprehend the theory, he had a more refreshingly direct phone call that started with "Nick, these people are assholes." He and Mark Dearborn had analyzed the responses like two FBI semioticians and were pretty sure they'd nailed the identities. Referee 1, they thought, was a scientist named George Dodd. Referee 2 appeared to be Heidi Hamm, a biochemist at the University of Texas. And Referee 3, they figured, was Gordon Shepherd, a Yale neurobiologist who had been working in smell for many years and was, judging from his publications, a devout Shapist. "If your paper was not reviewed by Shepherd," one of Turin's sources e-mailed him after reading the review, "it was reviewed by someone who thinks as he does."

Turin told Short that he believed Referee 1 to be Dodd and that he thought Dodd might have an ax to grind with him. Short shouldn't resubmit to Dodd. Short said, Hmm, ah, yes, well, mmm, right, and told Turin he wouldn't. In fact, Short agreed that they would submit to three completely new people.

Turin was also diversifying his weaponry and gathering ammo. He'd walked out the anatomy department's doors, crossed the quad to UCL's physics department, and forged a strategic alliance with the eminent physicist Marshall Stoneham. Stoneham had a patrician demeanor and a benevolent calm as deep as his scientific reputation, and he quickly developed a fascination with Vibration: Why, it was *marvelous*, this, *physics*, particles and quantum mechanics, inside a biological system? *Fascinating!* So, Lucka (Stoneham never quite remembered how to pronounce Turin's given name), how *does* this work exactly? Stoneham both wrote and called *Nature*'s editor in chief, John Maddox (whom he knew personally), to suggest the names of some suitable referees. Turin felt very good about all this. Maybe they'd actually get people who understood. . . .

On another front, the BBC had begun filming now, moving into high gear on the documentary, and Turin was waging skirmishes with producer Alison Baum over the simplification of his science. She was, calmly and politely but relentlessly, presenting it in a way she felt the public could follow it; Turin didn't see why the public couldn't follow "7-transmembrane G-protein receptors." But at every conflict they would manage to work it out, the producer bringing it down a few levels, the star balking (as stars do), everything slamming to a halt, and she gently leading him back to the A-B-C version, after which they'd roll cameras again.

Everyone was conscious that while *Nature* had to publish before *Horizon* broadcast (didn't they?), they were crawling toward publication in *Nature* while rocketing toward a national November 27 broadcast on the BBC of *A Code in the Nose,* as the documentary was now being called. Over at *Nature,* Short seemed so agitated about the BBC's broadcast—but so uncommunicative about exactly what it was that was agitating him—that Turin finally entreated John Lynch, who ran the *Horizon* science program at the BBC, to call Short directly. This was fine with Lynch, who, increasingly nervous himself about this timing question, was coincidentally at that exact same moment seeking Turin's permission to call *Nature.*

In fact, Lynch and the BBC had been uncomfortable about this tightrope-walking act from the start, Lynch in particular nervous that Turin would suddenly balk on the film if *Nature* hadn't published. *Nature* had priority, and everyone knew that. So Lynch had phoned Short after August: Here (he explained to Short) was what *Horizon* was up to, and was it very likely *Nature* would publish before their broadcast? Short, true to form, couldn't be pinned down on an answer. At first, what Lynch had heard him say was a flat: "If you broadcast before we publish, it will absolutely jeopardize the paper's publication in *Nature*." That was very bad; in the BBC's bunkers, Baum and Lynch and Rosin began an ongoing strategic huddle about *Nature*. They thought *Nature* would work with the BBC's time frame, but *Nature* seemed to be taking an incredible amount of time. (Baum told herself that, well, this was what happened with truly new ideas.)

The closer the deadline got, the more concerned Lynch was becoming, but the more diaphanous Short's position, too. Now Short seemed to be saying that it was *possible* that the broadcast wouldn't kill Turin's chances, but then it wouldn't help them, now, would it? And (Short let drop) they'd hit some snags on peer review. . . . Which didn't make John Lynch feel any better about Luca Turin. BBC science journalism hardly wanted to send *Horizon* out on some bridge *Nature* wouldn't cross. So Lynch sought to shore up his flank by establishing a strategic alliance with *Nature,* looking for an explicit association with the magazine to confirm that the science in Turin's Vibration theory was being taken seriously. Getting Short on the phone again, Lynch had a proposal: the final call would ultimately be Turin's, of course, but it might be nice if *Horizon* could append its broadcast with an official imprimatur of quality like "As published in *Nature* magazine." This smell paper of Turin's, said Lynch, had been in the works at *Nature* forever, it seemed (Short straightened his spine at this), and the BBC was going ahead with the broadcast, so . . .

Short was in his starchy-editor mode. We cannot hurry this process any more than we already have, he informed Lynch (who had not suggested that they had hurried it at all). They agreed in the end that *Horizon* was welcome to append at the end of the tape "Luca Turin's paper proposing the theory you have just seen has been submitted to *Nature*." Which, come to think of it, means nothing at all.

And when Lynch called Turin and asked, "Should we put 'As submitted to *Nature*' at the end?" Turin was so irritated that he said absolutely not, the Limey bastards. He said he didn't give a damn about *Nature*'s approval; his job was not to do their advertising. Lynch was ever so slightly concerned. There were questions. There were conflicts. There was a significant sum of the BBC's money riding on this thing. Was Turin sure about this? Lynch thought that the notion of appending "submitted" was a good thing. Turin thought it genuflected before *Nature*. (It did, of course, that was the point, but it nauseated him.)

On Saturday, September 9, 1995, Turin sent Stewart the draft of his rebuttal "With a few small bits still missing . . ." Having played the critic and the diplomat, Stewart's new attitude toward *Nature,* which he started expressing in no uncertain terms by phone and e-mail, was that if Turin had good evidence (and he did), and if the physics was correct (and it was), then the hell with all the blinkered, unthinking molecular biologists, Turin should stand his ground. Because the physics, Stewart was adamant, *stood,* damnit. "Thanks for the comments!!" Turin wrote back, but added with a bit of throat clearing (it was now he who was behaving diplomatically), "Most of them I have incorporated into the new version, though some I left out because, although I heartily agree with you ('fuck molecular biology,' for instance) my version is better matched to the impedance of the audience." ("Impedance" is an electrical engineering term referring to battery resistance matching load resistance—Turin meant he had dumbed it down for the idiots.) "I am rewriting the last section, which as you say is impenetrably obscure."

And then the final bit, on September 21, 1995, from Turin: "Here's one last thing I need: the abstract at the top. Can you help me improve it??" And the next day: "Thanks, much better! Let me know what you think." Then Turin copied the new version of the paper's abstract, calm scientific words masking an assault on everything molecular biologists and chemists thought they knew about the sense of smell:

I propose here a novel theory of primary olfactory reception based on a form of inelastic electron tunneling spectroscopy. The theory explains a number of facts about the relationship between molecular structure and smell that are very difficult to account for by receptor mechanisms based on recognition of molecular Shape. The molecular biology of the putative receptors in olfactory neurons is consistent with their being components of a biological spectroscope.

Which, when you came right down to it, just meant: Fuck molecular biology.

The next day, Turin sent *Nature* both his revised paper and his carefully diplomatic rebuttals to the first round of referee comments.

✦   ✦   ✦

IN SAN FRANCISCO, the BBC producers Isabel Rosin and Alison Baum were in the heart of the enemy camp, communing with the great guru of Shape. A man Turin had never met and yet knew intimately, John Amoore had for years waged active war (via journal, Internet, and international conference) against Vibration.

The problem for Baum—she was in charge, giving orders, worrying the details (the London crew was jet-lagged, groggy on California time; Amoore, an Englishman, had moved to California years ago)—was that she had to clear with Turin what she could tell Amoore about the theory. They couldn't just waltz in and give away its details, because it wasn't published. On the other hand, she was producing TV, she was nobody's baby-sitter, and they had to capture Amoore's emotional reaction to the theory on tape. Which meant she and the entire crew were stressed about the interview.

As the lighting people set up, Baum was prepping Amoore, whom she found a thorough gentleman. For Amoore, it was surreal. When Dyson had proposed his vibration theory in 1938, it had been just one more idea about how smell worked, and a very implausible one at that, and when Buck had found the receptors, which worked everywhere else by shape, vibration had hit the showers. Hadn't it? To Amoore, this boy—what was his name, Turin—he had an idea embarrassingly past its sell-by date (and Baum, though he was too polite to say so, was a deluded girl for giving it airtime). If Baum was aware of all this, she was also aware, through Turin, of the problems plaguing Shape. What *she* wanted was the struggle captured, visible, in Amoore's face, on videotape. She was prepping him while the cameras were focusing and they started turning on hot lights. She held her fire, guarding the crucial piece Turin had added to Dyson that made the machine work. They were rolling. She explained Turin's theory, and the dignified Amoore listened and replied, almost rhetorically, with just a bit of the impatience of the victor, "Yes, but what's the *mechanism* for this vibration theory?" What exactly made it work? Baum said, "Electron tunneling," and Amoore went very pale and completely quiet. He understood immediately the implications. For a moment he looked as if he were going to burst into tears. Baum prayed the cameras were getting this. They were. They quietly turned off the equipment while Amoore went outside for five minutes.

On a personal level, Baum reflected, she really felt bad for him, it was the man's life's work being assaulted and all that, but, on the other hand, she had to say that after all there just seemed, well, so many flaws with his theory . . .

Stewart, when Turin told him about it, frankly found Amoore's honesty—his acknowledgment, even if inadvertent, of the threat to his own theory—admirable. Only interpretable, Stewart commented, if he's a *real* scientist. And they were pretty rare these days. Turin agreed.

Then the BBC crew fell back to Britain and, on home territory again, turned their attention to the filming of Dr. Luca Turin, which he found amusing, if a bit weird. He filed the story with Stewart.

Date: Wed, 4 Oct 1995
To: stewartw@helix.nih.gov
Subject: ambient mayhem . . .

Re the BBC, madness in plentiful supply. They're going to interview me in the train on the way to Paris on Sun, there and back in 6 hrs! Half a first-class carriage (empty on Sun) is reserved for filming, donated by Eurostar (the channel tunnel train company). Last Saturday: all sorts of filming tomfoolery in different locations meant to impersonate my lab (different lab), my home (someone else's) and a bookshop in Lisbon (a bookshop in Leicester Square, actually) where I found a *great* 1964 book that helped me a lot (as you know, textbook writers still wanted to be understood in those halcyon days). The following week, Wednesday at Quest UK, Thursday and Friday in Paris (perfume stores and Quest France!!). This is going to be fun . . .

Apart from this, nothing new (thank God).

Sunday morning they boarded the Eurostar and started setting up in the narrow spaces in the cars, and the train eased out of its crystal cocoon in Waterloo station and whispered toward the continent, hurling itself into the tube below the sea. The crew thoroughly enjoyed filming Turin. He turned out to be a natural on camera, and they loved his energy. Baum and Rosin found him an excellent communicator of science, and he was perfectly willing, when they said, "Cut!" and stopped him, to rephrase things more simply. At least usually willing. They were in first class (which everyone loved), and the stewards brought some very good food and some even better wine, and his communication got better and better as the wine went down. He was eating these little exotic orangy fruit no one had ever seen before, and he said to the camera, "See? That's what you get in First Class, fruit from outer space." (They put it in the film.) On arrival in Paris they were unprepared for how hurriedly they had to pack all their equipment and rush to get it all off the train to get it through customs, dash madly around to Departures, lugging cameras and cables, and jump back on the return train in time to take off in the other direction for London. But they managed it.

Then the producers proposed something that made Turin extremely nervous. He had opened his big mouth.

Months before, during filming prep, Rosin and Baum had been grilling him on the theory, and he'd mentioned his little primary-smells test. Wait, they'd said, stopping him, what was that? Well, he'd basically mixed blue vibration with yellow vibration and gotten green vibration, only with smells. He'd taken the minty Left carvone and added to it an 1800 carbonyl vibration until the vibrational chord changed and the molecule suddenly smelled of caraway. Isabel Rosin had just loved this idea. (He'd grinned, proud.) It was perfect! she'd said. (Yep, he'd said, it was a really nice experiment.) Why, they'd do it in front of some perfumers and get it all on film! (Uh-oh . . .) Oh, don't worry! she said, it'll be great evidence for your theory. (Or, he thought, it would be the opposite; *he* had smelled the vibrational transformation to caraway, but he'd neglected to ever try it with anyone else, and what if it completely failed while the cameras were rolling?) So the whole crew got on the train in London again, the BBC with its crates of electrical equipment, Turin with his little mint carvones and some butanone in a plastic refrigerator container. This time they stayed in Paris, headed to the Quest lab, where the BBC had gathered three of the most highly respected perfumers in the industry: Maurice Roucel, Calice Becker, and Françoise Caron. They set up the whole thing, made him wait downstairs in the lobby so he couldn't sneak a huddle with the perfumers. Then they called him up and started rolling the cameras. Turin was so nervous he felt like an electric wire. The perfumers were interested but professionally detached.

He unpacked his little carvones and got out his smelling strips. (The cameramen crowded in to get the shot.) Quietly, he passed around the Left and Right carvones. OK, yes, they agreed that the caraway version smelled of caraway. And the mint smelled of mint. And (Turin's Vibration experiment) if you added an 1800 wave number to the mint? Maurice Roucel motioned to his assistant. Could she make up the mixtures? Thanks very much. She left. The clock ticked. After a few minutes, she came back, put the vials of clear liquids before them, and they started smelling. The 10 percent butanone mix? It still smelled of mint, they said. The 20 percent butanone, the carbonyl-rich potion with its nail-polish-remover smell? It still smelled of mint, they said, and glanced at one another. . . . In the BBC documentary, the camera pans in close on Turin's face, which is frozen in a tense smile. Forty percent butanone . . . 60 percent butanone . . . and suddenly, they said, "This smells of caraway." He had not said the word *caraway,* had not indicated in any way what would or would not happen to the smell. They were unanimous. Suddenly the smell switched. Well, they disagreed as to whether the jump occurred at 60 percent or 70 percent butanone, but there it was. The BBC producers were quite happy with the tape, it was terrific, oh they'd certainly be using it, nice little demonstration of the theory, and so on. They started packing up. Turin wanted to collapse on the floor.

He loved doing the looping—voice-overs—in the studio (he had to actually act a bit, saying "sulfur" in a convincing voice) and drooled over the Finnish Genelec monitor speakers. And from Nick Short at *Nature*, news, or at least a hint of it. "Nick also said," Turin wrote Stewart, " 'we've never had a paper quite like this one before.' Whatever that means, I like the sound of it. I put it to them that I needed a quick answer to turn around in time for Nov 27"— the scheduled date of the BBC broadcast—"if they rejected it. Nick said they would let me know 'very soon.' "

The wait was becoming worse. Turin, and everyone else, was feeling increasingly sure that *Nature*'s and the BBC's time frames were on a collision course. No one wanted to broadcast before publication. But perhaps the broadcast would be the same week as publication in *Nature*, and they'd do PR together; it would be great for everyone. That was what they told themselves, anyway.

❖   ❖   ❖

APPARENTLY, SAID TURIN one day at a talk he gave at Hewlett-Packard, survivors of the Hiroshima bomb had remarked that at the same moment that the bomb flashed, they smelled burning rubber. What was odd about this was that these people were miles from the blast site—which meant that though the light reached them instantly, it was impossible according to the laws of physics for any smellable molecules from any burned area to have gotten into their noses. So what were they smelling? Here was another fact: an atomic bomb gives off a very powerful and broad-frequency range of electromagnetic radiation, including infrared. (The flash we see is just the radiation in the visible spectrum.) Perhaps the burning-rubber smell was to those people's noses simply the infrared equivalent of the visible flash to their eyes. In other words, they were smelling vibrations released by the Hiroshima atomic bomb.

The Hewlett-Packard people listened quietly.

◆   ◆   ◆

IN THE SUMMER of 1995, Turin got a call from a Dr. Glenis Scadding, a doctor in London at the Royal National Ear, Nose, and Throat Hospital. She had heard about him through Jane Brock, she said. Scadding was a smell doctor. (Reading between the lines, Turin got that she was actually a very famous smell doctor, the smell doctor of last resort in Britain.) She was faced with a baffling medical case, that of a former nurse living in a rather remote part of Scotland who had already seen three neurologists. The woman suffered from a very rare disorder called cacosmia, whose symptom is that virtually all smells smell vile. Scadding was wondering if Turin might be able to help.

Janet Rippard first noticed the cacosmia sneaking up on her in 1992. "You know," she said, "when you leave the roast in the oven and you come back and the whole house just smells scrumptious and full of spiced roast smell? Well, ever so slowly, it went from a wonderful smell to something vaguely unpleasant, so slowly I almost didn't notice it." She was a practical Scotswoman and had no time for nonsense. "I remember eating ginger biscuits and saying to my friend indignantly, 'They've changed the recipe for these ginger biscuits! They taste like black treacle.' But they hadn't changed the recipe. What was changing was me."

Over six months, insidiously, her life turned inside out. The disease's initial effect was to make her astonishedly aware how social and how constant eating actually was. Wherever she went, people offered a drink, a cup of tea, cakes, and it was as if they were cheerfully holding up offal. Didn't they know it all smelled oddly vile? She suddenly began finding it difficult to walk into a supermarket, and the greengrocer's was worse. Restaurants were torture, but her husband wanted to go, and so she went, although she wanted to run away. It was like being in a sewer all the time. When she went to church, the ladies' perfumes gave off such a horrid smell she once had to flee Aberdeen Cathedral. Flowers were as bad. She awoke to find herself somehow, suddenly, living in a permanent noxious haze that smelled like wet dog, in some toxic trench laced with filth.

THE EMPEROR OF SCENT

Anytime they were making hay or silage on the farms next door, or when the tides washed the seaweed up on the beach four miles away on the North Sea, the smell was horrendous. When they drove by a farmyard and the pig or horse manure made the other passengers exclaim, "Oh, what an awful smell!" she'd notice absolutely nothing different.

Mrs. Rippard went to the local ear, nose, and throat surgeon in Inverness, but he didn't know quite what to do with her. He gave her a complete examination. Everything was normal. He did scans for cerebral tumors, and there were none. There's nothing we can do, he said apologetically. She saw another doctor. And another. He referred her to a clinical psychologist, who, baffled, suggested that Mrs. Rippard "go to the top of the tree," and so they arranged for her to see Dr. Scadding.

Down in London, Scadding did MRIs and other scans and tests and came up with nothing. After the ordeal was over, Scadding said with great regret that there was nothing else they could do, they had gone as far as they could go. In order to end Mrs. Rippard's suffering, Scadding suggested severing the olfactory nerve. She knew a surgeon in America who did the operation, so she checked with him, but then she went back to Mrs. Rippard and reported that the procedure was experimental and dangerous and had a low success rate. She felt helpless saying it. She happened to mention the case to Brock, and Brock told her about Turin.

Turin was doubtful. "I'm not a doctor." But Scadding said, This woman has tried absolutely everything, and we're about to section her olfactory nerve surgically, and so he thought, Well, OK, and took Mrs. Rippard's phone number in Scotland and called her up.

Everyone she met, Mrs. Rippard told Turin in that first conversation, had taken on a particular smell of their own, their hair, their breath. Every single person stank. *She* stank. She hated the way she smelled, unwashed no matter how clean she was. Stale. Sweaty and dirty both. And her life. . . . When they went for Christmas dinner, she had dry rolls. She could just manage a bit of Christmas pudding. The only things she could drink were very black tea and very black coffee with half a teaspoonful of milk. Lemonade tasted like engine oil. Orange juice was loathsome. She hated her disease; it was just unending torture, she said, unending torture. Turin frowned in concentration and asked her what did—and he'd name something, wood, beer, metal—smell like. Inevitably the answer was some shade of "Oh! it smells terrible, vile, horrible, it's like burning rubber, burning hair, fresh vomit, I can't stand it." She lived in a sterile prison of unscented soap. Turin wrestled every clue. He put them all in his head and thanked her, and hung up and chewed on it. He came up with exactly nothing. That was the first call.

A few days later, he phoned her again and asked more questions. He got in the habit, started calling her to demand, Could she smell this? Well, how about that? and then going away to think about it. "Can you smell acetone?" he asked one day. "Well," she responded crisply, "I don't know." ("Ah dooon't *nooo.*") "Haven't *got* any, have I!"

"Well, get up," Turin said, "and go to the chemist's and smell some." So the former nurse got up and went to the chemist's and smelled some acetone, and went back home and called down to London and reported to him that acetone smelled of . . . nothing at all. Nothing. (It's acetone that smells, strongly, of nail-polish remover.) He was a bit surprised (so was she), and he hung up and puzzled over the acetone, but if it held a key, he couldn't see it.

(Dr. Scadding had explained to Mrs. Rippard that Dr. Turin had some sort of new theory of smell, but Mrs. Rippard didn't pay it any mind.)

Mrs. Rippard couldn't bear to see people eating meat; it was, she said, as though the meat were running with pus. She couldn't eat any fruits or vegetables. For five years she had lived on a diet of whole meal bread, all-bran cereal, and boiled bleached rice. She could get baked potatoes down but not boiled potatoes, because they had so much water. As she made the tea, she had to hold her breath because the steam smelled foul. She would run the bath, and because the water was a bit brackish where she lived, she would retreat from the tub, gasping at the stench of it. But then in one of their conversations she remembered the fact that there were, actually, a very few smells that remained normal. Marmalade still smelled normal and nice, "the thick, dark variety, chunky, Ah moost seh, Ah've always been foond ah marmalade." Tonic water was also nearly right, and she could manage to drink that. *Huh,* said Turin. But he couldn't see a connection. They hung up.

Then one day she mentioned something else. He was asking her, for the nth time, about what the bad smells *smelled* like, and she interrupted him to say that, well, every so often, when she smelled something, it would smell perfectly fine for the very briefest moment, the normal smell, and then instantly it turned a vile, vile odor that was completely different from the normal one. And Turin had, as he called it, a brain wave.

Epilepsy is, essentially, uncontrollable reverb in the neural system. Normal neural systems absorb a stimulus and respond to it and then (crucially) damp the neural response down so that it doesn't simply go on forever. They wash the signal out of the brain and wait for the next one. The neural systems of epileptics, on the other hand, fail to damp things down. The brain receives the signal, and instead of processing it and then letting it drop, the brain lets it go on and on, even ratchets it up into a hysterical pitch. Epilepsy is neural feedback that won't end. Generally it is caused by some sort of physical damage to some part of the brain—scar tissue, say, from a head injury in an accident. What most people think of when they think "epilepsy," the bodily convulsions, are probably scarring of the part of the brain that controls motor function. And so Turin called Dr. Scadding at the Royal National Ear, Nose, and Throat Hospital and gave her his diagnosis: Janet Rippard had epilepsy of the brain, specifically of the first station in the smell pathway, the olfactory bulb.

Scadding thought about it. This is a long shot, Turin said, but antiepilepsy drugs are quite cheap and quite safe, so it wouldn't cost anything to give her those and see what happens. Scadding said that, well, they were going to sever her olfactory nerve anyway, they might as well try this. September 8, 1995: "Super fascinating about the cacosmic patient," wrote Stewart, who was following it all from Washington, "you should get her on phenobarb by the end of _today_." "Matter of fact," replied Turin, "she *will* be!!!!!!!! Glenis

Scadding acted lightning-fast last night and prescribed sodium val-proate." It was a common anticonvulsive used by millions of people for over thirty years. "She's starting immediately (nearest chemist is 8 miles away, the stuff will get there tomorrow am) and going on holiday on monday. Fingers crossed....." Scadding called Mrs. Rippard, who was about to depart for Cyprus. It was late October. Mrs. Rippard started taking the tablets in Cyprus, one tablet three times a day.

Nothing happened. Nothing happened in Cyprus, nothing hap-pened after she came back. For weeks, Turin would call Scadding and he would call Mrs Rippard and ask, What effect? and he would get the reply: "Nothing."

Then on a Saturday evening, December 16, Mrs. Rippard was sitting on her sofa when she suddenly wondered if there was some-thing different about the room she was in. She would have sworn the actual dimensions of the walls were changing ever so slightly, an alteration in the geometry of the space around her, the objects in it, and their relationship to one another. Then she realized, with a jolt, that she was smelling normally. People in that part of Scotland gen-erally start their evening peat-bog fires with coal, and the peat and coal fumes used to reek to her, make her mouth tingle horribly and her tongue go dead as if it had been anesthetized by the dentist. People were starting their fires. She could smell them. They smelled like fires.

Cautiously, she got up and started going about the house, smelling everything she could get her hands on, opening tins of things she hadn't smelled in years, biscuits and fruits and flowers and clothing. It all smelled as she remembered, and her memory triggered with each smell with a strength that amazed her. She couldn't believe it. She smelled water, opened a tin of pepper, then a jar of mayonnaise (but then closed it again very quickly; the may-onnaise smell took four months to come back), baked beans, and chocolates, which used to smell revolting. Now they smelled lovely, and she had one, and then she got some vanilla ice cream and started eating it (although that one took a tiny bit longer to come back properly) and drinking milk. She was over the moon. Her husband was watching television, and she didn't mention it to him because she thought, It *can't* be coming back! It *can't* be. . . . She was up and down all night. All these things she hadn't smelled in years. She went and dug the shoe polish out of a box and smelled it and smelled it.

The next day she decided to do the ultimate test and smell the one thing that had the vilest stench of all: cucumber. Any cucumber, even a single slice without the peel in a sandwich, would assault her with foul odors for hours. But she was in the middle of Scotland, and the nearest cucumber was fifty miles away, so she got in her car and drove fifty miles to buy a cucumber. She took it home, unwrapped it, cut it up, and fixed a nice cucumber salad on a plate. She leaned over it and inhaled. It smelled of fresh cucumber. She ate it.

The day after that she said, "Right. Perfumes now." She got in her car, drove to Aberdeen, went to a department store, and systematically smelled all the perfumes she hadn't been able to smell for five years. When she called Turin, he asked, "How do they smell?" She said, "Oh, they're wonderful." But then she told him some of the perfumes she loved, and he winced (her taste in perfumes was not exactly his) and raised an eyebrow and said, "Mrs. Rippard, there's still something wrong with your nose." He sent her a bottle of *Après l'Ondée,* Guerlain's 1906 creation. She loved it and wore it. On January 5, Turin e-mailed Stewart: "Hi Walter!!!!!! The 'fog' lifted (her words). I feel so good abt this I could cry!"

Dr. Scadding tried to reduce the sodium valproate dose, but the cacosmia came back, so she raised it again.

Scadding called Turin to ask if he wanted to meet Mrs. Rippard in person, as she was traveling down to the hospital in London for a final test before discharge. He found a lovely, solid, buxom woman in her sixties with, as he put it, "a twinkle in her eye and a sensible skirt—you know, former nurse and all," jolly and pleasant. Seeing her, he realized why it had taken so long for the sodium valproate to kick in. Mrs. Rippard was quite plump, and fat tends to soak up active molecules. It had to be saturated with the drug before there was enough to build up in the brain. She said to him, "Ach! Yerr a *cleverr* lad!" He was beaming. Scadding and her nurses were beaming.

◆   ◆   ◆

MRS. RIPPARD'S PERCEPTION of a difference in smell being a difference in physical space didn't surprise Turin in the least. "Well, of course. You wouldn't be surprised if a change in your eyesight or hearing changed the way you perceived the dimensions of the room around you. Smell is the same. It's about where you are and what relation that has to other things in time and space."

◆   ◆   ◆

ON OCTOBER 7, 1995, Turin collected his mail and found from *Nature* the responses of the second round of referees. He tore them open. They were even worse.

He spent a number of hours simultaneously numb and feverish. He thought seriously about dropping it, all of it, altogether—the theory, the experiments, everything. Then he decided there was only one thing to do, which was to grit his teeth and try again. He rallied and plunged into yet another response.

"I confess," Turin began his response to Short, "that the unfairness and inaccuracy of some of the referees' comments discouraged me to the point that I considered withdrawing the article from *Nature* and submitting it elsewhere." To start with, as far as Turin could tell, *Nature* had clearly resubmitted to the original Referee 1 despite Short's assurances that they wouldn't. "I have reexamined the paper that you sent me," Referee "1" had written scathingly (the "reexamined" wasn't too subtle) "and still find it unsatisfactory for exactly the reasons given in my first report." Turin, baffled, reminded Short that he'd agreed not to resend it to these people. Marshall Stoneham had *recommended* other people. Short replied that they had tried to get three completely new people, but the people they'd sent it to had said they didn't understand any of it and had sent it back. So out it went to the same three who had rejected it.

At least this time Referee 1 deigned to specify a problem: "There is virtually no attention paid to . . . how a system scans electron energy." "The answer is, of course," Turin snapped, "that no scanning is involved, as I made clear," and he once again quoted the paper's description of a fixed number of receptors covering the full spectrum of vibrations. This—and *not* "scanning"—was the goddamn physical mechanism. Turin was sick of it: "Referee "1" . . . claims that there is no physical mechanism specified in the [paper] . . . a claim that is patently false. This is prima facie evidence that either he has not read it or that he has not understood it."

Referee 1 then returned to saying that Turin had equated an electron-tunneling spectroscope with an optical/laser spectroscope. (Turin had explicitly done the opposite.) Referee 1 veered to take a wild shot at Turin's "specific examples" (the molecular shapes Turin had assembled whose smells contradicted Shape), complaining that they didn't explain how the mechanism would work—which was a job, Turin pointed out, that they were never intended to do in the first place.

Turin left Referee 1 for Referee 2. Referee 2 started with some throwaway sniping. (She—or he—insisted on simply repeating that "distance from the membrane was a problem, hydrophobicity notwithstanding," leaving Turin to note exhaustedly that 1) Referee 2 had once again forgotten to explain exactly *why* it was a problem [it wasn't] because 2) numerous experiments starting in the 1870s had shown that hydrophobic molecules—which smell molecules are—can not only quite easily cross membranes but regularly *did*.)

But Referee 2's primary criticism was of a piece of the machine Turin had proposed, a docking site—sequence HYCYPH—for the G-protein, the tiny bike messenger that got switched on when the smell molecule hit the receptor. The little G-protein accepted the information the smell molecule brought and raced off to relay the smell message to the neural highway that would lead to the brain. Referee 2 said flatly that the G-protein didn't bind to Turin's proposed docking site. So Turin took the critique to Mark Dearborn ("Look, the referee is giving me grief over this"). Dearborn looked at it and said, "Yeah, looks like Heidi Hamm." He pointed Turin to a 1994 paper in the *Journal of Biology and Chemistry* proving that HYCYPH was exactly where the G-protein docked. Which was, of course, extremely helpful to Turin. The thing was this: this

1994 paper had been written by Heidi Hamm. In the attached "Dear Dr. Short" letter that Turin sent with his rebuttal, he wrote "Heidi Hamm had, in a recent paper (attached), proved that my proposed docking sequence is involved. . . . If, as I strongly suspect, she is the referee, this means that she is having to ignore her own work, as well as basic physical chemistry, simply to obstruct my article." Dripping sarcasm, Turin generously provided for Short his docking site and Hamm's, neatly placed side by side. ("For comparison," he specified, as if there could be any other possible reason.) They were, of course, exactly identical: HYCYPH. (Much later, they concluded they'd read the tea leaves wrong, and Referee 2 remained an utter mystery.)

Referee 3 misinterpreted Turin's theory of binding, after which he posed an irrelevant question about whether the theory could be applied to other proteins. Referee 3 did have one legitimate question: If (he asked) Turin's smell receptors were of the G-protein class (and they were), and if all other receptors in this class recognized molecules by Shape (and they did), then how come only this *one* G-protein receptor would work by Vibration? Why would the smell receptors be the one exception?

Turin had a response: "Let me turn this question around," he proposed. Guess what: the receptors in our eyes that recognize light and color are also G-protein-class receptors—and they don't work by Shape. *They* work by being hit with photons and interpreting their wavelengths—which is to say, their *vibrations*. (It wasn't quite this simple, but the point remained.)

Referee 3 then turned, with open disdain, to Turin's "smell" evidence. (Referee 3 wrote the phrase " 'smell' evidence," his distancing quotes dismissing smell's reality; here was a guy who researched smell for a living, and he didn't seem to actually believe in it, like a biologist who researched color vision referring to some dubious phenomenon called "color.") This evidence, 3 simply dismissed out of hand—the enantiomer experiment, the metal carbonyls, the aldehydes, everything. "The very fact," commented Turin grimly, "that he puts the word smell between inverted commas . . . shows what little regard he has for this evidence."

"In summary," Referee 3 concluded, "the author has not adequately addressed the previous criticisms," and added as a final disparagement, "He still fails to present a compelling argument that his ideas have even a remote chance of being relevant."

Then there was Referee 4. A new referee. (The Turin camp triangulated on the semiotic details and guessed at Caltech's John Hopfield.) He opened his comments with: "I have read through the article by Turin, and the various referee comments and the rebuttal. In my view, the article does not have the slightest chance of being correct." He then mischaracterized Turin's electron-tunneling theory, criticized Turin for not explaining the "sweeping" of the electron-tunneling receptors (again, Turin wasn't proposing that the receptors "*swept*"), and ended the paper "must be rejected on its total lack of physical basis." Which returned directly to the central criticism of Referee 1, which Turin had already answered: the "physical basis" was *electron tunneling*. The referees seemed to be literally incapable of registering its presence on the printed page.

Perhaps most astonishing of all was the referees' complete lack of interest in the one thing central to the entire question: smell itself. He had offered to send them the molecules and allow the referees to smell for themselves. "I confess," Turin ended his letter to Short, "that I was taken aback by the fact that none of the referees availed themselves of my offer to furnish the smell molecules in question. Do they consider it beneath their dignity to deal with the most basic of all the evidence?"

Turin carefully checked the physics again with Stoneham, across the quad, who thought that, well, there was one criticism from referee 4 that might be valid. (It involved the question of how easy it was for the electron to spew energy at things other than the smell molecule and would you or would you not thus get an accurate reading; Stoneham and a younger UCL physicist were busy looking into it.) Nevertheless, Stoneham still backed Turin up. Basically, the physics that Turin proposed worked. Trying to be helpful, Turin even wrote a suggestion to Short that, given the paper's speculative nature ("It's not *actually* speculative," he said to Short on the phone, "it's *different*"), perhaps *Nature* would want to protect itself by publishing it under some sort of category like "Hypothesis." And he very carefully took pains to end his letter on an upbeat note: "I take this opportunity to thank you for the fair- and open-minded treatment I have received from you in the course of this long and at times stressful process."

He shoved it in an envelope on October 31, 1995, and mailed it to Nick Short.

✦   ✦   ✦

FRANÇOISE WAS FOLLOWING all this quietly, watching what it was doing to him. She was the curator of a photography collection, and one evening, sitting in her living room in Paris, she told him a story. It was about the invention of stereophotography, in which two pictures are taken at slightly different angles, put in a device that separates them, and then presented, one picture to a person's right eye and one to the left, allowing the person to see in three dimensions. The man who invented three-dimensional stereophotography was an abbot. Because he was French, his dearest dream was, naturally, to present his invention to a *comité* of the illustrious Académie des Sciences, the ultimate legitimizer of French science, and to win its blessing. So he brought his equipment before an august committee of three people. The first was blind in one eye from birth and thus could not, by definition, have stereovision. The second had extreme strabismus—was cross-eyed—and thus could not, by definition, have stereovision. The third was his worst enemy. The committee, said Françoise, rejected the invention.

She just thought it was relevant. He appreciated her saying so.

✦   ✦   ✦

IT WAS NOW early November. *Horizon* was still aiming for a broadcast on November 27. *Nature* still hadn't said a word. Test of nerves.

Bits of intelligence surfaced erratically. On the phone, Short revealed that *Nature* was getting a new editor in chief, a man named Philip Campbell. So, said Turin, and what did Campbell feel about the paper? Short murmured something that translated as: Who knows.

Turin and Stewart spread their meager entrails. There were, it appeared, some good omens. A few days later, on November 6, 1995, Turin sent Stewart an impatient but upbeat e-mail.

> Here's some interesting news from *Nature* via the BBC: Nick Short away all week in Boston, took the manuscript with him, no decision taken yet. [*Nature* editor] Barbara Cohen said to the BBC that "for every (!) person saying it's crap, there's another saying it's great" soooooo . . . . . . they're still "considering accepting" (gasp, first time I hear _that_ word) "it as a 'Hypothesis,' but don't get your hopes up etc etc." This pussyfooting around with a let-out clause is typical *Nature,* but as long as they publish it I don't care if they call it "Manic Ravings" or whatever else.

And suddenly the *Horizon* broadcast was upon them.

◆   ◆   ◆

THAT EVENING, EVERYONE was to congregate at Isabel Rosin's parents' home, a beautiful apartment just south of Hyde Park. Turin left for the party in a taxi with Françoise, gripping a bottle of Moët et Chandon Brut Imperial. Rosin had invited around forty people, including, from the Shapist camp, Charles Sell, who regretted he couldn't come, and Sell's Quest adjunct Karen Rossiter, who could and did and was, to Turin's perception at least, cold to him. Given that he was attacking everything to which Rossiter had devoted her professional life, he wasn't entirely surprised. There were lots of BBC people, some French embassy people, Rosin made food, made sure the champagne was flowing, Alison Baum brought her mother. In the apartment, he stood drinking and eating just to calm down, people buzzing around him, tension mounting. At eight o'clock the TV was turned on and the *Horizon* logo materialized on the screen, and there he was: a scientist named Luca Turin and his new theory of smell. He had already seen the program several times, so he wasn't really watching. (Linda Buck appeared, talking about the receptors. She didn't look very happy.) He estimated afterward that he had had two bottles of champagne, he could barely stand up, and he wasn't even drunk. Fifty minutes later, the show finished and forty people turned their heads to look at him. Then he and Françoise said their good nights and got in a taxi and went home.

Two million people watched. And his life changed.

First, there were the phone calls. R. V. Jones, assistant director of the Royal Air Force Intelligence Section during World War II, author of the wonderful book *Most Secret War* and one of Turin's gods, called out of the blue just to offer congratulations. Turin gripped the phone. Then came word from Jana Bennett, a big shot in BBC science. She had liked his performance. Bennett was quickly followed by a beautiful gilt invitation: the BBC was inviting its contributors—and Turin—to a party on the tenth floor of the BBC complex in White City, London. Turin figured it was some big party, so he invited Jane Brock to tag along, put on his party clothes, and they set off.

They were in the lift when he started feeling strange. They were standing next to Judi Dench and the TV anchor Esther Rantzen. The elevator opened on the tenth floor, and everywhere were people he saw on TV every night. Ben Elton was chatting with Jeremy Paxman. He and Brock walked past Charles Wheeler and Clive Anderson. He wound up standing near the wall, trying to make himself as inconspicuous as possible, until he saw Jeremy Clarkson, who'd done a BBC piece on cars that had showed Icelanders repairing their SUVs' tires by exploding them back onto the rims with lighter fluid. He went up to Clarkson and said, "I loved that section on cars and Iceland!" Dawn French turned around and said, "Yes, Jeremy, when are you going to fix my car?"

He was sidling up to the director general of BBC2 and asking, Do you happen to know if the producer of the documentary on Yugoslavia is here? (he'd really liked it; the DG peered round the room and murmured I don't *think* so . . .) when Jana Bennett came up to him. She opened with Oh, Luca, glad to see you, and then, to his surprise, she said, We should do programs—you're a born scientific communicator. He swallowed and explained that the reason he'd been good was that it was his baby. Ninety-nine percent passion and one percent amateur dramatics. She said politely, Well, let's think about it. He left the party in several states of shock.

The proposal came quickly. The BBC wondered, informally, if he'd like to do a series on the supernatural. The supernatural? He replied that frankly that was like shooting fish in a bathtub, that it was generally second-rate footage of second-rate phenomena, plus every channel was doing it. The whole world was one giant *X Files,* it wasn't even his field of inquiry. No thanks. That was the end of his TV career.

Turin also got a surprise visit from the chief editor of *Chemical Senses,* a publication that sat well below *Nature's* heights in the scientific-publication pantheon but was still a respectable science journal. The editor, Steve van Toller, had seen Turin on the BBC and been fascinated. Did Turin have a moment to chat? Certainly he did. What about? About publication, it turned out. Might Turin, van Toller wondered, be interested in publishing his paper in *Chemical Senses*?

Well . . . Turin was certainly flattered, and pleased, but no, he was really counting on *Nature's* taking the Vibration paper. Naturally he appreciated van Toller's offer. Of course, said van Toller quite amicably, handing Turin a business card. If Turin did have any trouble with *Nature,* van Toller would put the paper in "under," he added "my authority."

Ah, said Turin, not knowing exactly what "under my authority" meant. Thanks. They shook hands. Turin filed the card away somewhere.

Then there was a different kind of impact, more radioactive. The UCL anatomy department Christmas party was a lavish affair with hundreds of people, held under the bushy eyebrows of Geoffrey Burnstock, anatomy's head. Turin was talking to everyone and having a great time. He saw a colleague, a man he knew was a friend of Linda Buck's, so he went up forthrightly and asked him what he'd thought of the *Horizon* program. Buck's friend replied that it was the worst piece of shit he'd ever seen. How dare Turin pose as an expert on smell. Turin blinked. The guy kept going. A few people began turning their heads. Turin said that, well, since this conversation wasn't very rational, he'd shove off, and left for another group. The guy followed, broke in, and said that he knew more about smell than Turin did. Fine, said Turin. They were an inch away from coming to blows. Someone said, Look, you guys, take it outside. Your story's crap, the other scientist said, you know nothing about the molecular biology. You haven't read the paper, replied Turin. You want to read it? *Fine,* said the man and left. People looked at each other and then looked away.

A few days later, Turin rather grimly e-mailed the guy. Did he really want to read the paper? Turin received the following reply.

> Date: Fri, 8 Dec 1995
> To: l.turin@ucl.ac.uk
> From: xxx@ucl.ac.uk
> Subject: Re: olfaction paper
>
> peace and love Luca—I would love to read the manuscript—I am sorry I reacted so violently, but it is one of my many character defects. Thanks very much for your kind offer—I can't wait to see it,
>
> all best,

And then this:

> Date: Sun, 7 Jan 1996
> To: l.turin@ucl.ac.uk
> From: xxx@ucl.ac.uk
> Subject: Re: olfaction paper
>
> Happy New Year Luca,
> I thought the paper was a terrific read, very provocative and interesting—everyone in the lab has had a look at it too. There does seem to me a big gulf between the smelling experiments and receptor occupancy conclusions. I imagine that, like pain, smell is an interpretation of a range of activated receptors. I also don't see how you can get the receptor to read the molecule without its rigorously using shape, vibes or no vibes. So as you can see I am still a sceptic. I just don't see why you need such a complicated theory (electron tunneling), and I think much more direct experiments are necessary. If someone finally matches a specific odorant to a receptor, then I am sure you can resolve this in a matter of months, and make me eat my words (or not as the case may be!).
>
> all best,

At least there were pleasant encounters as well. Dr. Christopher Zeeman called Turin and said brightly, "Hello, this is Christopher Zeeman, you haven't heard of me." Turin said, "Christopher Zeeman? Created catastrophe theory? Five-dimensional spheres? World-famous mathematician?" Zeeman, delighted: "Oh yes, you've heard of me!" Zeeman had called (he'd seen *Horizon*) to suggest that Turin take part in "one of these Royal Society things," a series of exceedingly prestigious and exceedingly stuffy scientific poster exhibitions of new ideas. Zeeman was thinking that Turin could maybe show off two molecules with the same shape, different vibrations, and different smells. Enthusiastically, Turin responded that Marshall Stoneham had just set up exactly that.

The Royal Society "thing" was an exhibition called *Frontiers of Science*. Like everything Royal Society, it was the prestige of prestige: once a year, twelve scientific exhibits were created for the event by twelve scientists ("twelve *lucky contestants!*" commented Turin dryly) who were chosen to present their science. During the day, children and the public. At night, the august fellows of the society, their guests, and royals. White tie.

How to make his little posters stand out. The big labs had complex exhibits, vast, all sorts of electronic bells and whistles. Turin's, in the event, was the most low-tech entry there, although visually it was decent because his mother had done the graphics on her Mac. His assistant was Désirée Gonzalo, a neuroscience master's student. She'd asked him, What should I wear? He'd said, Well, it's formal. Do you have a black dress? She arrived wearing a beautiful smile and a long black dress slit, it seemed to him, up to her navel. Never had so many men been so interested in smell. Not that he minded. He didn't. He was entirely in favor. A man a few feet away avidly pressed Gonzalo on a detail of electron spectroscopy. "Well," she began doubtfully, "I think Luca should tell you." "Never mind Luca!" the man barked. "*You* tell me!"

Turin, on the other hand, was wearing a part from an old radio. Along with "white tie," the invitation had said "medals and decorations," so he had plucked a large, red, Russian-built resistor from the electronic debris in his office and pinned it on his formal clothes. He explained to everyone who asked that it was "La Médaille de la Résistance."

Onlookers not inspired by Gonzalo, however, were appalled. A humming cloud of disapproval ebbed and flowed angrily, and it centered on the little vials of smells that Turin had brought. This wasn't, said the buzz, real science, it wasn't appropriate, this was stuff that *smelled*. A man in white tie planted himself like a side of beef before the exhibit and bellowed, "*Young man, I don't believe this!*" OK, said Turin, smell a Sulfur and then a borane. He held out a bottle. The man sniffed. It smelled of Sulfur. "OK!" he boomed. "*That's the Sulfur—now let's smell the borane!*" Turin removed his fingers and said, Look at the bottle. It was the borane. No Sulfur. "*Fine!*" bellowed the man and swept off. That was when Aaron Klug, famous Cambridge University scientist and esteemed president of the Royal Society, approached. "Some little guy," said Turin, "who looks like Woody Allen without the jokes, hung with a medal the size of a dinner plate and the determined grimness you see in Holocaust survivors." With his Central European accent, Klug announced, "I am Aaron Klug. I have put a pencil mark next to your name in the program." Turin was alarmed. The buzz looking on was holding its breath. Klug had two flunkies behind him with, Turin thought, those expressionless faces that pass for cool at Cambridge. Klug said in a flat but not necessarily hostile tone, "Can you explain this to me?" So Turin started taking him through the posters. Klug was saying "Yes" and "No" and "Hmm" and "Yes" and "Hmm." Then he asked to smell Turin's molecular examples. Turin handed him a molecule and asked: What is it? "It's Sulfur," said Klug with a tone that said, "Obviously!" Turin smiled and explained that it was a borane. It had no Sulfur in it at all. But it had, on the other hand, the same vibration as Sulfur. At which point Klug actually smiled. He said, "I like this. Do you have a reprint?" Turin gave him one, and he walked off with his retainers. Turin thought, Well, at least that's over.

He was patiently baby-sitting his posters when Colin Blakemore, the esteemed head of the Department of Physiology at Oxford University, came up to him to say (with what seemed to him a combination of relief and incredulity), "Sir Aaron actually liked your exhibit!"

That's nice, said Turin.

The following morning, a woman in the press office at the Royal Society said to him, Sir Aaron liked your exhibit! By this time, Turin was saying, Yes, fine, I've heard, in a clipped manner. She gave him a look and said, So you don't know what happened? No, he didn't. Ah, she said. *Well.* Well, the fact of the matter was that when Sir Aaron saw that Turin's Vibration theory had been put into the exhibition, he'd ordered it removed. The only reason it hadn't been was that tens of thousands of expensive, glossy programs had already been printed up.

Oh, said Turin, really, and wasn't sure how to feel about this. He knew it didn't feel good.

❖   ❖   ❖

FOR CHRISTMAS, HE went to the Continent.

Date: Sat, 23 Dec 1995
  To: stewartw@helix.nih.gov (Walter W. Stewart)

Hi Walter, back from Rome and off to Paris. Tried to call a couple of times to say hello, will be at Françoise's till Jan 2, then back here. Everything OK. Rome great, but a tad provincial, St. Peter's uglier than hell, the religious equivalent of the head office of Chase Manhattan. Rented a moped for a couple of days. That was fun.

❖   ❖   ❖

AFTER ALL THEIR worrying, *Nature* had had no reaction at all to the BBC broadcast. No "Yes." No "No." Which was OK (no "No" meant a still possible "Yes"), but Turin became so frustrated that he assembled his mounting grievances for Short. It was January 22, 1996.

Dear Nick,
Another week has gone by with no news, making a total of eleven since I sent you my replies to the referees' comments. I appreciate

that, were it not for your personal interest and fair play, things would have never got this far. I also realise that, as you said, my paper poses unusual problems and has not been served well by the refereeing process. However, I'm sure you can imagine how dispiriting it is for me to sit and wait with no definite deadline for an answer one way or the other.

He had given a talk to the British Society of Perfumers in a hotel in North London, a very English affair with a generic red and a generic white in rented glasses and lovely people, as only the British can do. When he arrived, everyone was already half drunk and in a jolly good mood, and he gave a talk distinguished by two ten-minute power blackouts, during which, to everyone's delight, he continued talking in the pitch dark and saying, "Next slide," which they greeted with hilarity. He told them he'd been trying to take different vibrations and add them to each other to build a chord that would have a certain smell. Like vanilla. He'd been messing around, adding benzaldehyde's vibrations to guaiacol vibrations, and—Turin announced this momentously—he'd made of them a mixture with a lovely vanillin smell! At which point some old guy opened his mouth and said, "So what's new, we've been doing that in soap since forever." Turin said, "Excuse me?"

It turned out, Turin later informed Short, that functional per-fumers, faced with the problem that the vanilla odorant vanillin dis-colored soap, had for years been giving their soaps a vanilla smell by mixing these exact two smell molecules, neither of which smelled of vanilla at all by itself and neither of which was *shaped* like any other molecule that smelled of vanillin. The Shapists, Turin said to Short, would argue that the receptor was feeling part of the guaia-col's shape and part of the benzaldehyde's, but Turin's caustic re-sponse was: How *interesting* then that when you put together the vibrations of guaiacol and benzaldehyde, which just happened to sum to the same vibrations as those in vanillin, the shape was com-pletely different and yet the smell happened to be *the same*? And that was, what, Nick, pure coincidence?

A few days later, his tone had turned furious. He'd picked up *Na-*

ture and read an article by Henry Bourne, a G-protein expert at the University of California at San Francisco, whose data entirely supported Vibration. This time, the gloves were off.

Date: Fri, 26 Jan 1996
Subject: message to Nick Short

Hi Nick,

I was looking today at the latest issue of an obscure and erratic (not to mention slow) journal called *Nature* and saw the structure of the G-protein trimer. Henry had told me it was in the pipes, and I was impatient to see where "my" proposed docking bit fitted in. It turns out my bit is a) well exposed to the outside and b) not a million miles from the binding site!! Which makes it that much more plausible.

Short sent no response. And then he did. Turin, almost audibly gritting his teeth, told Stewart that Short had made the referees back down on most of the points, but two minor things—Short wouldn't specify further—remained, on which the refs had declared themselves incompetent and suggested two other judges. At Turin's request for a time limit, Short promised a final answer by March 7, though it occurred afterward to Turin that he hadn't specified the year.

March 7 went. Nothing. On June 5, Turin wrote Stewart, "The matter has now been referred to Philip Campbell (Maddox's successor, i.e. Nick Short's boss!!) I _hate_ the wait!!!!???"

Two weeks later, pacing the floor of his torture chamber, he was reaching a psychological limit. He called Short and drew a line in the sand. He stated flatly that their stupid system of only fast-tracking papers overtly competing for other prestige journals (*Science* and *Cell,* to name them) was making sure that truly original stuff took a permanent back seat. Short agreed. Turin then stated that since Philip Campbell would be acting on Short's recommendations rather than the paper's (now huge) file, Campbell should just read Short's letter and come to a damn decision, fast. Short agreed to this as well. So (with some surprise at his own daring, taking a deep breath) Turin stated—this was the ultimatum—that he would be coming to *Nature*'s offices on Monday at 5:00 P.M. to collect *either* the paper, to take it elsewhere, *or* the paper's acceptance.

At 3:00 P.M. the following day, his frustration boosting his resolve to follow through on this brinksmanship, he e-mailed Short. He kept the tone light:

> Hi Nick!
> As advertised, I'll come round at 5:15–5:30. I'll be bringing a bottle or two of Sauternes to celebrate :-). I hope *Nature* stocks glasses . . .
>
> all the best,
> luca

Within five minutes, Short called him, sounding shaken, to say he'd just spoken to Philip Campbell. (Well, thought Turin, so this is the way to make things happen.) Campbell couldn't come to a decision till Thursday lunchtime, and, Short said (ruefully, it seemed to Turin), he couldn't stop Turin from coming to snatch the paper away but wished he wouldn't. Turin considered this, then went for broke. Upping the ante, he told Short that he wouldn't pull the paper on one condition: Short, for once and for all, must tell him *what his recommendation to Campbell was.* Short finally relinquished his reserve and admitted that he had recommended acceptance of the paper, though published as "Hypothesis." *Nature* did this about once a year. But Campbell had the final say. Fine, said Turin. Campbell had till 5:00 P.M. Thursday, and Turin would bring the Sauternes. Short said, What if the decision is no, should Turin bring the wine? To which Turin replied that whatever the outcome, by that point they would both need a stiff drink. To this, Short agreed.

Thursday—June 20, 1996—Short did not call Turin. Turin called Short. The air was simultaneously frozen and electrified.

Short: We're turning it down.

Turin: Why?

Short said evasively, Well, it's Campbell.

Bear in mind, Turin noted crisply, that two days earlier you told me that you had recommended that Campbell accept the paper.

Well, said Short, it's Campbell.

They immediately sent him a fax confirming Short's news: *Nature* magazine was officially rejecting Luca Turin's paper proposing a new Vibrational theory of smell. It was now 330 days since the paper had been officially submitted. Somewhere in this, Nick Short happened to inform Turin that the almost year it had taken was a *Nature* record for the process. Great, said Turin.

Mildly delirious with either anger or relief, Turin and Stewart now broke open their carefully constructed arsenal: they were going to try to reverse the rejection. As an opening salvo, Turin fired off an e-mail SOS to Stoneham, a personal friend of Campbell's. All was, it seemed, not lost; Stoneham was sufficiently roused to arm himself immediately with fax machine and telephone. He radioed back:

> Date: Fri, 21 Jun 1996
> Subject: Re: smells!
>
> Dear Luca,
> Thanks for the disappointing news. I am just about to fax Philip, and will phone after about an hour (my bet he is well protected even from those he knows well). Happily, there is one straight error of fact in the referee report (if true, superconductivity wouldn't happen, nor would it be needed because metals would have no resistance).
>
> Let's hope it works.
> Marshall

Turin was fortified. In fact, Stoneham now impressively prepared to drag into the fray Nevill Mott, a Nobel Prize winner for his work in solid-state physics at Cambridge and one of the truly big guns in physics. In the United States, they had another major piece of artillery, Nobelist Marty Rodbell, the codiscoverer of the G-proteins, who had indicated support.

But when Stoneham phoned Campbell, Campbell deftly outmaneuvered him. Campbell said that oh, of course, the problem was not with the physics, no, not at all, it was the *biologists* who thought Turin's theory was garbage. Stoneham, a bit nonplussed (he wasn't a biologist, couldn't judge this), relayed this to Turin, and Turin said immediately that he didn't believe it, given, first, that Short had told Turin he was sending a positive recommendation on publishing and, second, that Referee 4's critical thrusts had concerned *physics* (criticisms Stoneham had parried), not biology (which Turin could defend against because he was a biologist). But the offensive line was crumbling now. Stoneham, who had made a valiant tactical effort, felt fatally blocked by *Nature*'s official position. Of course, *Nature*'s official position apparently didn't coincide with *Nature*'s (baffling) *unofficial* position, since on June 27 Stoneham got a letter from Campbell saying that the rejection "doesn't mean I think Turin's thesis is wrong."

And the big guns simply didn't fire. Rodbell was occupied and never entered the battlefield. Nevill Mott, like a king in chess, turned out to be so big as to be simply undeployable. Stewart had exhausted his ammunition. And Turin was finally worn down. In an e-mail whose subject line reflected his now heartfelt viewpoint on the whole matter, Turin wrote the epitaph to the *Nature* affair:

Date: Fri, 21 Jun 1996
To: stewartw@helix.nih.gov
Subject: the state of science

Great quote from a colleague: "The scramble for career advantage among scientists amounts to a race for the best deck-chair on the Titanic."

After a year, that was it for *Nature*. The paper was dead.

◆   ◆   ◆

MARSHALL STONEHAM APPROACHED it all thoughtfully. "They sent it out to some referees who may have been sensibly chosen," he said, "but they obviously had misunderstandings. A referee can go off on a tangent, thinking you're talking about something you're not talking about at all. It's happened to me. They're not immoral or incompetent. *Nature* had to decide: Are we going to take this article which may be regarded as extreme in some quarters or are we going to do the safe thing and reject it? And they chose the safe thing."

Turin had a grittier comment. "I think I was just an unknown from UCL. If it had come in with Yale letterhead, they'd have put in the attention it would have taken." He shrugged darkly, turned away. "But then, the scientific peer-review process itself . . ." Turin was wearing the grim, tight smile he gets when very angry. "One of my colleagues calls peer review 'peer preview' because one of the things about getting to be a big-shot silverback is that you get to see all the best stuff a year and a half before everyone else. Why does all the good stuff come from the 'best' labs? Is it only because those guys are that much smarter? Hardly. They're legal inside traders. They get to see all this stuff, and by definition no one ever knows who they are, so they're protected. It's *lovely*."

Stewart, for his part, reached a firm conclusion: "These were obviously people who didn't want to see the theory published. Look, any worthwhile journal ought to take a skeptical position, and *Nature* is entitled by its mandate to reject almost everything because it can be published in a specialty journal. I refereed *Nature* for a year, and I found that you could reject just about anything as either trivial or too specialized or simply untrue, and that leaves not a whole lot that you needed to think hard about. But Luca's is exactly the sort of paper *Nature* should publish. Their mandate is the most interesting thing that's happened that week in science. And most papers should say something to every scientist, which is a hard goal. When you're polishing the finding of one more gene, that's not really it. What's interesting enough that everyone ought to sit and think about it?"

✦   ✦   ✦

IN A WAY, Turin now experienced a strange release. "Fear," he said, "is a powerful motivator for scientists one way or the other." He had been afraid of one specific experiment, twisting every way he could to avoid it, because it was an experiment that would, quite simply, make or break his theory. It was about isotopes.

You can think of isotopes as different versions or flavors of some elemental atom. Coca-Cola Classic is a fundamental element of popular culture—basic, ubiquitous, indivisible. But this basic element comes in different versions: Diet Coke (the sugar has been extracted from its molecular structure—literally—and replaced with aspartame, so this version of the element Coke is lighter than the regular version), Caffeine-Free Coca-Cola Classic (same structure, just stripped of caffeine, so again, lighter), Cherry Coke (the basic element, plus cherry added, so this element is heavier), Diet Cherry Coke (lighter sweetness structure, heavy cherry added), and so on.

Atoms come in different versions too. Each isotope version of an atom (an isotope of, say, Carbon) differs from the regular version (regular Carbon) by how many neutrons it has in its nucleus. (In Greek *isotope* breaks down to *iso,* same, plus *topo,* place—as in *topography*—and thus means "same location." All isotopes of an element sit on the exact same square in the periodic table.) The basic version of an atom of Gold (Au, number 79 on the periodic table) is perfectly balanced at 79 protons, 79 neutrons, and 79 electrons. But atoms of Gold come in "isotope" versions, each of which has exactly the same number of electrons and protons (79). The difference is the neutrons (77, 78, 82, and so on). An isotope version has a different number of neutrons packed into the nucleus. (Ions are similar to isotopes except that ions are about how many electrons there are—more or fewer electrons than normal, which gives you a plus or minus charge—whereas isotopes are all about how many neutrons there are, which gives you elements of different weights, various High-Fat, or Super-High-Fat, or Low-Cal, or even Totally Fat-Free, versions.)

Take Hydrogen (H). The simplest of elements, it has one electron (a negative charge) and one proton (a positive charge). Two things are interesting about Hydrogen. First, it's the only element that has no neutrons. None. And second, since the electron is a tiny little Tinkerbell of a particle that zips around weighing virtually nothing, basically the entire weight of the Hydrogen atom is in its one big, solid proton. Which means that Hydrogen is the one atom where, if you add a neutron to it, you'll be *massively* changing its weight, basically doubling it.

Like regular Coca-Cola, regular Hydrogen (H) comes in a normal and an extra-heavy version: one electron and one proton, but with one neutron added, too. This Hydrogen isotope is Deuterium

(D). Heavy water (D_2O) is just H_2O whose Hs have been replaced with heavy Ds, literally heavier water. (Pack in yet another neutron? You've now got a Hydrogen isotope called Tritium. It weighs three times as much as normal Hydrogen, but its nucleus is unstable and Tritium is radioactive.)

Turin was concerned by all this for the simple reason that Hydrogen's shape is exactly the same as Deuterium's. Externally, isotopes are twins because their identical electrons zip around in an identical way to form identical shells. But internally the extra, heavy neutron in Deuterium makes a huge difference in the vibrations; they vibrate much more slowly. If the Shapists were right, isotopes, which are shaped the same, should smell the same. But if smell was Vibration, isotopes should smell different because the vibrations are different. So Turin was predicting—whether he wanted to or not—that you'd get an "isotope effect," two molecules that smelled different even though shaped *exactly* the same.

And if he did the isotope experiment and it didn't work—if he went and smelled two isotopes and they smelled the same—he'd be dead. Which was exactly why he had been dodging it.

Turin picked up his dog-eared Aldrich catalog and started searching for a candidate isotope.

When you build a molecule out of Hydrogen isotope atoms, the molecule is said to be "deuterated." Turin found that Aldrich sold only thirty fully deuterated, heavy-weight molecules, and they were all rather nondescript odorants, mostly solvents. Aldrich had no economic reason to make more: deuterated molecules are used in nuclear magnetic resonance imaging machines, a tiny, specific market, and Gucci and Dior couldn't be less interested in a deuterated cedarwood. On top of that, Turin saw, they were expensive.

He found, to his irritation, that Aldrich no longer listed the deuterated compounds separately, so he was flipping pages backward and forward when he glimpsed acetophenone. His eyebrows flew up. He had, completely by chance, recently been idly perusing the new perfume chemistry catalog of the industrial giant International Flavors & Fragrances, and he'd happened to notice that IFF sold acetophenone as a perfume molecule. The great Steffen Arctander, author of the immense two-volume encyclopedia of odorous chemicals, describes it as "a pungent, sweet odor in dilution resembling hawthorn or harsh orange blossom type. The effect in perfume is generally a flowery one, coumarin-like [haylike], warm, slightly animal, powerful." Perfumers use it when they want an orange-blossom effect (orange blossoms grow the molecule naturally). Since it was used in perfumery, Turin figured that it was probably a strong odorant. It was also nontoxic. It was also stable in air. Well.

He hurriedly flipped to the right page, checking isotope . . . ? isotope . . . ? There it was. Aldrich happened to make acetophenone in an isotope version. For whatever reason. He had his test. Smell the before-acetophenone, the regular stuff with H. Then, courtesy of Aldrich's chemists, who had been busily taking out the light Hydrogen atoms in the acetophenone and repacking it with heavy Deuteriums, smell the after, the deuterated acetophenone with D. Turin picked up the phone and ordered the H and D versions and set the phone down again and managed to exhale.

For a day or so he puttered around the lab, half working on various things, his mind at high rotation but only vaguely connecting with the objects before him.

The molecules arrived through the post. Turin shut his door.

He ripped off the wrapping and pulled the two containers out of the Aldrich package and carefully cracked open (it was in a sealed glass vial) the H version. He smelled it. It had a slightly gluey smell, like artists' rubber gum, a toluene smell.

He cracked open the D version, leaned his nose over it. It smelled—fruity instead of toluene, lighter. Different. Turin slumped in his chair, rejoicing.

He called up Charles Sell at Quest. Sell, said, coolly, "Impurities."

Well, said Turin grimly, they could resolve the impurities question easily enough. Could he put the two through Quest's gas chromatograph? A gas chromatograph would tell decisively if they were smelling impurities or the molecules themselves. Certainly, said Sell coolly, come on Tuesday. On the morning of Tuesday, July 23, 1996, Turin arrived at Quest, south of London in Kent.

A gas chromatograph smeller is a rather amazing machine. It is essentially eighty meters of thin silica tube wound up inside an oven, which gradually heats the tube as a steady stream of odorless argon gas is passed through it like a conveyor belt. Put a complex sample of chemicals into one end of the tube, and the sample's components will break apart (the oven heats them and they boil off), separate, and travel through the tube on the conveyor belt of helium. The trick to it is that the components break apart at different times and thus travel at different speeds, which depend on their boiling points: the light, low-boiling ones rush first onto the gas belt, the heavier molecules lag behind, and the heaviest follow last, each separate, each one coming along in its own time and place. In about fifteen minutes a needle starts registering peaks interspersed by flat baseline as the separated molecules come out the end, and at each peak, you stick your nose into a place on the machine and smell them as they pass by, one by one. Every single peak as it comes by is absolutely, completely pure. When you smell a molecule coming out of a gas chromatograph, you are smelling *only* that molecule. GC smellers are somewhat expensive, and perfume companies are one of the few places you find them.

At Quest, Turin found the body language tense. Sell and Rossiter and their colleagues had written learned articles on smell as Shape, and their bosses had invested millions in smell as Shape. He was holding either proof or disproof of all of this, and they were all perfectly aware of it. But they didn't want to show it, so it was all coolness and surfaces. Sell, at his computer, glanced up to see Turin, and then waved a benign hand at Ken Palmer, who had just appeared. Palmer was a Quest institution. The senior lab tech who, among other things, ran the GC smeller, he was around fifty, a plainspoken man with a strong South Counties accent and a legendary sense of smell. One of the more famous Ken Palmer stories people told was that, just for a lark, he had taken an adult-learning course—analytical chemistry—in which at the final exam each student was given five little vials of chemicals and asked to analyze each with the lab techniques learned in the class. Palmer simply cracked each one open, smelled them, and wrote down their correct chemical structure by their odor. "Ah, Luca," murmured Sell, "right, the GC, Ken, could you, right, yes, fine, cheers." Turin had always enjoyed a good relationship with Palmer. "There's a sort of traditional English support for the underdog," Turin explained it. "Ken likes that I'm just breezing in, flouting all the knowledge these perfume magnates profess to have."

Palmer, too, was fully aware of the implications of Turin's test. And from years of working at Quest, he knew H-acetophenone's smell perfectly by memory. So he didn't bother with the H version, simply put the D-isotope in the machine, flipped it on, made a few adjustments, and chatted with Turin for fifteen minutes. At 10:03:49, the needle started jiggling. As the various impurities and other junk floated past, they became quiet. Then the needle really jumped, and the pure isotope started coming through the tube on its silken conveyor of gas, and Palmer stuck his nose in it and inhaled, smelling the completely pure D-acetophenone. He turned to Turin and said, "My God! That doesn't smell like acetophenone! It isn't gluey at all, it's much more fruit and bitter-almondy!" Turin and Palmer were electrified. To make sure, they put in the H version. It smelled like glue. The difference was subtle, but the isotopes definitely smelled different.

They went up to Charles Sell's office. They sat down. Turin's legs were jumping with excitement. Palmer, as was proper in England for a lab tech in the presence of his university-educated boss, was standing quietly back by the door, watching closely. Sell finished dealing with some business on his computer screen, then turned his attention to them. So, he said, how was it then? Turin opened his mouth, but Palmer jumped in: "Charles, they smell different!" Palmer handed Sell the smelling strips. Sell held each up to his nose, inhaled. He was framed against the large glass factory-like window of his office overlooking the Quest buildings, with their chemists and their millions of dollars of machines and computers and their immense vats of chemicals outside. Sell, to Turin, appeared mildly bored. Hmm, yes, said Sell, they smelled different. Not hugely, but different. Right, well, anything else they could do for Turin?

Turin blinked. Here he was, almost jumping out of his skin, and Sell was simply not reacting. There is no earthly reason that these two molecules should smell different except vibrations. Palmer was agitated. Sell was not reacting. It was surreal. Sell's computer sat quietly, having relaxed itself into the screen saver, a ribbon of words that calmly unfurled itself. The screen saver read, "Listen to advice and accept instruction, and in the end you will be wise."

Turin walked out of Sell's office and stood stock-still for a moment in complete shock. He came around enough to thank Palmer profusely for his help and saw that Palmer felt this was a big occasion, that he was excited too, although it was Quest, and it was England, and the emotion was kept carefully in check. Palmer went back to work, and Turin turned down the hall.

He went to see Karen Rossiter. Rossiter, from a working-class family with little experience of universities, had pushed herself up through Quest to earn a Ph.D. in chemistry. Her dissertation was on the way Shape determined a molecule's smell. She was sitting at a computer ten times more expensive than his, with an immense screen. The computer's purpose was to display molecules' shapes and then list their smell profiles and to search for the link between their smell and their shape. Turin casually said to her, "You can turn off your machine, Karen. H-acetophenone and D-acetophenone smell different." Rossiter understood the implications. "Oh, right," she said. "So, you off then?" and went back to work at her computer.

That's it, thought Turin. You perfume scientists have just witnessed from orchestra seats the end of Shape, and there has been no acknowledgment whatsoever from any of you that your world has exploded.

Turin left Quest, took a taxi to the little Kent station, and got on the train back to London.

◆   ◆   ◆

AND SO TURIN picked up the phone and called Steve van Toller of *Chemical Senses*. This is Luca Turin, he said. So, look, you said if I had any trouble with *Nature* . . .

Of course, said van Toller pleasantly.

So, uh, said Turin, they said no. Does your offer still stand?

Van Toller took the paper. No more referees. (Turin asked if *Chemical Senses* wanted the *Nature* referee reports; van Toller said, in effect, No, who gave a toss.) No waiting, no negotiating, no jockey-ing for position, which was, in the event, what the phrase "under my authority" turned out to mean.

Van Toller's one bow to the referee controversy (or to the singu-lar nature of the paper, depending on your point of view) was that the article was published under the heading "Original Research Paper." It is the only paper *Chemical Senses* has, in its history, ever published this way, and it was van Toller's way of distancing him-self from a theoretical work. But he took it. Turin wrote up the acetophenone evidence and put it in the draft and sent it off. *Chemi-cal Senses* received the paper on July 31, 1996. Steve van Toller published "A Spectroscopic Mechanism for Primary Olfactory Re-ception" on September 30.

❖   ❖   ❖

THERE IS ONE other way of getting into the pages of *Nature*.

A "scientific correspondence" is a small thing, basically just a let-ter to the editor, nowhere close to a real, self-respecting "paper," just something a *Nature* editor might publish if he were so inclined. Turin started writing one about the isotopes.

He sent Short a description of the different acetophenone smells and (to back himself up) the traces from the Quest chromatograph. Short passed it on to another nameless referee.

The referee wrote back:

> I read with curiosity the . . . item you sent. It felt like going back 30 years to the dark ages of Wright's vibrational theory of olfaction. We have been there before, and luckily the field has emerged to the sanity of regarding olfaction as part of biology. We are extremely content with [Shape's] hypotheses, many well-proven. . . . Going back to the world of ad-hoc physical theories that ignore the vast body of knowledge of general receptor science is truly unnecessary.

That was it for *Nature*.

PART
II

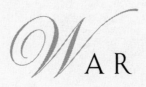

AR

V

✦

COMPANIES

HEORETICALLY, TURIN'S SMELL theory could make some people very, very rich.

The first nibble from the private sector materialized just before the BBC broadcast in an e-mail. It was from David Gallagher, the friendly English Oregonian with CAChe Scientific, which had just been bought by a British company named Oxford Molecular. The e-mail's subject was "Smells like an opportunity."

CAChe Scientific
Oxford Molecular Group

Hi Luca
We are working on some opportunities with some fragrance companies. Would you be interested in signing an agreement with Oxford that gives you a royalty on all sales or deals that come out of it? The opportunities could range from a few hundred K to several million pounds (it's too early to know just yet). Something like a 5% clear royalty on all revenues is typical for this sort of situation, and Tony Marchington is agreeable to this. Let me know what you think.

regards,
Dave

Marchington was a cofounder of Oxford Molecular. OxMol's interest in Turin's research was clear: OxMol sold software programs—two in particular, called Sybil and Tsar ("Structure Activity Relations")—mostly to huge drug companies like Bayer and Schering-Plough, for "rational drug design": the drug giants used the programs to predict the pharmacological effect a molecule would have when it hit a receptor. The programs predicted this effect by the shape of a molecule of Prozac or Percodan, and because drug-receptor interaction *does* in fact function by Shape, the programs worked for drugs. The neat trick OxMol wanted to manage was to sell their programs to the perfume Big Boys, who would attempt to use them to predict a molecule's *smell*. But the evidence indicated that they wouldn't really work in that role, so no sale. OxMol's bosses immediately understood—Gallagher had told them about the guy in London working on smell—that if Turin's theory was correct, and if they licensed the predictive algorithm at its heart, Oxford Molecular's smell-prediction software would actually perform, which meant that the Big Boy who bought the program would eat the others for lunch and royalties would be flowing like water to Oxford Molecular.

And to Turin. He was excited. Maybe he'd make some money out of this.

They sent him a contract, and he went over it, feeling strange. He asked Stewart to eye it, "in particular their proposal in para 1 of page 1, that my consultancy be exclusive in my part to Oxford Molecular in *all areas of software and databases associated directly or indirectly with my research.* I think that's a bit too open-ended, don't you?"

OxMol invited Turin to give a lunch talk at their offices, which he did. (They then asked him to leave the room so they could discuss him.) Yes, they were interested. Could he meet them at Heathrow in between flights? He did, twice (they were flying first class).

He waited. He didn't hear anything else from them.

◆   ◆   ◆

YOU THINK YOU'VE smelled every smell by now. You think you more or less know the full range, the rich, velvet perfume of daylilies at the West Sixty-seventh Street Korean market to the stench of rotting fish sloshing under a Gulf of Mexico pier. How could there be more? The fragrant eau de toilette of ripe mango on hot asphalt, rancid palm oil, and raw sewage bathing Manila's open-air markets. The iced February wind in Wyoming over frozen dirt at midnight, where you can smell the surface of the moon. The instantly recognizable stench—electrical, plastic, foul, unique—of the RER trains in Paris. Sliding glass door, steel light pole, aluminum elevator, and the other metallic nonscents of Tokyo. The smell of Colorado pine on warm rock in summer. The alarming Agent Orange smell of chemical warfare when the photocopier breaks and the poisonous toner spills out and your nervous system goes on alert. The public toilets of Buenos Aires, which smell of the 1950s. The scent of ozone in the lightning just before the rain starts pulverizing the earth, throwing the dust in the air, then sluicing it violently away and the small plant stems snap green and raw. (You've even smelled the ones you haven't smelled, from movies, from legend. World War I's deadly mustard gas smells strongly like mustard, the lethal war gas phosgene, $COCl_2$, has a pleasant smell of new-mown hay, and the poison cyanide smells nicely of bitter almonds.)

You think there are a certain number of smells, and you've smelled them. You're wrong. There are, like undiscovered continents filled with unimaginable animals, millions of hypothetical molecules yet to be created, millions of atomic structures that exist, thus far, only as mathematical possibilities, which we will create. Take all possibilities, Carbons multiplied by double bonds multiplied by isotopic versions of Oxygen, methyls attached to propyls bonded to ethyls, and the numbers skyrocket. This is the math of the old tale of the Indian sage who was asked by the king, "What shall I give you?" The sage replied, "Put one grain of rice on the first square of a chessboard. Then put two grains on the second square.

Then four on the third." The king laughed and agreed: "But this is nothing!" Then the sage said, "And so on." By the last square on the board—the sixty-fourth—you're at something like 2^{63} grains of rice, which is more rice than there is on earth. Within the astounding number of fragrance molecules left to discover, there are going to be gorgeous smells, breathtaking, mesmerizing scented wonders we can't imagine today. Not all the molecules you can design on paper are actually makable. Some will fly apart. Some will melt, some will collapse or explode. But some will cohere and will smell. And what will they smell like? No one has any idea at all. And no way to calculate or predict them, at least for the moment.

A molecule was found in the 1960s in the laboratories of Camilli, Albert & Laloue, endowed with a very strange smell. Some describe it as "oysterlike." Turin describes it as "halfway between an apple and the knife that cuts it, a fruity turned up to a white heat." They named it Calone, after the initials of the firm. Another molecule came out in 1980, also with a strange smell. Turin: "Wet concrete and musk with a fruity, spicy note. Called Cashmeran. Weirdest damn thing. It's a molecule that changes colors all the time." Both molecules have made piles of money for their creators.

If Turin is right about smells being vibrations, you shouldn't be surprised that there are thousands of smells you've never smelled: it's the same with light. In 1709 the Englishman John Herschel laid a prism in the sun, and the prism spilled its rainbow into the air: violet to blue to green to yellow to orange to red. Just past the red, where the rainbow ended and there was nothing, Herschel placed a thermometer. The thermometer heated up. Herschel thought: There are colors of light here that are heating it, colors I have never seen.

These are colors that have no names, colors we can't imagine. Invisible colors (the over 99 percent of all photons vibrating outside the visible range), zillions of photons generating zillions of shades and hues. All electromagnetic radiation is color.

The Big Boys in their giant industrial kitchens know there are new smells to be found, wonderful, mesmerizing, undreamt-of fragrances, scented wonders for which we will pay any price. They know that the smell-prediction algorithm, which will make all the new smell molecules you could desire, is a machine to grind out gold.

◆ ◆ ◆

ONLY IN JANUARY 1996 did Luca Turin, for the first time, attempt an actual prediction of smell.

Stewart and Turin had started daydreaming about industrializing Turin's discovery. They figured this meant creating a company, so Turin trotted over to see his head of department and put a few questions to a few friends in the corporate world and then sent an e-mail to Stewart that "by the end of the week, you will be a co-director of 'The Fragrance Prediction Company Ltd' with offices in London!! UCL gave the green light this morning, and is a (minority) shareholder." Turin loved doing graphics and logos, so he'd soon be "sending some slides to Quest with our logo—attached—!!!!!!!! Meaningless so far, but very exciting nonetheless. As they say, even dwarves started small."

But Turin and Stewart talked it over the next day and made a strategic decision to postpone the Fragrance Prediction Company, first because there was no point in setting it up until they had some clients. And second because they needed investors. The thing was, the company's logical investors were its clientele—the Big Boys: IFF and Quest and Takasago, Givaudan Roure and Haarmann & Reimer and Firmenich—and Turin had to get a fix on what it would be worth to them. Precise figures were impossible to pry out of them, but he estimated that if each molecule, both the few good ones and the useless thousands, was now costing them (he put all his clues together and came up with a number) $3,000 to make, their savings in molecule production alone would be $3 or $4 million a year, while costs for testing and so on would plunge. When you added in increased efficiencies, the savings in salaries of all the chemists you'd summarily round up and fire, the savings from shutting down the labs of all the chemists you'd fire, not to mention the devastating commercial coup over your blindsided, cowering competition and the rocket that this would put under your share price, the figure could, within a few years, be billions. They could, of course, try to get a company funded on a shining possibility, but they decided to hold off until they'd developed the secret engine driving its heart. That engine was an algorithm, and that, Turin started to build.

An algorithm is simply a mathematical formula with which you calculate something. (The question came up of patenting the work Turin had done at UCL. Algorithms are notoriously difficult to patent, and the patents, if granted, are even more difficult to enforce: how do you prove someone has been using your formula if they say they haven't? Better to keep it quiet.) An algorithm can do anything. If you want to count cattle and the only information available is the number of legs, you count the legs, plug this information into the algorithm—which is "N legs divided by $4 = X$"—and out pops the number of cows. Assemble your information ("here are the vibrations and partial charges in this molecule"), plug it all in, the algorithm (this one infinitely more complex than "N legs divided by 4") crunches the numbers, and you get your answer ("this molecule will smell like dried shrimp shells and peppermint").

We have, deep inside of us, a smell algorithm, created by the Greatest Engineer: evolution. The algorithm is a way for the brain to plug in a constant inundation of incredibly complex information and get a result. Turin knew there was one—all scientists agree on this—simply because that is exactly what the brain does with hearing and vision: the human brain uses, every split second, without breaking a sweat, two breathtakingly complex algorithms. In vision, you have only three receptors covering the spectrum of wavelengths, and yet the brain uses an algorithm for vision that gives you thousands of distinguishable colors. The vision algorithm, worked out by Edwin Land, the inventor of Polaroid film, is what allows a Polaroid camera to make sense of all the millions of pieces of photon-vibration-frequency and light-intensity information and turn them all into a three-by-five snapshot (and why Polaroid makes the "Land camera"). In hearing, thousands of tones cascade into the ear, and huge chunks of the cochlea vibrate, *and yet* with its algorithm the brain is figuring it all out and giving you sharp pitch discrimination, separating the peaks, giving you voices and notes and sounds. Utterly brilliant mathematical precision, applied every millisecond. If Turin was right about smell, at the instant of conception nature downloads into each of us a copy of its proprietary smell algorithm, which derives smells from vibrational data, just as it downloads a copy of its vision algorithm (Evolutionary Version 3,000,000,000.0) and its hearing algorithm (programs designed to run on *Homo sapiens* neural hardware).

Why did it take Luca Turin until now to try to predict smells? Because of the difference between theory and practice. Or, if you'd like, proof and prediction. Or, to put it still differently, because Turin had now reached his limits of the understanding of science and gone through the looking glass, had entered the netherworld on the edges of quantum physics.

Creating a theory holding that we smell vibrations and actually applying that theory to the practice of predicting smells are two completely different enterprises. The question to ask for the first, to prove the theory, was: "Can you do experiments showing that smell is vibration?" Which is to say: Can you put together a group of facts that you just can't explain any other way? And the answer was, yes, the boranes and isotopes and so on were just that, facts that only Turin's theory could explain. That was a science problem.

But the multimillion-dollar prediction question was this: "Why do *this* particular molecule's vibrations smell of rose—*and how can I, purely according to theoretical principles, predict which hypothetical vibrations in some hypothetical molecule will smell like rose too?*" That was ultimately an industrial problem, a process problem, and it was more complicated by a factor of, say, one thousand. Suppose you prove that we smell vibrations. Great. It means almost nothing for predicting the smell of some brand-new molecule no one's ever smelled. Why? Because every vibration in the air, which makes a sound when it hits the cochlea in the inner ear, has two important aspects, a frequency—how many times per second it vibrates back and forth, which gives you a tone, an A flat or a G—and an amplitude, how *loud* that A flat or that G is. And every vibration of every bonding electron has both these aspects, too. Measuring a bond's frequency—"Is it an A flat, a G, F sharp?" (Is it wave number 386.187 or 2955?)—is, as Turin said, "a piece of piss," just throw it in a spectroscope or calculate it. Measuring the loudness of a molecular vibration (the amplitude, how *strongly* the vibe will be felt by the nasal spectroscope) is virtually impossible, and the reason for that couldn't be simpler: we just don't have the technology yet, either to replicate the measurement in the lab or to calculate it accurately. The amplitude is determined by the "partial charges" on each atom of the molecule, and at the moment we have no way to measure partial charges. Or rather the technology we do have to do this is ridiculously primitive and notoriously inaccurate. *That* is mostly a physics problem. And even if you could measure them with some instrument, you wouldn't know how the *nose* was doing it. How in the world were tiny receptors made of cells detecting partial charges? That's mostly a biology problem. All of which means that you could prove the Vibration theory entirely, *prove* it definitively—but because you didn't have the technology to measure amplitude, you still couldn't *predict* for Givaudan whether some molecule would smell of fresh green Aspen bark or burning hair. You could have a million dollars from your Nobel Prize in Chemistry for smell work and not a penny from any prediction-software royalties.

Which was why predicting smells was low on Turin's list.

But he squared his shoulders now, grabbed a molecule, and tried it. To create the smell-prediction algorithm you have to know three things (all are obligatory).

First, you have to calculate each vibration of the molecule. This gives you a readout showing all the molecule's vibrational peaks from wave number zero to wave number 4000, the standard mountain range of crests and valleys. This one is not too tough.

But, second, you now have to find the precise height of every single vibrational peak (which is the intensity or springiness of that bond).

And third, you have to find something called "pitch discrimination," the breadth of each peak, a better way of saying that being,

"How separated will each of these guys be from its neighbors, and can you actually tell them apart or do they just blur together?"

Turin's problem with all three was, again, technology.

For number 1, you could take the molecule and point your infrared spectrometer at it and measure its vibrations' frequencies—except that often spectrometers can't separate each vibration, if they're too close together, so you get the wrong answers. Or you can just calculate their vibrations mathematically, although the precision in doing this is directly proportionate to how much time you take to do it. If you want to calculate the frequencies in ten minutes, the computer will do them to the nearest 10 percent, which is to say that your data will be garbage. If you want the nearest 1 percent, it'll take the machine twenty-four hours, or two days, or three. And .01 percent? There's just no known method that will do that; we know, today, the masses of the atoms to five digits of precision, but what determines wave numbers is also the tautness of bonds, and our quantum chemistry methods aren't that good yet. It takes immense amounts of time and calculating power to do a single molecule, and even then we don't have anything like a fine-grained photograph.

For number 2, finding the height of each vibration's peak, the problem is that it is flatly impossible. More precisely, it is all drastic approximations and blind guesswork.

And number 3 is a question—telling the peaks apart—that doesn't at this moment in our scientific abilities and human technology have a good answer.

Still, Turin was too intrigued not to try to cobble the algorithm together in a rough version. He shopped for models, selecting an off-the-shelf tunneling formula that physicist C. J. Adkins had created. He got on a train to Cambridge to go see Adkins and show him what he'd done with his formula, removing (Turin cheerfully admitted) all the bits he didn't understand. Were those bits, well, crucial? Adkins squinted at it from one direction and squinted at it from another and said that hm, yes, well, good enough as a start. Couldn't do better. Not with the present state of the art. Scattering intensity too damn tough to calculate. ("It's an 'active research area,'" sighed Turin to Stewart, rolling his eyes, "meaning: 'Stay tuned.'")

On January 20, 1996, Turin e-mailed Stewart his first crude recipe: "1)," he dictated, "calculate partial charges using dumb but apparently efficient Huckel method." Steps 2 and 3 concerned checking out each atom's motion in each vibrational mode and multiplying by the partial charges. Step 4 was "replot the whole spectrum thing"; 5 was to divide it all up into chunks to do stats. "(How)," Turin queried incidentally, "(does one represent points in 8-Dimensional space, btw?)" And "6) serve warm." He added: "Keep this strictly to yourself for the moment, it could be worth some dosh" (money).

Turin's smell algorithm, by the way, is

$$\sum_{i=1}^{N} q_i^2 x_i^2$$

where x_i are displacements (usually given as Cartesian displacements in x, y, and z) and partial charges q_i are calculated by the chemistry software. That is the secret formula. But an algorithm demands something. These tiny mathematical machines, especially the newborn ones, are voraciously hungry.

Unlike other mathematical formulas, algorithms need to be fed data to make them grow strong, just as a newborn child's brain needs to be fed massive amounts of stimuli for its neural organization and development. The baby algorithm's food was correlations. The correlations were between the vibrations of molecules (alpha-octyl cyclopentanone's unique chord) paired with reliable odor profiles ("sweet and oily-floral, mildly balsamic odor"). Each vibration-smell correlation makes the algorithm more intelligent, stronger, more accurate. Once it knows that *those* molecules have *these* vibrations that correlate with *these* smells, it starts understanding how to predict vibrations it has never seen before. So it needs correlations from thousands of molecules, millions of molecules.

The correlations sat inside databases. The databases belonged to the Big Boys.

✦   ✦   ✦

TURIN'S PUBLICATION IN *Chemical Senses* elicited almost no reaction whatsoever. He had assumed it wouldn't. Still.

At least in this vacuum there appeared one entirely unexpected use for his theory. It was delivered via the radio.

Turin was cleaning his apartment one afternoon and listening to Radio 3, what he, a classical-music junkie, refers to with gratitude as "the BBC's amazingly expensive, elitist, and wonderful classical station." Radio 3 was playing an absolutely glorious piece of music he'd never heard. He waited as it ended, ready to bomb the BBC if they didn't give its name. They did: "Lento" by a composer named Howard Skempton. Turin had never heard of him. He went out and bought the only Skempton CD he could find (the only one that existed), which included the twelve-minute piece for full orchestra called "Lento," and perusing the liner notes saw that Skempton lived in Leamington Spa, near Coventry. So he called him up.

He was, he told Skempton, doing a course called Practice and Philosophy of Science at UCL, to which he invited anyone he pleased. Turin believed that musicians were more rigorous than scientists. The structure, the rules, the pure math. Would Skempton come and give a lecture on science and music? Skempton would be delighted. He arrived in the class on his appointed day. The lecture started; Turin put on "Lento," twelve minutes long. There was complete hushed silence in the basement seminar room.

When Turin explained his theory to Skempton, the composer was fascinated, particularly by the idea of smells as frequencies. "Ah! Like *aural* tones." Well, yes. "You mean, as if you smelled *notes?*" Well, yes, actually, said Turin. "Well!" What if, Skempton suggested, they collaborated on a musical piece based on contrasting smells. Turin thought about it for an instant. They would transform the vibrations of Molinard's *Habanita* into musical vibrations. *Habanita* is based on vetiver (a grass from the Caribbean; its roots provide an oil that contains, among other things, a molecule called vetiverol) and vanilla. Turin proposed the vibrations of fourteen or fifteen of the perfume's electron bonds—which meant fourteen or fifteen wave numbers—and with Skempton translated them into sound frequencies. ("Easy, you just keep the ratios of the numbers equal but shift them all into the audible range.") Skempton took the notes and enthusiastically set out to use them to create a piece. "The question," Turin said to him excitedly, "is will it sound like vetiver and vanilla."

Post-*Nature,* he was forging ahead. His personal life was ambiguous. "Françoise not v. happy about us," he wrote Stewart, "sort of periodically sick of me and my supposed aridity, went through a bad patch but now better. I love her dearly, but we really are tuned to different frequencies." Speaking of which—"My favorite composer (and now friend) Howard Skempton is writing a concerto for accordion, oboe, and strings based on vanilla and vetiver to be premiered next March!!!"

He was still trying to put his theory out there. Acrid flares of hostility echoed back to him. Mark Dearborn happened to attend a conference where the illustrious Yale smell researcher Gordon Shepherd was speaking, and Dearborn stood and said, Dr. Shepherd, there's a new theory of smell out there. The author is Luca Turin, and it has to do with molecular vibrations. Never heard of it, said Shepherd (with, Dearborn told Turin, evident distaste). Where was it published? *Chemical Senses,* Dearborn said. Shepherd gave a thin smile. Oh, he said sarcastically, that'll increase the readership of *that* journal.

Turin tried to put the incident out of his mind, but it bothered him.

❖　❖　❖

FRANÇOISE BROKE UP with him, or he with her, half by accident. Her life was in Paris, her museum job, which she loved, was in Paris, as were her numerous brothers and sisters, she spoke halting English, and after five years of skirmishing and negotiation, both parties were exhausted in their mutual camps. His friends were telling him that she loved that he was entertaining and great at dinner parties, she loved his irrational optimism, and (he was aware) the fact that he was lost in admiration of *her*. But she simply didn't care about the science. It won't work, Luca. She was in love with him, but never with the science. He was lonely in London, but it was the loneliness of very few people understanding what you do. And this included her.

He'd started reacting to her, if not entirely consciously, he'd been "rocking the boat," intimating that perhaps he just needed a little break, and Françoise sent him a fax that said in that case it would be better if he didn't call her or see her. He read the fax and didn't call her or see her. Which was of course the wrong thing to do, and that was that.

And so he was alone. Except for a woman, named Desa Philippi, whom he had met when he sat next to her on the Eurostar. They were conversing by the time the train pulled out of the Gare du Nord. She was, she told him, an editor of modern art books with a degree in art history. Inwardly, Turin rolled his eyes (art history, Christ! The intellectual soft stuff . . .). She was German, with long silvery-blond hair and a methodically passionate manner. They heat-edly debated modern art, and Turin soon reached the conclusion—which, always generous, he immediately shared with her—that here was a battle of two utterly incompatible, diametrically op-posed worldviews: breakneck nineteenth-century romanticism (him) versus modern realist pessimism (her). He told her that as far as he was concerned, there was no goddamn reality that he would not, at any time or any instant, trade for a workable dream, dreams being what make one happy. They got to Waterloo Station and parted. Despite the conversation, he gave her his phone number, which he believed in doing with great-looking women, and she called.

On one of their first dates, they went to the Royal Opera House at Covent Garden to see *Palestrina,* by the relatively little-known composer Hans Pfitzner. To Turin, *Palestrina* was beautiful because it is about the moral dilemma of a man who is a musical Galileo, a man who is in touch with the heavenly music of the spheres. The powers that be want him to compose music as propaganda for the church, to act upon the masses, and he refuses, he wants to be left alone to listen to the voices of angels, he doesn't want to take part in the visible church. Should he be in the world or not? Then the souls of ten dead composers appear to him and say, Write the music; God's voice will be heard no matter who commissions it. And so he writes beautiful music. This high-calorie, overblown romanticism moved Turin so much he cried like a fountain all the way through Act I. As the curtain came down, he turned to her, blowing his nose, and asked, What do you think? And she said, Oh, typical piece of turn-of-the-century German kitsch. Which was, Turin readily admitted, perfectly true, except that his favorite novel happened to be Henry Rider Haggard's *She,* which was Wagnerian symbolism in an Edenic Paradise laid on with a trowel. With great effort, he controlled himself.

Then he fell in love with her. This did not, in any way, cut down on the sword fighting. Philippi: "I'm the classicist and rationalist and Luca is the romantic in the nineteenth-century velvet fog with lots of heroes. Our early dates from hell were all about heroes and antiheroes. My antiheroes are Montaigne and Nabokov and Kierkegaard. His heroes are Michael Faraday, the greatest experimental physicist of all time, Diogenes, and Clément Rosset." Turin: "Talent. I don't care about talent. Nabokov is talent. Who cares. What I care about is having something to say. And not how you say it—this notion that literature is form is absurd. The ideas are what matter."

And then there was a sea-change. It happened because he went to a movie theater in Clapham and saw *Titanic,* which changed his life. "One of the most fantastic movies ever made," he said, "for a whole bunch of subliminal reasons. A meditation on death, on how easy it is to die, this cold water, the ship is brand-new like the twentieth century, it has no patina, it was modern, you can smell the paint in all the scenes in the movie, electric light was new, and you feel that." To him, the *Titanic*'s story was about what people do when faced with great difficulty, but as Wagnerian saga, done in a truly straightforward way, with no distancing at all, just as Wagner would have done it. All the symbols, utterly real: the great ship, great might, the iceberg, the gleam, the green freezing water. It came at the right time for him. He realized, he said, that he had only one life, and he had to live it. He left the theater sobbing. He had a connection to Philippi that was stormy but vast and real.

✦   ✦   ✦

AT EXACTLY THE time that Turin began looking to hitch his theory to one of the Big Boys—who could not only help him prove the theory but feed his infant algorithm—the Big Boys came looking for him.

Each of the fragrance-molecule-manufacturing multinational corporations is made of a pair of Siamese twins, one aesthetic, one scientific. Each twin is inextricable from the other and yet utterly distinct.

The Scientific Siamese Twin is each Big Boy's chemical-research side. For Turin to calculate the vibrations of a thousand molecules on his little Mac atop his messy desk and then carefully match each with its correlating smell profile was not just agonizingly slow; it was preposterous. It would be like one person building the pyramids. The Big Boys had immense R & D budgets, miles of aluminum glass labs, and armies of chemists churning out molecules in their scientific factories. And they had been doing this for decades. The treasure they had thus produced—proprietary, industrially classified molecule-and-smell data—was ensconced deep in electronic caverns guarded from competitors' prying eyes. He needed these databases, pure, raw, abundant, lovely data, heaping piles of analyzed molecules, big ones and small ones, simple and complex ones stuffed in files and on hard drives. Each molecule they created had two things, its structure, which Turin could translate easily into vibrations, and its "smell profile," smell's language, the descriptors they had painfully and with excruciating care (it was the essence of their business, after all) assembled for each molecule, which one was "sweet, rosy fruity, honeylike," which one gave "sweet ethereal floral but also herbal woody, and dry."

Vibration-language combinations. These were the secret codes, and he needed them. He needed to feed them to the algorithm one by one till it had thousands in its mathematical belly, reached critical mass.

Then there was the Aesthetic Siamese Twin. Each Big Boy employed a perfumer upper caste, separated from the molecule jockeys down in their labs. These creatives translated the briefs and directives sent them from the Fifth Avenue offices of Tommy Hilfiger and Helmut Lang into the scented potions that went into the little bottles. The perfumers in their towers in New York and Paris and Geneva were connected by a common blood flow to the molecule pushers, used in their potions and elixirs the materials the white-lab-coated sorcerers created, the elixirs to entice and land contracts from the alarmingly groomed, gelled, tinted, black-clad representatives of Gaultier and Prada and Comme des Garçons. They were intellectually and temperamentally removed, their plush offices far from the grit down in the molecular-construction sites and atomic smelting pots of the drab lab buildings. Yet—because they ruled perfume's aesthetics, because it was up in their hushed towers that each new molecule was auditioned, evaluated, whispered about, and either lived or died—they were the true crucibles of fragrance, the directors of the potions Turin loved, and the determiners of which molecules were given a chance to make money. Yes, the smell algorithm's power would be harnessed by the chemists, but ultimately it would slave for the perfumers.

At that moment, by pure coincidence, Turin found an open door to both downstairs and up. Both of Quest's twins were beckoning to him from their different sides (in this case, either side of the English Channel; the perfumers in Paris, the chemists in Ashford) and he began a strange bifurcation of tasks, working for Quest in two ways, neither twin having any idea that the other had engaged him for its own purposes.

Yves De Chiris, head of Quest's fine-fragrance division in Paris, and the other perfumers throughout the industry had first known Turin's name through his perfume book. Then the journalists who covered the perfume industry began calling him, and quoting him—*Votre Beauté* and *International Cosmetique News*—which meant the general media started calling—the *Times* of London and so on—and his name started popping up even more frequently. His growing ubiquity derived from the precision of his analysis of perfumes and the startling honesty of his opinions. Turin had little patience with pop perfume journalism. It tended to elide into New Age pablum, undergirded by prurient urban sex-mythology, both of which he openly despised, dispatching them like a cheerful executioner. His candor made some of the journalists call more often, though others, used to overheated, precious, and cloying copy from domesticated "critics" who loudly praised certain houses and quietly received nice little perks in exchange, found his lack of tact shocking and disorienting. "I'm interested," a nice young reporter (American, female, so earnest, so sincere) asks via e-mail, "in why you think we wear fragrance." He replies, "Because it's the most portable form of Intelligence." Exactly what she was hoping for! Now for some teasing, delicious little smell sound bites. She dangles one of her experts before him, like bait before a trout. "Margaret Spencer, a sensory psychologist, says it's a matter of sexual advertising."

She waits for an equally cunning strike from the trout. The trout merely raises an eyebrow. "One function of fragrance," Turin responds with equanimity, "which is established beyond doubt is to allow pop psychologists to talk endlessly about sex in polite society."

Well. Next question. "Jane Franken, a consultant," she continues, "says perfume is 'aspirational.' We crave to be richer, prettier, sexier, than we are."

Turin, blithely, and quite on the record: "A trite comment from a woman who made a lot of money from dull fragrances and plans to carry on."

"Do you suppose something like *Vanilla Fields* or *Angel* appeals to both the sex and the food drive?"

Once again with the sex. Turin replies tersely, "*Vanilla Fields* is a low-calorie banana float which appeals to the mentally obese."

When she tries mixing in science—"Torie Lefton, a medical physiologist at Duke University Medical School, postulates that since chocolate releases opiates in the brain, it might be that its scent does too"—Turin, who considers this pseudoscience, replies, "Tells you more about her than about perfumes. . . ." And cheerfully signs off with "All the best, Luca."

Quest's De Chiris sent word that they were interested in hiring him to act as a sort of Outside Evaluator for their perfumers, a commentator on their work, a suggester (now, *this* he found interesting) of novel uses for the new and sometimes baffling, weird smells the chemists manufactured, and a general oracle of trends in perfumery. That was the basic job description. Was he interested? Yes, he certainly was.

So they started whisking him down from London and into Quest's protected heart in Neuilly, outside Paris, to smell the new molecules still smoking from the anvil. What did Dr. Turin think of this one? What of that one? (They asked him what to do about the smell of Dove soap, and he suggested a really nice iris synthetic they had. They seemed to like the suggestion.) And could he think of any *use* for these new molecules, there was this one—here, this vial. Odd, isn't it? Bizarre, yet interesting, wouldn't he say? (What *would* he say?) Most of these were newly minted but commercially disappointing Quest captives, branded molecules owned exclusively by one company. Quest had a huge economic incentive to make its captives big stars, but there were problematic captives, the ones no one in-house could think what to do with, how to mate them. So they sent them to him in velvet boxes to evaluate, each in a small, emerald-colored vial with a *Q* on it, the bottles laid out like Mikimoto pearls. He sampled them with avid interest, as if working through a box of exotic chocolates.

"This one's a single molecule. At the end of a meal when you've made a mess of your plate and you dump a banana skin on top of the rest? Banana skin in a trashcan. One of the perfumers at Quest told me it smells of vomit. I can see what she means. It's *precisely* the sort of mixture between main course and dessert that would only happen in vomit.

"Here's the nth molecule that smells of chrysanthemum, which is to say funereal, which is to say like a chemistry lab, because chemistry labs smell like chrysanthemums. Surprising, but so it is.

"This one smells like a garbage can in Manila: hot papaya with cheap nail varnish.

"This one has an impurity of butyric acid." How did he know? He shrugged, made a face: "Feet, smells like feet." (He motioned impatiently at his feet.)

"This one is a pineapple, but it's an unsmiling pineapple."

Then they asked about perfumes. They sent him forty-two fragrances, the best-sellers in masculines and feminines, and they asked him to write a memo. Tell them what he thought—everything, the trends, the ingredients. Read the future.

He smelled them all and went away and thought about them and came back and started writing, in French. The result—"Note to: Quest Perfumers, December 14, 1996"—is as frank and revealing an inside view into the thought machinery of perfume creation as one can find. It is also decidedly bleak. "Perfume," he told them straight off, "is going through what smells to me like a bad patch."

He began his analysis with women's perfumes. "Most appear to be inspired by eating disorders." This, in his view, was particularly grave given that one of the most important schools of perfume composition historically (he named Guerlain) is in reality an offshoot of haute cuisine. The secret of Jacques Guerlain's success was his ability to make women literally mouthwatering. In his great perfumes of the Golden Age—Turin named *Mitsouko, Shalimar, L'Heure Bleue*—Guerlain had created abstract olfactory desserts, hovering in the air, and it was all about food. Add some choice floral notes (the armloads the florist had just dropped off at the servants' entrance, the caterers hurrying to arrange them before the guests arrived) and some woody notes (the floors had been freshly waxed that morning), and from the little Guerlain bottle came the smell of a well-to-do bourgeois interior at evening through which wafted the portents of an excellent dinner party.

Today's modern school, he contrasted bluntly, "is inspired by the hospital rather than the home. After a bulimic phase (*Poison,* etc.) and its procession of high-calorie confections, we are now riding the crest of an anorexic phase (*Eau d'Issey* and its countless imitators ad nauseam)." More than twenty recent perfumes belonged, in his view, to this "bloodless" school whose signature was Calone with backnotes of bleached florals in which you were hard put to smell anything except musk, and a pretty sterilized musk at that. He'd had, he sniffed, to keep a smelling strip of Guerlain's potent *Jicky* at hand to verify he hadn't become anosmic. What kind of perfume neurosis was this? "It is well known that anorexia involves a concern about internal cleanliness, i.e., what comes out no less than what goes in. No 'animal' notes, as the polite euphemism goes, and no earthly delights either. Furthermore, it is now possible to connect one's own little phobia with a worthy cause commonly known as 'concern for the environment.' No pollution, please, either in Antarctica or on my skin."

He sighed. This cleanliness obsession was perfectly captured in the absurd story you heard (true? false?) about Issey Miyake having supposedly asked BPI for a perfume smelling of water. It showed, Turin wrote, that Miyake's genius had its limits, not because the idea was bad but because it was impossible. Water has no smell, and absolute cleanliness smells of absolutely nothing. The reference point of Calone, he sniffed, was "a low-calorie meal served on a stainless steel tray."

So it was a bad time. Ah, but! There were two routes out of the present rut. "Abstract art," first. And "nouvelle cuisine."

The abstract school of perfumery, said Turin, had its roots in two all-time greats, Coty's *Chypre* and Chanel's *Chanel No. 5*. These two giants set the standard for perfumes without any obvious natural reference point and enabled the autonomous development of perfume as Pure Art. From distilled garden roses, we were suddenly amidst synthesized Carbon atoms. It was like jumping from Delacroix's neoclassic people with arms that looked like, well, human arms into a nonhuman, natureless Kandinsky world of triangles, dots, and machine-tooled blobs. Either you could do it or you couldn't; Turin noted the rumor that Jacques Guerlain, the master of perfume as natural haute cuisine, tried to adapt the abstract *Chypre* to his own taste, never succeeding. Hardly surprising, Turin shrugged. Like asking an expert pastry chef to excel at inorganic chemical synthesis.

And then, of course, there was the true reference of *minimalist* abstraction, the stupendous *Chanel No. 22*. The most striking thing about it, wrote Turin, was that this formula was seventy-five years old, and it was as if it had been created yesterday. They should use its magnificent powdery whiteness today in a different context. How? "Let me start with a self-evident statement: Mugler's *Angel* is brilliant, at once edible (chocolate) and refreshingly toxic (caspirene, coumarin)." Mary McFadden's *Gold,* which Quest had also created, restated *Angel's* basic concept in a less gaudy way. How about creating a perfume in which chocolate—"(without vanilla)" he added pointedly—met mint against a background of *Chanel No. 22's* powdery aldehydes? He loved the mint-chocolate harmony of Bendicks candies, which "has always struck me as daring, almost but not quite 'wrong.' I can easily picture a *Chanel No. 22*–After Eight mints hybrid, perhaps with a note of caspirene taking advantage of the latter's ambivalent mothballs-rum or mint-molasses character." The difficulty would be in the dosage of the sweetness of this confection, but a competent perfumer should be capable of it.

Then to the nouvelle cuisine school of perfumery. Now, the first great explorer of this olfactory territory, in Turin's view, was Ernest Daltroff (1870–1941), the genius behind Caron, and what, he wondered, might a modern version of Daltroff's memorable mimosa–black currant creation *Farnesiana* smell like with a more fluorescent black currant and a less mawkish mimosa? Similarly, perfumers had been quoting the hothouse pastel of *Royal Bain de Champagne* right and left, but no one had really *committed* to this direction, namely "overripe fruit headed for the bin." The chemists had more than once welded atoms together into a nice rotten fruit. What about it?

For newness, they could look to Quest's own perfumer, Maurice Roucel. The best recent creation in Turin's view was Roucel's *Tocade* "which proves one can make something new with something old and something borrowed. I feel that its manifest chic lies in its skirting close to biscuit and Turkish delight without ever saying so clearly. *Tocade's* rose note is slightly iridescent-metallic; one of the olfactory features of molecules containing a cyclic ether bridge (epoxides or dioxolanes as in the molecule Karanal) is a bright dryness equivalent to a musical 'sharp.'" Take that molecular spell and weave a good perfume out of it the way you'd build a good Sauterne, by balancing out a great deal of sugar with an equivalent amount of dry acidity. There was any amount of molecular magic at their disposal. *Sublime* (Jean Patou) provided a good example of this, with its intensely sweet amber note decorated by cedroxide (and vetiveryl acetate?), though the overall effect lacked some filling in. They could wave a chemical wand over their classical compositions by using the C-O-C note in its pure state as found in Karanal. Look at *Rive Gauche,* brilliantly rejuvenated by a pinch of just o.5 percent Karanal. And how about the food-inspired epoxide compositions, like strawberries plus pepper (phenylethylglycidate, another epoxide + elemi).

They should by all means steal from the greats. Germaine Cellier, whom Turin revered—"genius perfumer of Roure after the war, onetime model, drop-dead beautiful, dyke, and leader of the 'brutalist' school of fragrance composition: a simple and striking accord, and the gaps skillfully filled in by quiet notes"—what, he asked, would *Bandit* be like if Cellier were to compose it today? Be daring. Isonitriles smelled horrifically vile. And yet: he was, he confided to them, pestering Anton van der Weerdt and Charles Sell to wait for a Friday evening, steel themselves, take some nice perfume nitriles (violette nitrile, agrunitrile), and (as unbelievable as it sounded) make isonitrile versions of them. His Vibrational theory suggested, he said, that they should be potent, greener, more peppery.

Now, men's fragrances. Again, devastation everywhere one looked. Turin divided them into three styles: "faded gentleman," "raging queen," and "young buck." There was always, he duly noted, the delicate problem of male perfumery. Unlike women's fragrances, which were practically obligatory, many felt that men's fragrances lived under the constant threat of the famous question posed by Prince Emmanuel Bibesco, who after a lengthy inspection tour of a friend's mansion filled with relentlessly tasteful objects settled exhaustedly into an armchair and asked: "Very good, but why not nothing?" Indeed, the faded gentleman was almost invisible: no "sillage" or perfume "wake," a discreet smell up close, and that suggestive only of immaculate cleanliness. Add the melancholy that comes naturally to understated heroes, and you'd simply lost it. He listed *No. 89* (Floris), *Lords* (Penhaligons), *Mouchoir de Monsieur, Eau d'Hermès.*

So how to modernize them. Well, one might shift men's fragrances "surreptitiously" toward recast women's classics. Yes, men's fragrances had always erred on the side of comfortable dullness, which Turin held an underrated British virtue. But times had moved on, and a little recklessness was now welcome. They already had some women's classics that skirted the masculine: *Rive Gauche* and the green chypres *Y, Jolie Madame, Vol de Nuit, Diorella*—"(the real *Eau Sauvage,* in my view)" he said—were just waiting for some guy to discover them; stick some masculine camouflage in the head-notes and a cleaner drydown, and you'd have terrific masculines. "The excellent reconstruction by Calice Becker of *Vent Vert* shows how it can be done," he instructed. "As I write this, I am smelling the legendary *Iris Gris* and *Ambre Antique,*" and why in the world were sweet violet ionones so curiously absent from recent men's fragrances (except *Grey Flannel* and *Givenchy Homme*)?

The "raging queen" style mostly delivered hefty fragrances "and, curiously, overlaps with a butch Saddam Hussein tendency which, no doubt, helps export sales." What he liked here was the rough virility of the clichés of the fifties (*Aqua Velva*) or the seventies (*Azzaro pour Homme*), and it seemed to work better very down-market. "In my opinion only women can wear these without being faintly ridiculous." And as for the "young buck," Turin wrote, there were imitations galore of *Cool Water, Van Cleef, Drakkar Noir,* and *Azzaro pour Homme.* "Dihydromyrcenol and ambroxan are, I am told, on the way out." So what worked? *Havana Reserva* was presentable, but the unisex efforts (*CK One, Paco*) were a muted medley of recent hits, and the male anorexics (*XS, Miyake*) "insignificant."

New ideas? Antisnob to the core, Turin ended by steering their gaze toward functional perfumery: Tide laundry detergent and the stuff the shower-gel and hand-cream people were doing. Patricia de Nicolaï's scented candle was "good enough in my opinion to start a minor religion from scratch." Fine-fragrance perfumers, watch out.

The Quest perfumers received the memo with interest. The relationship was getting stronger, and then a reporter called from Paris, from the French magazine *Votre Beauté.* Would Turin do an interview with them? Sure, what'd they want to talk about? About, among other subjects, the house of Dior, upon which Turin opined forcefully that Dior were all scoundrels because they had had their classic fragrances redesigned by accountants. This he stated plainly and on the record. *Votre Beauté* quoted him, identifying Luca Turin as a Quest consultant. It happened to be at that exact moment that Quest was hoping to win a significant brief from Dior, whose Paris executives read the *Votre Beauté* article. Dior called the head of Quest in Neuilly, and Turin was immediately fired. This ended Turin's activities on the perfume side of Quest.

Walking very, very fast on a London street Turin said, "Dior is run by lower life-forms. It is run by second-rate accountants. These are people"—he gathered himself to deliver this, as if passing a microscopic gallstone—"who use a thing called 'afffff-ter shave.' *First-rate accountants* would see that it was to their advantage to keep the quality up."

At lunch near Tottenham Court Road, he explained, "The financial temptation to dilute perfumes is almost irresistible. I mean, if you can make your *oudh* go twice as far. . . . Instead of using ten kilos you use five, and given how much this stuff costs per gram, the temptation to futz is just irresistible. It's why Guerlain and Chanel and Jean Patou are so great. Not necessarily expensive perfumes. Just great ones that are never, ever diluted. No tricks, no cheating, no cutting corners." He sighed. "But today all bets are off. When the big fragrance firms take *L'Air du Temps* and wreck it by having an accountant redraw the formula to take out the expensive ingredients and substitute cheap ones, what they are doing, among other things, is depriving thousands of people throughout the world of the thrill of the memories that are infused with *L'Air du Temps* because unless it is the same smell, it won't trigger. The pale new reflection may be, intellectually, objectively, a reflection. It may carry sort of the same top notes, that musk in the base, and rationally you can identify the similarity—but your brain stem isn't electrified. Memory isn't triggered. *L'Air du Temps* used to be much more intense, raunchy, strange. And they kept everything that it had in common with its contemporaries and removed everything that was different. There's a lot less benzyl salicylate. It's a very peculiar note, almost a wintergreen oil. So now it's just like a dozen other fragrances. The ingredients of the *L'Air du Temps* that you can buy off the shelves today are cheaper. It smells more chemical."

He drums his fingers on something. "I have an ancient sample of the real stuff." He bought it in North Carolina, at JR Perfumes, intersection of I-95 and N.C. 70.

The professionals conserve perfumes under refrigeration in lightproof aluminum containers, since light is the main damaging agent of perfume. You should always store perfumes in total darkness. The official word, from Jean Kerléo, the chief perfumer at Patou for the past thirty years and the director of the Perfume Museum in Versailles, is that perfumes keep for two or three years. Turin disagrees; he's smelled "perfectly good things" that were seventy to a hundred years old. So he admits they don't smell *exactly* like they did the day they were manufactured, but in his opinion you absolutely get the idea. He once found, in a good antiques store in Moscow, an extremely rare perfume, *Le Parfum Idéal* by Houbigant, made in 1900. The formula had disappeared from the face of the earth, and no one knew how to make the stuff. The perfume was in an exquisite, unopened Baccarat crystal bottle, and it had lived through the revolution, two world wars, Lenin, Stalin, and Khrushchev. He paid a hundred dollars for it. The woman who sold it to him thought he was crazy to pay so much. It was probably worth a thousand. He donated it to the Perfume Museum, and they managed, through gas chromatograph smellers, to reconstruct Houbigant's formula. They gave a bit of the perfume back to him. "If," says Turin, "you ignored the first minutes because the top notes were slightly fatigued from the journey, the next three hours were absolutely sensational, three hours that showed you why this perfume *made* Houbigant." The house is allotted by some a small, crucial role in changing French history. During the Revolution, Louis XVI and Marie Antoinette were trying to escape the guillotine, dressed as ordinary citizens, and were apprehended in Varennes. "The legend," Turin says, "is that they exited the carriage, acting natural, and she descended in a breathtakingly heavenly cloud of Houbigant. That's how they caught them and cut off their heads. No ordinary Citizen had that fabulous shit."

The only revenge Turin could exact upon the accountants was through his perfume guide. Like a Michelin reviewer removing a star from a chef's cuisine, in his most recent guide he peeled away the heart beside *Chamade,* "for," he wrote, "Guerlain found it appropriate to destroy the finale by adding a synthetic note—incongruous and pale—to the drydown. *Arrière toute!*"

◆   ◆   ◆

AT THE SAME time, Turin was pursuing Quest's Scientific Twin, the manufacturer of smell chemicals. Here the stakes were much higher.

Turin had created his theory chatting with Charles Sell. Now, he was trying to sell Sell on potential olfactory alchemy—and the industrial decimation of Quest's competition—through Vibration. Turin made a proposition. To create the algorithm, Quest would give him its precious vibration-smell correlations. Quest, in turn, would control that algorithm. Think about it, Charles. They could whisper their wishes to the algorithm, which would disappear back into its bottle to reemerge with the new lilac, the new marine, the new mesmerizing smoky Oriental, to transifix the customer at the counter. (Turin, incidentally, for his part would get not only a working algorithm but absolute proof before God, Man, *Nature,* its peer reviewers, and every biologist, chemist, and physicist on the planet that his scientific theory was correct. And at that point, all of them plus the angry people at Christmas parties could be damned.)

Sell, in his cool, English way, was interested. He proposed to Turin that they conduct a series of tests to determine whether or not the giant multinational would bet on Turin's horse. Turin would, Sell noted, have to sign a confidentiality agreement, keep strict secrecy, et cetera, et cetera. Yes, yes, said Turin hurriedly, and got his hopes up.

He went down to Quest's headquarters in Ashford. On the back of an envelope, Sell drew five molecules. This was the first test. They were Quest Research Molecules that Sell's team had synthesized, and so of course they were, Sell made clear, secret. (Of course, said Turin, of course.) Turin had never seen them before.

Sell, sphinxlike, told Turin he had to answer two questions. First, by calculating their vibrations, Turin would have to tell him which of these molecules were woods, which musks, and which ambers. What, in other words, was each molecule's odor "character"? Second: Which of these smelled strong and which weak? The strong-weak question Turin had never given any thought to, and it surprised him.

Turin took the five of them back to London and carefully fed their structures one by one into his computer. He set MOPAC loose on them, and MOPAC gave him their tunneling spectra, and he then launched a little piece of software he'd created, and it translated the spectra into vibration frequencies. There were the vibrational fingerprints of each molecule.

He then sat down and took a hard look at what he had. He immediately saw that two of the five had a feature he'd come to associate with musks: the spectrum between wave numbers 500 and 1000 was positively jammed with vibrations. Woods, by contrast, often had a peak at 500 and a peak at 1000 but in between more or less nothing, a valley between two mountains. But he had a problem, and that was language, the fact that people have great difficulty applying descriptions to smells. Even perfumers used the word *wood* to describe odors that were pretty different. So he made a logical request of Sell: "Give me the 'reference' musk, wood, and amber," which was to say, what did *Sell* consider the molecules that best represented those odors? The reference musk, replied Sell, was cyclopentadecanolide, wood was cedrol, and the amber would be Jeger's ketal. Turin now had his benchmarks, so he could compare the smells consistently. He looked at the vibrations of each reference and compared them to the vibrations of the five. And, yes, the vibrations fit. He started labeling the five molecules. He reflected, with some excitement, that with access to only five Quest molecules and their corresponding descriptors, he was starting to create his algorithm.

He faxed the odor characters to Sell. (He also took a sort of wild stab at guessing each one's odor strength but didn't put much stock in it.) He waited eagerly for a reply.

Sell called back. He was typically laconic. "You're better at identifying smell character than smell strength," said Sell. Which, to Turin, meant first that he'd done not too badly on odor character (that was exciting), and second, that there was no acknowledgment of this from Sell. So he hadn't gotten strength. He'd never *thought* about it before. It was as if Sell were saying, "You're better predicting the location at which gold is buried than the depth." But he kept this to himself and asked how many of the odors he had gotten correct.

Oh. Yes. Right. He had gotten all five correct. Just from their vibrations.

One for one. Sell proposed a second test.

This time, he gave Turin ten compounds and five reference smells. Turin took them home and started putting them into his computer and calculating wave numbers and so on. But the problem here was that he had ten smells but the electronic topography for only five references (this simple fact made it a very different test from the first one). And he started getting lost. He sweated over it for weeks, but he often found himself right in between the references, and he just didn't have the maps to get himself out. He named the ten molecules and sent them back to Sell, but word came back from Quest that he'd only gotten half of them right, about 50 percent, which he could have gotten by pure chance. Turin noted that if you had only five references and ten spectra, you were swimming—some molecules were equidistant between two references, and what were you going to say? Was it rose or was it magnolia? Anyway . . .

One for two. Sell proposed a third test. Take three molecules smelling of lily of the valley, said Sell. Sell reached across his desk for some scrap of paper and simply sketched them out. Turin was awed; Sell could draw thousands of molecular structures purely from memory without a glance at any database. Each of the three has an alcohol group, said Sell, sketching them in. Replace all three alcohols with a methyl group, said Sell, and only one of them still smells of lily of the valley. Which one was it?

That, it turned out, was a piece of cake for Turin because it so happened that alcohol-group vibrations were easy to calculate. Turin cheerfully ran the molecules' vibrations, predicted one of the three, and went back down to Kent to lay it before Sell. Sell looked at it and said, Ah, well, yes, he'd gotten it right. But then he added that perhaps Turin had looked them up, the odors of these three, because they were, it happened, public domain? Turin (clearing his throat) said that, first, he hadn't—he'd done the vibrational calculations like he was supposed to, thanks—but, second, even if he *had* looked them up, the point was (he pointed at the three spectra sitting on the paper) *the vibrations gave this answer;* you didn't *need* to "look them up."

Two for three. Sell appeared to be interested. He suggested that Turin draw up a proposal, a plan for collaboration between Quest International and Luca Turin, so that they could delve into this weird theory more deeply. Now they started talking money, research funding. Quest would supply salary, lab, and a vast database of aromachemicals to feed to his hungry algorithm. This would basically be gruntwork, taking Quest's data and grinding out wave number–smell correlations, which is what he would do at Quest over five years, feeding the results to the algorithm.

In exchange, if it worked, Quest would get a license to print money.

Turin costed out a five-year plan, arriving at £150,000 a year of Quest's money, which included his salary (£65,000 annually), computers, equipment, assistants, and so on. All signals were good, Sell was showing enthusiasm in his controlled way, and Sell's boss at Quest, a Dutch chemist named Anton van der Weerdt, seemed on board.

It all came down to a presentation. On October 8, 1997, Turin got on a train to Kent. They picked him up at the Ashford station in a gleaming Jaguar and drove him to Quest's immense offices. He walked into a sterile conference room to find van der Weerdt, Sell, and a manager whom Turin had never met before.

It was van der Weerdt, Quest's chief R & D man, who presented Turin's plan to the suit. He spoke, although not in detail—the men who ran Quest knew nothing of computational chemistry, or physics, or biology—about the possibilities if this gamble were to pay off. How much? the man asked. (How much would it cost them?) Three-quarters of a million pounds, said van der Weerdt. The figure hung in the air. Money, they understood. The three Quest men looked at one another.

The accountant spoke up. This was, they could all agree, a significant amount of cash. And, naturally, it was only the company's chemists who could truly evaluate its potential. The accountant turned to the chemists. Are you truly behind this? Turin looked at them. Well, said van der Weerdt. It was certainly *interesting,* this vibrational idea, this new theory of smell. He seemed less than fully convinced. Turin looked to Sell. Sell said nothing. Turin thought: It's dead in the water.

Stomach-turningly, the cynical thought materialized like black smoke in his mind. There was one little catch here. The Big Boys' chemists would naturally greet the prospect of Turin's algorithm with all the joy with which textile workers greeted the Industrial Revolution's spinning machines, which eliminated their jobs and their livelihoods. "They're perfume chemists," Turin realized. "They're going to help me create a machine that replaces them? Nope. Perfumery is not a research-driven industry. If it were, the people running these companies would have degrees in chemistry. They don't. They have degrees in poetry from the University of York."

When the meeting was over, they thanked him politely and showed him the door. He walked out of the Quest building and stood in a state of shock in the driveway waiting for his ride. A tiny Ford drove up and stopped, and he squeezed himself into it and felt that pretty much summed things up. Later, Quest contacted him to say they'd turned the plan down.

❖   ❖   ❖

ALMOST IMMEDIATELY THERE was another Big Boy suitor. Givaudan Roure, the Swiss giant, had been picking up signals, and now Zurich called. The people at Givaudan were quite interested; could they test this theory? Sure, said Turin. Marvelous, they would start setting up the process, get him a contact person. In a little while, they called. His contact would be one of Givaudan's fragrance chemists, a Pole named Jurek Bajgrowicz. Immediately, the problems began.

Turin had met Bajgrowicz at a lecture he'd given at Givaudan and had found him unremittingly hostile, huffing and puffing through the talk to everyone's annoyance—not surprising, since Bajgrowicz had devoted his professional life to supporting Shape and would, if Turin's theory was right, probably lose his job. (Turin had begun looking at everything in terms of whose interests were threatened.) He had, in Turin's view, proffered questions with the politeness of a man offering hand grenades with the pins pulled. At the end, Bajgrowicz had said, Let's face it, Luca, neither of us understands smell. In front of thirty people, Turin had replied, You don't for sure, but maybe I do.

Turin now communicated all this to Konrad Lerch, the head of scientific R & D at Givaudan and Bajgrowicz's boss. Look, the guy had a conflict of interest, said Turin, and therefore Turin couldn't see why he should be the contact. Givaudan reacted with fury, saying that, first, this was a collaborative effort, second, all their chemists were involved, not only Bajgrowicz, third, Bajgrowicz was Turin's contact because he was the most knowledgeable man, and, fourth, Bajgrowicz was Turin's contact because they didn't want to upset Bajgrowicz. Well, OK, but Turin sure as hell didn't like it.

And then there was Givaudan's insistence on his signing a strict confidentiality promise not to reveal the formulas of Givaudan's molecules to anyone. He had no problem with this, other than the fact that it was of highly limited usefulness. Everyone knew that if the formulas fell into a competitor's hands they weren't worth much without their matching descriptors: "leather," "harsh," "sweet," and so on. Here was a formula. Great—so what was it, and was it worthwhile spending weeks of time and thousands of dollars on it? And in any case, getting a molecular formula is like being handed a photograph—but *not* a recipe, not the "how to"—of a very complex French entrée. It's described as having beef and a red wine sauce. Well, fine, but how do you *make* it? Was the beef sautéed in oil or butter? Was there a wine marinade? (If a marinade, how do you make the marinade?) (For that matter, how do you make the wine?) Was it childishly easy or fiendishly hard? You could get a molecule's structure, see your quarry *right there,* sitting on the page, the Carbons here, an amine group there. But you don't necessarily know two things. You don't have any idea how to build it. (Start with an amine? End with an amine? The standard rule of thumb is that for a really tricky molecule, if you give it to four different process chemists, you'll get back four completely different ways of synthesizing the thing. Or none, and you'll never figure out how to make the thing.) And you also don't know (oh, yes) what it smells like, which is to say that you have no idea whether you should even bother with the thing at all. Yes, a smart chemist and a lot of effort could probably produce the entrée. But Givaudan was basically insisting he sign a promise not to reveal coded messages.

Now, the instant you have the descriptors, the language key, then these molecular structures become extremely sensitive commercial information. But they weren't giving him those.

Of course he signed.

The test arrived from Zurich on November 16, 1997. Dear Dr. Turin, read the letter from Bajgrowicz, very interested in your theory of olfaction. "We would like to evaluate its possible application to the difficult task of designing new odorants." OK, so Turin had told them the theory couldn't yet predict what a compound would smell like, but it *could* tell how close that molecule would be to Thai Basil or Turkish Rose (to some "reference compound"). (Bajgrowicz added that if Turin wanted to "provide us with even more convincing proof of your theory," they'd added a third series of compounds he could take a shot at.) With Swiss precision, Bajgrowicz stipulated that since Turin's passing the test was a *conditio sine qua non* for Givaudan's collaborating with him, Turin would get no payment. And he stated with no subtlety that the structures of the compounds were secret, any use or commercialization illegal. And that was it. He looked forward to the "hopefully convincing" test results and signed "with best regards," from Jurek Bajgrowicz.

Fine. Turin opened the test. Part I was a series of molecules sketched out structurally. He had to calculate their vibrations and answer the question, Which of them were musks? Part II was a rather strange molecule and eight almost identically shaped molecules (stereoisomers): Which of the eight were sandalwoods? Fine. Part III was: Which of these twenty structures is closest to Givaudan's "reference amber," its standard amber?

He got to work. He noted with interest that Part I was like the Quest tests except Givaudan also wanted him to tell them which were odorless—easy enough. Part II, with the eight stereoisomers, he couldn't make sense of because when he calculated the spectra he didn't find much difference between them. But Part III he found "the real thing." They had given him a sketched-out reference amber and a whole scad of other ambers, and he was supposed to say which were the closest. He'd have no problem saying, "That one's going to be closest to the referent," but ranking them by distance was going to be tough because of the Catch-22: he didn't have the vibration-smell correlation data he needed to develop the algorithm he needed to give the Big Boys the answer they needed to forge the alliance he needed to get the data he needed to develop the algorithm. But he spent days, running them through three different methods of calculation, and the methods coughed up one of the molecules as definitely being closest to the reference amber. So he sent his results to Switzerland and said, For Part I, here's what I think, for Part II, I can't really tell, but if I had to answer I'd say this. And for Part III, which was really interesting, here're the closest couple of ambers, and in this case I'm really pretty sure I'm right.

The next thing he got was an e-mail popping up in his computer saying, The results are quite disappointing; those molecules don't smell like what you said they'd smell like.

Turin was pretty disappointed himself (and mystified; how had Part III gone so wrong?), but he figured that when Givaudan gave him the right answers, maybe he'd be able to fix the problem. And maybe it was just the eternal language problem, that the adjectives and nouns he'd used weren't those used by Givaudan. So he e-mailed back: Really a letdown, but so it went, could they please let him know the odor profiles—were they "citrus," or "metallic," or "green"—of the molecules, or better yet send samples so he could judge himself, and he'd try to fix it.

He got a message back: Sorry, can't do that.

What? Turin called Switzerland. Hang on a second. We agree to do this test, I spend all this time doing all these calculations, you tell me they're crap, you don't tell me which ones are right and which are wrong, and now you won't let me check whether the odor profiles are correct? The Givaudan representative replied, snottily, that their odor profiles were quite correct, thank you, they had been determined by Givaudan's perfumers. Turin replied that he didn't give a damn if their odor profiles had been determined by the pope because he had long experience with the problem of different people matching smells to words. *He* wanted to smell them. Otherwise the whole test was a cipher, and no one really knew what it meant.

Nope. Sorry.

He phoned up Bajgrowicz. They managed to have a civil conversation. But Bajgrowicz said: No molecules. Sorry.

He tried sending an e-mail to R & D head Konrad Lerch.

Dear Dr Lerch,

I sent preliminary results to Jurek Bajgrowicz 10 days ago, and he informed me that the results were "somewhat disappointing."

It also emerged from conversations with Jurek that GR has at the present time no intention of disclosing to me the odor profiles of the compounds I calculated, much less allow me to smell them. Had I known this in advance, I probably would not have taken part in this test run. The reason is that odor profiles are frequently in error and subject to interpretation. One lesson I have learnt in the last couple of years is to _always_ smell things for myself. I am sure nothing more than a confidentiality agreement is needed here. I am sure you will agree that a scientific venture such as this one can only be entered into in a spirit of mutual trust and openness.

In order to show you that I am sticking faithfully to my end of the bargain, I have decided to send you the complete data set arising from my calculations rather than merely the results. This will allow you and your chemistry staff to appreciate the difficulties involved in spectral interpretation, and, I hope, to discern patterns that I, in my ignorance of the smells of the compounds, am unable to see.

all the best
luca

Lerch merely passed the e-mail to one of his chemists, who called up hopping mad at Turin for violating protocol by corresponding directly with his boss. Turin replied briskly that Givaudan Roure's internal politics were not of primary interest to him and hung up.

Silence for a week. Then out of the blue Turin received a letter dated January 28, 1998. It was from both Dr. Konrad Lerch and Dr. Jurek A. Bajgrowicz (Givaudan, Corporate Research, Ueberlandstrasse 138, CH-8600 Dübendorf, Switzerland), and it simply and summarily canceled the arrangement. It began nicely enough (thank you very much, Dr. Turin, for the calculations, and so on) and informed him that his answer had been analyzed by Bajgrowicz's team. And the result? "Your answers are too ambiguous, and in most cases in disagreement with the olfactory descriptions provided by our perfumers." Translation: He'd gotten the smells wrong. *(Huh? . . .)* And no, they wouldn't tell him what the smells actually were, and no, they wouldn't let him smell them himself. The deal was off. Moreover, "we still have no proof that it is the vibration and not the shape that determines the odor. The results do not allow to decide in favor of your theory. Under the circumstances we are unable to propose you any collaboration." Sorry. Givaudan would like to recompense him "at least partially" by a contribution of £1,000. (Could he please send them an invoice so they could prepare a check.) The letter ended, "With best regards."

Turin didn't want a "contribution" of £1,000. *He wanted the damn smells.* He didn't trust Bajgrowicz even to report his results accurately to his bosses. Turin didn't, he made clear, particularly trust scientists even when there was nothing at stake, much less when one had his butt on the line. Also, perfumers create odor profiles by *analogy*. If you've only ever seen blue and someone gives you turquoise, said Turin, furious, you're gonna write down blue even though it's also green. Each perfume company had its own culture of odor description, "and when you turn smells into words it's always dodgy. There's the famous business of phenylacetic acid. Some people say it smells like piss, some people say it smells like honey. You'd hear this, you'd kick the whole thing out of court, but in fact, guess what, urine and honey happen to be very similar smells, and so the words are tricky. Also, I thought for my own benefit after I put in a fucking month of work I wanted to get something out of the test. Suppose I was entirely wrong. Fine. I wanted to know where I was wrong. I wanted feedback because feedback is valuable."

But that was the end of that.

◆　◆　◆

ONE DAY TURIN was talking on the phone with Yale biochemist Mike Lerner, telling him about his Vibration theory, and Lerner said, Fascinating—after all this trouble we've had getting the smell receptors to work, can I draw Randy's attention to it?

Randall Reed was a Johns Hopkins molecular biologist who had worked under Lerner and was one of the biggest names in olfaction science in the world. (He was an expert in the smell receptors.) Turin, impressed and hopeful, said, Sure, great, by all means.

Turin waited a few weeks, then picked up the phone and called Reed. Reed answered. It was a miserable conversation. Turin found Reed doing "this monosyllabic impression of a scared rabbit, this tone Americans put on when they're afraid someone is trying to sell them insurance."

"Hi!" Turin opened in his usual enthusiastic way: "This is Luca Turin!"

Reed: Yes?

"Um—so are you familiar with my theory?"

Reed: Yes?

Well, uh—so he was calling to, you know, touch base. Mike Lerner thought Reed might find the new theory interesting—could Turin help in any way? Perhaps they could even collaborate!

They then went through a torturous slog in which Turin tried to make a connection and Reed gave no information. Turin hung up, baffled.

The next thing he knew, he got a phone call from Mark Dearborn in North Carolina. Dearborn had just received a call from Dr. Claude Klee, a researcher at Duke. Klee had no idea that Dearborn and Turin were buddies, and she had mentioned casually to Dearborn that she'd just been to see Reed. She said, You know, Randy is working on this absolutely amazing theory of smell. Really, said Dearborn, and what is it about? That smell, said Klee, is vibration!

Dearborn, caught off guard, blurted out, Oh, I know all about that, my friend Luca Turin is the author. And (Dearborn now told Turin) Klee just shut down. He'd pursued it, but she had changed the subject. So Dearborn, a bit bemused, was phoning Turin to say that, well, he was sorry, he'd blown it without having found out what was going on. But according to Klee, Reed was working on *Vibration*.

Turin decided straightforwardly that he'd just send Reed an e-mail.

>Date: 2/2/98
> To: randy_reed@qmail.bs.jhu.edu
>From: l.turin@ucl.ac.uk
>Subject: grapevine
>
>Dear Dr. Reed,
>I hear through the grapevine (no indiscretions committed, I assure you, only a series of coincidences) that you may have been testing my theory. Is this so, and if so can you tell me anything about it? I hasten to add that I am not collaborating with any mol. biol. group on this; my inquiry arises out of curiosity and a desire to help if I possibly can.
>
>all the best,
>luca

He figured Reed would just hit the "Reply" icon and fill him in. A standard, open, honest exchange between scientists. And he was eager to discuss the paper (he'd housed it on the Web, www.physiol.ucl.ac.uk/research/turin_l/chemical_senses_complete.pdf). But there was no reply. He found this strange. He also found it incredibly rude and scientifically unprofessional. What to do?

He waited a few weeks. Nothing. He cleared his throat and sent the same e-mail again, sticking at the top a friendly "Hi! did you receive this message I sent you some time back? Thanks. Luca."

Still no answer. Turin was thoroughly ticked off but thought, Well, maybe Reed's been out of town. Maybe he hasn't been getting his e-mail. So he called Reed's secretary and asked, "Has Dr. Reed been at his office these past few months?"

Yes, she said.

"Does he read his e-mails?"

Every day, she said.

He never got an answer from Reed.

The whole episode depressed him. He'd worked so hard on this, and the big guys in smell with the big positions at the big universities wanted him, he felt, to "evaporate." He blinked, trying to put up a brave front. "Fuck 'em!" he said, honestly wounded and incredulous. "I mean——" He cast about for what he felt. "I mean, I'm getting used to it, but I still don't think that's the way science should be conducted. What Mark Dearborn, the bitter realist, would say to *that* is 'Yeah, Luca, and that's why I'm a full professor and you're just a junior temporary lecturer.' But I don't care about being a junior lecturer. What I care about is that unless you play the game in a real asshole fashion, you're screwed. Mark would laugh at me and say, 'Why should Randy talk to you?' I'd respond, 'Because it's in his scientific best interest. Because it's for the greater glory of God. Because all of us scientists are supposed to work together.' "

❖   ❖   ❖

AT LEAST A few things were going well. Agnès Costa sent him a business proposition. Costa was a young, attractive, wealthy Frenchwoman who ran Fragonard, a small French fragrance house (her family's), and divided her time between Paris and her mansion in the south of France. She had become aware of Turin who knew how, but from Fragonard's fabulous Paris bunker, she proposed his making a pitch to design one of four new fragrances. If he was interested. Sure he was interested.

He phoned up an English perfumer named John Stephen. Stephen was a guy Turin enjoyed hanging out with, a relaxed daredevil who flew his own plane and drove powerful motorcycles very fast. He was also a perfumer. Stephen and Turin proceeded to win two of Fragonard's four briefs, so Costa said that since Turin was working with her, they should spend some time tossing ideas around. She flew him to Nice for a jaunt on her yacht, the *Trois Soeurs,* off the Côte d'Azur. Under a brilliant Mediterranean summer sun, he boarded the yacht, chatting with the other guests. They set sail out onto the blue water, and somewhere into the hors d'oeuvres and the first glasses of wine Turin realized, perfume being a close little world, that he was sitting next to Konrad Lerch's boss, Geoff Webster, the new, American head of Givaudan Roure.

Webster, for his part—he was a powerful executive type, paradigmatically midwestern-looking—didn't realize that Turin was Turin till halfway through the main course, and when he did, he was quite interested. (He had, apparently, heard terrible things about this "vibration guy.") They talked perfume businesses, and Turin, reading between the lines, realized that his smell experiments with Givaudan had been going on during a very high-tension corporate merger that was going to wind up with the firing of hundreds of employees. Christ, big surprise no one wanted to touch him. He decided not to push the Bajgrowicz-Lerch affair, although he did make the pitch for Vibration. Webster listened amiably, seemed intrigued. But nothing came of it.

◆　　◆　　◆

BACK IN LONDON, Fred Adkins, a consultant to University College London, called to tell Turin that he now had a third Big Boy suitor. Turin, perennially hopeful, said, Yeah? Adkins had pitched Turin's theory to Takasago, the Japanese molecular-fragrance giant. Takasago seemed enamored.

Takasago's people would like to meet Dr. Turin. Could Dr. Turin arrive soon? Could they receive Dr. Turin at Takasago's New Jersey plant? Dr. Turin, for his part, was sufficiently intrigued to try another trip to the commercial altar. With about a billion-dollar annual turnover, Takasago had several interesting captives— Ambretone for one, a musk that smelled quite nice and was even more nicely profitable. Takasago wanted out of him a machine to make more.

For the dowry, Turin proposed low upfront research costs footed by Takasago (for him and a lab assistant) with a big financial payoff in case of success—he would get royalties. If it didn't work, Takasago would have lost basically nothing.

In April 1998 Turin flew to New York City and from there departed for New Jersey and Takasago's headquarters. He hit it off with the new chief chemist, Andrew Lupo. Also he had a conversation with another chemist there, to whom he said, "Shape is crap" and got the response, "Yeah, we know." He was quite pleased.

When it was over, he took a bus back to New York and flew home. He never heard from Takasago again.

AUTHOR'S NOTE

*Y*OU MAY HAVE noticed by now a strangeness, a journalistic imbalance, in this account. It comes from something I myself noticed only gradually.

The default of the serious reporter—it's certainly mine—is to present both sides of a story. You generally realize at some point, at once indefinable and crystal clear, past the initial excitement but short of true understanding, that you've stumbled into a story. I happened to meet Luca Turin because the Eurostar from Paris to London was twenty minutes late. We were in line in the Gare du Nord, and we started talking about the finale of *Mission: Impossible*. Where they fly some helicopter into the Eurostar tunnel? "Oh yeah, sure," said Turin, "although of course that's physically impossible." Really? "Problem with air mass." How's that? He explained it, using his hands. So, I said, he was a physicist then? "Biophysicist." What was he researching? "Smell. And vibration." As we got on the train, I asked for details. The point arrived just before Waterloo.

So you scout out the view of the side through which you stumbled into the story (because you inevitably enter through one side's point of view), understand it thoroughly, learn its arguments, and then you decamp for an equally thorough stay in the enemy lands on the other side and *those* opinions. After that, you go away and synthesize a balanced presentation from the two sides.

It is therefore disorienting, almost surreal, to enter a story through one side and then, gradually—I thought I must be imagining things—find that that side is so loathed by its opponents, so vilified by and toxic to them, and so axiomatically unworthy in their estimation of serious consideration that they actually refuse to share their own view with you. Or are so unremittingly hostile that their attempts to do so fail to qualify as "thoughtful," which amounts to the same thing. Or proffer a critique so tendentious as to be substantively worthless. Which leaves you, as a journalist, in the bizarre and infuriating position of knowing, or assuming, that there's a second, legitimate side but having effectively no access to it. I began this book as the simple story of the creation of a scientific theory. But I continued it with the growing awareness that it was, in fact, a larger, more complex story of scientific corruption, corruption in the most mundane and systemic and virulent and sadly human sense of jealousy and calcified minds and vested interests. That it was a scientific morality tale.

The response to Luca Turin's controversial theory embodies the failure of the scientific process, both as an ideal and in the day-to-day functioning of prestigious scientific organizations like *Nature* or, for that matter, the giant research mills at the Big Boys. Turin once grimly opined to me that the reason Geoff Webster, CEO of huge Givaudan Roure, couldn't rationally evaluate Vibration—and thus Givaudan's true corporate interests (I met Webster at a Fragonard perfume launch in Paris, and he insisted to a group of us that smell was definitely shape)—was not Webster's fault but the fact that "he has to listen to some Shape-chemist dwarf in Zurich with an axe to grind." I discounted this as hyperbole. I wound up agreeing with it as analysis.

Start with the fact that the most objective, thorough, scientific criticism Turin's theory has gotten, the one that normally I would use as the journalistic foundation for presenting Shape's point of view to you, is contained in the four peer reviews from *Nature* magazine, on the basis of which *Nature* rejected Turin's paper. Reviewers 1, 2, 3, and 4 remain anonymous. The scientists that Turin and Stewart identified by deduction—Dodd, Hamm, Shepherd, and Hopfield—deny authorship, as they would arguably in any case be obligated to were they in fact the authors (such is the system), and *Nature* naturally will not divulge that information. Because of the way scientific peer review is set up, this meant I couldn't ask Referees 1 through 4 anything. All I had to work with were the reviews themselves. The problem is, the reviews are incoherent.

I first went over them in detail with three scientists in the Turin camp, whom I knew and whose expertise covers the three fiefdoms inhabited by the paper, chemistry, physics, and biology: chemist Walter Stewart, physicist Marshall Stoneham, and biologist Mark Dearborn, all esteemed in their fields. Their analysis ultimately agreed with my own, which is to say that as far I can tell 1) Turin's Vibration paper's respective chemistry, physics, and biology are entirely scientifically viable as such and 2) the *Nature* peer reviewers' comments—as well as those of Philip Campbell, *Nature*'s editor in chief—relied on patent tautological criticism. To reiterate their gist: the biologists said the chemistry was wrong, the chemists said the problem was the physics, and the physicists said the fault lay with the biology. This is not to mention the casual, obvious, often grotesque inaccuracies filling their readings.

I incidentally note for the record that I have, by no means, always seen eye to eye with Turin during the process of reporting this story. I told him when we reached Waterloo that I wanted to write about him, a prospect he greeted with pleasure. It was a friendly beginning to a professional relationship, and during the four subsequent years of reporting, the relationship almost ended several times. Turin at various moments told me with fury that I knew nothing about science, rejected my assessments of him personally and professionally, demanded "total control" of the manuscript "so that," he said, "if I don't like a single word in there it doesn't get published," and threatened to withdraw his cooperation entirely from the project. He doesn't like or agree with all the opinions I've expressed here, nor with all my characterizations, particularly of him. Turin's partisans, notably the scientist I've called

Mark Dearborn (who was by turns difficult, negative, patently hypocritical when he felt it served his purposes, and "completely paranoid," his own descriptive of himself and one I fully agree with), at times actively warned Turin not to cooperate with me and withheld information. Walter Stewart took half a year to return my e-mails requesting an interview. This hardly endeared them to me.

But in the end what matters is the data, which is to say the facts as far as they are discernible. The Vibrationists gave me data. Had the Shapists given me, or had I uncovered, plausible counterdata demonstrating that Turin's findings were flawed, or could be explained away, or were factually inaccurate in favor of Shape, I could not have written the book. I tried, repeatedly, to go over the *Nature* peer reviews with the Shapists. There turned out to be simply no *there* there.

Initially, there was the Shapists' behavior. If you're familiar with the field, you have already noticed that the opinions of several of its major scientists are absent here. To give a taste of why this is so: I called one of the most highly respected senior olfaction researchers, someone I'd been assured would be an able intellectual match for Turin, at his prestigious New England university. The instant I identified the call as concerning Turin's theory, he immediately said, "This is off the record" (Why? "That's my business"), which meant that I could print none of it. He then launched into a diatribe against Turin's paper. It consisted of weak criticisms I had already heard countered convincingly by the Turin camp, one of which was answered by a graphic in the *Chemical Senses* paper. I pointed that out.

"I haven't seen that graphic," he snapped.

I paused; the graphic is central to the paper. I asked, You have *read* the paper, haven't you? "I don't need to *read* the paper," he said sharply. Well, I asked, would you please read the paper and then speak with me about it? "I don't have time!" he said, "I'm busy." I started to say something else, but he hung up. This is one of the world's preeminent Shape scientists. I cannot recall previously having come across a professional willing to attack, on or off the record, a paper that he had, in fact, not read; virtually every Shapist I attempted to interview did exactly this.

It was, at least, an education in human nature. In Coorg, India—this story is coming up—a group of us took a break from the smell conference we were there for and went on a short hike in the jungle. I caught up with a molecular biologist I'd been hoping to talk to. (We'd exchanged maybe four or five pleasantries up to that point.) I opened politely with the statement "I'd like to get your opinion on Luca Turin's theory." Her face iced over instantly. What about it? I said I wanted her scientific assessment of it. "You're writing about this?" I'm writing, I said, about Turin's Vibrational theory, yes. She looked directly at me and spoke crisply. "So basically, if he's right, he's a genius and we're all assholes working on garbage. Right?" She turned her back to me. She never spoke to me again about the theory, nor did she ever provide me with a scientific critique. She was not unique. I never got completely used to it.

The fact is that the neurobiology she and others are working on is not garbage. But she's not stupid. If Turin turns out to be correct, the Nobel for smell—and everyone is betting there will be one—will almost certainly be awarded for the discovery of this astounding biological mechanism rather than for describing the system's wiring and plumbing, the receptors and neurons. In the sense of winning a Nobel, if he is right, she is indeed wasting her time. That's the way the scientific rewards system goes. To refuse to discuss the theory's scientific merits is another proposition entirely.

What signifies in the end is the lack of Shapist scientific ammunition. The battle between Shape and Vibration is not over, and I categorically do not (and Turin, equally, does not) suggest it is. Though Turin has provided fascinating and convincing *preliminary* evidence, there of course has to be independent confirmation by other labs before Vibration is accepted. However, if the question in this story is "Should Luca Turin's theory, as any such theory seriously propounded and regardless of whose vested interests might be threatened, have been given fair and serious consideration by the scientific community?" or, more pointedly, "Was *Nature,* in relying on ego and emotion and incompetent analysis, professionally remiss in not publishing Turin's paper?" then the answer seems to be clearly: yes. It isn't merely that Shapist data was always transparently weak. (One Shapist told me that the metallocene experiment Turin had put in his paper was worthless because the nickel fattens up the molecule more than the iron, and the receptors could feel this difference in Shape. I took this to Turin, who pointed out that background thermal movement constantly changes the molecule's shape ten times more than the nickel does. I then took this back to the Shapist, who, literally, changed the subject.) But as I say, it isn't merely the weak data. It comes down to something even more basic: almost none of the critics of Turin's Vibration paper ever actually read it.

When I reached G-protein expert Heidi Hamm on the phone in September 2000, she explained at length that Turin's paper was wrong. So I asked her if she had read the paper. No, she said, she had not. I asked her if she would please read it. Irritated, she said that she would not, she was busy. I noted that criticizing a paper one hasn't read is considered tricky, factually speaking. Her response was that she didn't need to read it since it was wrong on its face. She then ended the conversation.

I called Randall Reed, one of the biggest olfaction scientists. First, he commented ad hominem of Turin, "Well, some people thrive on controversy" and said that he, Reed, didn't believe in Vibration. But he didn't believe in Shape either. He wrote off Strong Shape and then, immediately, Weak Shape: "Linda Buck believes we feel parts of the molecule," but this, he said, couldn't work. Why? Simple, he explained. The Weak-Shape theory ("feel parts of the molecule") is the three blind men feeling the elephant, and whatever part each one feels is added to the others and—voilà, that specific combination is the smell. This can't work for the completely obvious reason that if you say OK, there's a receptor for the specific shape of aldehydes, for straight long-chain carbons, and for alcohols, you have a problem: mixtures. Mix a four-carbon alcohol with an eight-carbon aldehyde, and then mix an *eight*-carbon alcohol and a *four*-carbon aldehyde; both of them have an alcohol group, an aldehyde group, a four-carbon chain, and an eight-carbon chain—and there would be absolutely no way you could tell those apart by their shape. They would have to smell exactly the same. And in fact, said Reed, they smell completely different. Ergo, Weak Shape doesn't work.

(I asked him what they smelled like, but he laughed uncomfortably and said, "Well, you'd have to ask a perfumer.")

"I sort of don't know," said Reed, "what the critical test of the Turin hypothesis would be, really." I suggested to him that the critical test would be simple: finding two differently shaped molecules with the same vibration and asking, "Do they smell the same?"

The following then happened. Reed said that, first, he didn't know how Turin calculated vibrational numbers, a strange comment given that the method of their calculation is standard. Then he asked how Turin defined "what is the same vibration," which was even stranger; again, the calculation method is standard and objective. (This is like asking how someone would define the frequency of a photon vibrating at 483 nanometers. The answer, of course, is 483 nanometers.)

"Also," Reed said, "I'd ask Turin this: How can you have two molecules that have different atoms but similar shapes? If they have different atoms, wouldn't they have different shapes automatically?" This is a question of basic chemistry, but Reed is a biologist, not a chemist, and—and this is not at all rare—apparently was unaware that there are examples everywhere of same-shaped molecules with different atoms inside them.

He then said, "I'd also ask him: When it comes to smells, what is a 'very similar smell'?" Here was, once again, a smell scientist simply not believing that mint smells like mint, which is to say not believing in the objective reality of smell. He ended by saying, "Buck believes in Weak Shape. Turin would go the other way and say Vibration. I fall in the middle. I believe a given molecule may fit a number of receptors, that the molecule puts its hands all over the odorant, it feels every part of its shape, but it's not always a perfect fit." Which was to say: a) I don't know how smell works, but b) I think it's Weak Shape, which c) I just disproved. That was my conversation with Dr. Randall Reed.

When I called Linda Buck, I started by asking her about Turin's theory, and she immediately said, in a very serious, guarded voice, "I would be very, *very* careful. This theory was around in the 1950s and was disproved."

But inelastic electron tunneling was not around in the 1950s and could not have been disproved.

"I was," she says, "pretty upset about the BBC program because they didn't tell me that it was going to be promoting this theory to its audience. There is, as far as I'm concerned, no evidence for this theory at all. It's all based on a few correlations. It's imaginary. From what I understand, people who understand the physics part of this theory don't think it makes any sense either."

I responded that UCL's Marshall Stoneham and C. J. Adkins of Cambridge, among other physicists, have spent quite a bit of time on it and find the physics solid. Buck seemed not to hear. "I was just reading about this group that doesn't believe in evolution," she said, "and they think that aliens put us here on earth. You can't refute it absolutely, but I doubt it's true. This isn't a theory of olfaction. This is an entire theory of biology itself."

Buck is phenomenally knowledgeable about the smell field. She talks with precision about all sorts of things, the molecular biology, pseudogenes; she cites all the big names in smell, Eric Moyers and Anne Houston and Stuart Firestein. And it's all very interesting, but none of what Buck talks about addresses the central question: How do we smell? What exactly is the smell receptor recognizing? Ask her directly, and she gives a categorical answer: "The shape." How? Again, categorical: Weak Shape. Yet when she heard Randall Reed's quote about her believing in Weak Shape, she appeared, oddly, to change her mind. She laughed, not happily. "I don't know why Randy would say that because that's not what I think." Yes, she admitted, she once threw out a suggestion that the receptors were fixing on several different shapes of a single smelly molecule. "But we won't know exactly what they're feeling until the structural biologists tell us," she said, adding, "I don't really hold to the [Weak-

Shape] theory." Which was to say that she didn't know *how* the receptors measured the shape, but she knew *that* they measured shape.

Well, then . . . Turin? "I've never met Turin." Grudgingly but honestly: "I've heard he's a bright guy." Hardening a bit: "I mean, if there were a compelling argument, I'd certainly listen to it, but I haven't heard one."

But what, I asked, did she think of the arguments Turin presents in the paper?

Buck said evenly: "I haven't read the paper." Which meant, I pointed out, that she had not read the argument of the theory that she believes "imaginary." She responded (not pleasantly) that she had "heard a lot about it." She said several times that she'd "heard a lot about it."

OK. What if I sent her the paper to read? She demurred tersely: No. Thank you.

Well, would she read it on the Web? I started to give her the paper's URL. She cut this off. She was busy. She had other things she had to read.

But, I said, she'd stated that if there were a compelling argument, she'd certainly listen to it.

She laughed rather irritably and said, "Well, I'm writing a grant." Then she said good-bye and hung up the phone.

I called Ken Palmer, Charles Sell's lab tech at Quest who had performed the isotope experiment and had confirmed that the two acetophenone molecules (same shape) smelled different. I needed to fact-check Turin's account of the episode, and Palmer confirmed it over the phone. A day later, on July 15, 1999, I received an e-mail from Palmer's boss, Charles Sell. Sell conveyed Ken's "uneasiness" about my citing him as an expert "since he has to deal with perfumers every day." When I told Turin about this, his concise comment was "Please, the perfumers don't give a shit about this," a conclusion I'd immediately reached on my own. Palmer didn't speak to me again.

But the rest of Sell's e-mail illustrates perfectly the quality of Shapist arguments. He went on to explain his underwhelmed reaction the day that Turin and Palmer laid the acetophenone-isotope affair on his desk. Yeah, he said, I know Luca thinks the acetophenone experiment we did for him proves his theory. But it doesn't. (Why not?) Simple, said Sell: "There could be other explanations." See, the vibrations Turin was getting by hitting these two molecules with infrared light was not, Sell wrote me, the only thing different between them. Hit them with nmr (nuclear magnetic resonance) spectra instead, and you'll get an even bigger difference in vibration. (Hm!) "As far as odour is concerned," wrote Sell, take out Hydrogens, put in Deuteriums, and you change the thing's chemical properties. Replacing *all* the Hs with Ds "will change the rate at which it will undergo keto-enol tautomerism," as well as affecting the desire of lone pairs on the oxygen toward hydrogen bonding. Any of this could make the receptor smell the acetophenone differently.

At first blush this sounds like a legitimate scientific argument. But then you realize . . . that, scientifically speaking, you can *always* come up with other explanations; the point is coming up with one that fits the data. When you actually looked at what Sell was saying, you found an immense amount of . . . nothing. Or more precisely, everything, an infinitely expanding number of infinite possibilities. Sell had proposed that nuclear magnetic resonance (NMR) might "possibly contribute" to a difference in smell, and Turin's succinct, and logical, reply was "If Charles can prove to me that we do NMR spectrometry with our nose, I will carry his luggage to Stockholm to pick up his Nobel. That's the NMR Theory of Smell, and Charles is welcome to propose it, but this is the first I've heard of it. Why stop at NMR? If you shine a neutron beam at deuterated acetophenone, it'll be absorbed more readily than nondeuterated. There: that's Turin's Neutron-Beam Theory of Smell! Great! I'm happy with that! What does it mean? Who knows."

It wasn't that Sell was wrong. It was that if one followed his logic, which was to cite every possible reason, one would end up arguing that smell could have been installed in our heads by the aliens who put us here on earth. Why not? Turin replaced Hydrogen with Deuterium in the molecule acetophenone, which had the same shape, and yet he and Palmer found a *difference* in smell. Sell argued that it wasn't Vibration by noting that changing Hydrogens for Deuteriums "changes chemical properties," which, he proposed, may change the smell chemically. OK. But he failed to note one fact: you can take bacteria, replace every Hydrogen atom in their microscopic bodies with Deuterium, and they'll live perfectly normally. Which is rather astounding and which dictates that any difference in either shape or chemistry in these isotopes will range from infinitesimal to nonexistent (while the smells, notably, are different). Sell's logic, more to the point, prompts one to ask, So what's *your* theory of smell then? And that, for Turin, is exactly the problem.

Charles makes all these criticisms, criticisms that imply alternative theories, but then never bothers to follow through on any of them. I was at Quest giving a lecture and told the group about ferrocene and nickelocene. Charles said, "Oh, but they have different electrochemical behavior." Which means that if you made batteries out of ferrocene and nickelocene the voltages on the outputs would be different because they have a different electron affinity. Well, fine. True. We all know that. AND??? *How does that relate to smell?* Because if smell turns out to be not Shape, and not Vibration, but Electron Affinity, then that's fascinating! But—ah!—Charles doesn't have any evidence for the Electron Affinity theory of smell. All his alternatives to Vibration are different, and none are linked, theoretically or experimentally, to any of the others. Which is called desperation. So I said, "I usually say that Shapists don't have enough of a theory, but the problem with you, Charles, is that you have too many." He just straightened his spine in his seat while everyone laughed. No wonder he loves me.

Turin's personality certainly played a role in the reception of his science—a problematic one. It is a difficult personality, not at all by intent (entirely despite it, actually; he is completely well-intentioned) but simply by nature. Under all normal circumstances, and when he is taken seriously scientifically, he is delightful, articulate, cheerful. People perceive him as intimidating, or arrogant, or combative, or insensitive because he is also these, in the blink of an eye, when contradicted or blocked. His fury at his colleagues' refusal to examine his work—Why, he asked, didn't they ever invite him to their big smell conferences in Boston and Los Angeles, the cozy colloquies where they got together to listen to one another?—comes out in bitter sarcasm. Also in recalcitrance. Turin is simply incapable of playing by someone else's rules if he doesn't see their use. Which then compounds their refusal. But the field's unwillingness to examine his data is, as far as I can see, ultimately based, entirely, on vested self-interest and bad science. And the data, in the end, is what counts. Every once in a while, accidentally, they showed their hand. I was asking Tim Pearce, an engineer at Leicester University who builds artificial noses (primitive machines that use conductive polymers to trap and detect molecules), about the refusal to look at Turin's theory. He responded calmly that it was "because there's a history involved." He rather clearly meant: We've been slaving away, and suddenly he just waltzes in here? "There've been over a hundred years of study in smell, and when somebody comes along with no history in the subject and then suddenly *announces* that there's a solution to all of this that everybody's overlooked, there's bound to be a reaction."

Pearce added, "Turin's been talking about this for a long time, but I don't think any data have been published."

I pointed out that in fact Turin had published a paper, in *Chemical Senses*.

Pearce shrugged and said, "As far as I know, it's very thin on data." But he hadn't read it.

Sometimes they were even more obvious. I was having dinner in the Café Latin in Paris with a young, very sharp executive from the Big Boy Givaudan and after a tense twenty minutes or so of discussion of Turin he stated, grimly and simply, *"Mes chefs, s'ils le voient, ils le flinguent."* If my bosses ever saw him, they'd shoot him.

I placed my first call requesting an interview to Dr. Richard Axel's lab on Thursday, August 20, 1998. There was no response. I left another message on Monday, August 24, 1998. Nothing. When I mentioned much later to one prominent olfactory scientist that I'd tried five or six times with no result, he snapped, "Richard never returns anyone's calls" and looked away.

Sir Aaron Klug of the Royal Society formally declined to be interviewed, twice. As for Nick Short at *Nature,* I began phoning him in the spring of 1998. Since Mr. Short was always in meetings, or away from the office, I would leave messages from New York with polite voices in London—my number, my name, and the name of *The Atlantic,* for whom I was working on an article on Turin. Yes, they would give Mr. Short the message. Yes, Mr. Short would return the call.

Mr. Short never returned a call. Not one. I began writing this book.

VI

+

INDIA

*I*N THE SPRING of 1998, Turin was invited, finally, to an actual scientific smell conference. The conference organizers wanted him to present his theory of Vibration on December 2, 1998. The interesting wrinkle was that instead of some plush university biology department in California or Germany, this conference was to be held in Orange County, in rural southern India, at a resort in a tiny hill station called Coorg.

The conference was organized by the Tata Institute for Fundamental Research, the Indian equivalent of Los Alamos and NIH combined (TIFR does both molecular biology and physics). Turin was delighted, and a little nervous. The invitation said that Eric Moyers, a world-famous smell scientist, was scheduled to attend, as well as two postdocs from Richard Axel's high-powered lab, and the microbiologist Marcel Postain, whom the *New York Times* turned to for quotes on smell. Turin would be giving a forty-five-minute presentation like everyone else, although it seemed that almost all the others were neurology and biology people, not chemists or physicists, and as usual he was the oddball. He'd never been to India, so starting off in the jungle—apparently the conference would be in the middle of an elephant preserve—would be interesting. And he felt a little nervous about what level of science the Indians did (would it be up to snuff). But what he felt most was: *Finally.* A conference.

In early October, Turin started preparing his talk, choosing the slides, trying to fit everything in. He really wanted to take them something to smell, maybe the acetophenone and its isotope, but no, the difference in smell between the two was too subtle. The carvones were too light and perfumey (same problem). The boranes too deadly. But he couldn't find anything else. He'd reached a state of tense frustration when, on October 5, he was ransacking the *Journal of Organometallic Chemistry* and tripped over a paper by a German chemist. Dr. Ulrich Wannagat of Braunschweig University had spent his life messing around with things called silas.

In the periodic table, atoms with similar chemical behaviors are grouped together. Column IVA houses, in descending order, Carbon (C), Silicon (Si), Germanium (Ge), and Tin (Sn). And the reason Silicon, Germanium, and Tin behave similarly to Carbon is that they share the same shape: like carbon, they make four bonds to their neighbors. Like Carbon's, those bonds are arranged tetrahedrally. What Wannagat had been doing for years was tweezering Carbon atoms out of molecules and putting Silicon atoms in their place. And then—wait a minute—*smelling* them, because he happened to be using fragrance molecules, and in fact (Turin couldn't believe what he was reading) the guy had considerately made sila versions of all sorts of perfume molecules, roses, violets, jasmines, musks. (And Germanium versions, and Tin versions.) Take linalool ("light and refreshing, floral-woody with a citrusy note"), yank out one Carbon atom and install a Silicon atom in its place. You got, reported Wannagat, a fragrance more hyacinth-like, sweeter. Find some methoxy groups, rip out the C and stick in Si, and you go from "camphoraceous, radish" to "minty, honey floral." This got you to the most interesting part: C, Si, Ge, and Sn versions of these molecules all had different smells *and exactly the same shape.*

Or, to be precise, the same shape but each on a slightly larger scale. Put in a Silicon, and it makes the same-shaped molecule, only a touch larger. But the vibrations are *massively* different because you've both massively upped the mass (Carbon's atomic weight is 12, but Silicon's is 28), and changed the stiffness of the bonds. Wannagat had even been so exquisitely thoughtful as to submit every single one of his creations to a perfumer at Haarmann & Reimer in Holzminden, Germany. His paper was titled "Odoriferous Sila and Isosteric Compounds: Comparative Odors of Homologous Organoelement Compounds of Group IVA (C, Si, Ge, Sn)" and in its abstract, Wannagat had actually written (now this was just breathtaking): "Noteworthy are the strong differences of odor in the system $C_6H_5CH_2El(CH_3)_3$ from C via Si and Ge up to Sn, standing fully contrary to the postulation of Amoore whereupon smell qualities are only controlled by size and shape of molecules." Please.

Turin had no idea who this person was, but he was very, very good. He immediately went on a mission for more Wannagat papers. With every new paper, it just got better and better. In the abstract of "Isosteric [same-shaped] Compounds According to the Hydride Principle of Grimm in the Range of Linalool Scents," Wannagat had written: "Therefore the theory of Amoore, after which only shape and size of molecules are ruling their odor qualities, must be called in question." The man was taking careful, repeated aim.

To verify all this, Turin would have to smell these molecules for himself. But how to get his hands on a carbon molecule and its sila version? Wannagat had retired, and his samples had all gone AWOL, so this required ingenuity. He wound up searching a peculiarity of Aldrich Chemical's founder, owner, and head, Alfred Bader. Bader, a distinguished chemist from Harvard, became concerned in the 1970s that a lot of odd, rare chemicals made for scientific experiments were being lost when their creators retired, so he went around buying strange molecules from retired chemists and stockpiling them. The result is a massive molecular flea market called the Aldrich Library of Rare Chemicals, which contains some valuable antiques in good repair, a few weird surprises, and some honest-to-God treasures. You pick through it.

Turin heaved the library's gigantic catalog onto his desk, flipped to the sila compounds, and began systematically going down the line for ones that he figured should smell—smaller stuff, uncharged, and reasonably stable. Whenever he found a candidate, he then had to try to find its Carbon mate. In the end, he found exactly one single pair, one of each. He bought them.

On October 21, the pair of molecules arrived, one Carbon and one Silicon twin, shaped exactly the same. He opened them up and sniffed.

The first was 1,1-dimethyl cyclohexane. Take that molecule and replace the first Carbon atom with a first Silicon atom, which makes it a sila. This was the second molecule, a 1,1-dimethyl sila cyclohexane.

And the smell? The Carbon twin smelled camphoraceous with a tiny bit of eucalyptus. The sila twin smelled of a very unpleasant green, cut grass with a nasty edge. They smelled absolutely different.

Turin was jubilant—at last he had an example that was not deadly poisonous, one he could actually give to people. The India conference was only a few weeks away, and he had the Carbon and sila molecules put in two little plastic containers, one red, one orange, to pack in his carry-on. Molecular show-and-tell.

◆   ◆   ◆

THERE WAS ONE creepy thing involving silas that made him shudder when he recalled it. He'd come across the silas before, actually, long ago. The silas had almost suffocated his theory in its infancy. Or not the silas exactly but the way the Shapists had dealt with them.

Just after he'd found the 2500 vibration-borane-sulfur smell connection, as he was gluing together the first pieces of his brand-new theory and looking around nervously for evidence that supported or (God forbid) contradicted it, Turin had found in *Chemical Reviews* (1996, vol. 96, no. 8, pp. 3201–40) a massive study of the smell literature. It was by Quest's Karen Rossiter. "You know how," he said, "when you're reading something, and you're tense, you sort of don't really want to know . . . ?"

In the review, basically a Shapist manifesto (she had pointedly titled it "Shape-Odor Relationships"), Rossiter had actually commented on Wannegat's astonishing findings, which were, to Wannegat, so clearly anti-Shape, but she'd gone about it this way: she had first noted (accurately) that the Germans had taken twenty different Carbon molecules and synthesized twenty Silicon twins for them. Then she had stated (accurately) that all twenty Silicon versions smelled different from their Carbon twins, seventeen of them smelling completely different except that (Rossiter pointed out accurately) in 3 cases they didn't smell *all* that different. (The C and Si carvomenthenes, for example, smelled pretty similar.) She had then written (here's where it started getting tricky) that, well, *sometimes* they smelled different and *sometimes* almost the same. Which was, given the score of seventeen to three, not *exactly* accurate. And then Rossiter had calmly written this sentence: "Those examples where the odor of the sila analogue is similar to that of the carbon counterpart are interesting anomalies for vibrational theories." The three contradicted Vibration.

And he had been so nervous that all the air had gone out of him and he thought, "Oh *shit*. This is very bad." He'd dropped the silas. He'd shoved them as far as he could under the carpet of his subconscious, forgot about them, and that way was able to go on.

But now he remembered where he'd seen Wannagat before. He rushed to grab Rossiter's review and reread it furiously. And he realized that Rossiter, "bless her dishonest little soul," had worded it in such a way that he, Turin, in sweating what he might find, hadn't focused on the fact that, first, the Carbons and their silas *all* smelled different *100 percent of the time,* whereas their shapes were virtually identical 100 percent of the time. The three she cited smelled different, and so contradicted *Shape*, not Vibration. And second, the seventeen molecules that had dramatic differences in smell *devastatingly* contradicted Rossiter and Shape. Which he'd been too emotional, in his vulnerable moments, to get through his thick head. She'd simply thrown out the 85 percent of the evidence that was most damaging and finessed the 15 percent that was left. "I guess," said Turin flatly, "it's 'The best defense is attack.' She knows you can't explain them by Shape. She immediately goes on the offensive."

✦ ✦ ✦

IN THEIR LIVING room in North London, three days before leaving for India and as the tall windows fade from dark red into grayblack, Philippi is preparing pasta for dinner and Turin, in a dark T-shirt, is fiddling with his expensive stereo. On the coffee table lies a book, *Symbiosis in Cell Evolution: Microbial Communities in the Archean and Proterozoic Eons* by Lynn Margulis. "So Margulis proposes this theory," he says energetically, "that eukaryotes arise from a symbiotic fusion with ancient bacteria, and that's how we got mitochondria, the things that live in our cells and burn the oxygen that powers us." Philippi holds out a chopping knife, and he gets up, trots over, takes the knife. "The thing is, the theory had actually been around in the 1920s, beautiful books were written on it, but it was discarded as ridiculous, trash. What am I chopping?"

"Parsley," she says, pointing.

"Margulis brought it up to date and pushed it like hell. They ridiculed it, and her. It was crap, garbage, blah blah. Now her symbiosis theory is the classroom standard. And everyone knows that mitochondria were created from bacteria. What's the parsley for?"

"Puttanesca," she says.

"For spaghetti?" (He uses an Italian accent when he says *spaghetti,* just as he always pronounces *vetiver* Frenchly.) She nods. "Oh, but she was *reviled,*" Turin says happily, chopping. "And—I love this!— she starts every chapter with a quotation from someone who said that symbiosis was crazy."

At the dinner table, Philippi serves the *spaghetti.* It's squirming all over the place. She laughs. "It's the wooden spoons," she says.

Turin raises his eyebrows. "It is a poor craftsman who blames his tools," he quotes dramatically.

She gives him a crisp look. "Lift your plate," she says. He lifts it obediently, grinning.

✦ ✦ ✦

TWO DAYS BEFORE India. Howard Skempton has invited Turin and Philippi to the premiere of a piece of his, to be performed by the

English Chamber Orchestra. They arrive at Queen Elizabeth Hall on the South Bank by the Thames, next to the National Theatre, and wave to Skempton and his wife, who are behind a small roped-off area, being interviewed, talking to music-industry people. Skempton, a small man with a gentle demeanor, beaming quietly, motions them over excitedly. They accept champagne. Skempton introduces Turin to one of the hall's administrators, a brisk blond Englishwoman. "Ah," she says, taking his hand. A crisp accent. "So *you're* Luca Turin, the vibration scientist."

"That's right," says Turin. "Biophysicist."

"I understand it's your theory of smell Howard used in a piece."

"My theory of smell," he nods pleasantly, "as applied to audible frequencies."

"Ah." The faintest frown passes over her face, a slight tightening of the features. Inquisitively: "You're *French,* originally."

"Yep."

A beat. "But you have an American accent." Her eyebrows are up, waiting for the explanation. It was a question. "Uh-huh," says Turin affably, sipping the champagne and looking around cheerfully as if she had said that the sky was blue. She waits an instant, then does a silent "*Right,* well then," and is off to greet other people. Turin explains to someone that for the Skempton piece, they'd had to translate from one human sense to another, translate the smell-able vibration range—wave numbers 0 to 4000, according to Turin's theory—into the hearable vibration range, which runs from the lowest sounds we can hear, at around 20 hertz, up to near 20,000. "Actually, middle A is 440 vibrations per second today," he notes, "although the Baroque A was a few vibrations lower. We've sharped everything." And were the vetiver and vanilla audible in the piece? "Absolutely. Absolutely."

The buzz of anticipation fills the entry hall. The chime sounds, and everyone begins moving inside. Turin absently hums the chime's pitch, moving with the crowd. "An A," he says to no one in particular. As he and Philippi find their row and sit down, the first violinist rises, strikes an A on the piano for the orchestra to tune by. It is the same note.

The program begins with a piece by Schnittke, "Concerto for Piano and String Orchestra," a series of disharmonic tensions, excruciating drawbridges leading between weird ravines, a music of sharks, sleep, and anxiety. Its basic components have been imbibed by every film composer of suspense. It swells, and then dissolves into a single platinum filament in the very dark room. "Wonderful," whispers Turin. After this, a startling contrast. The Mozart, by comparison (Piano Concerto No. 11 in F, K. 413), sounds dully traditionalist, Baccarat-manufactured schlock.

During the intermission, Turin and Skempton talk eagerly. Turin: "Impeccable playing. You hear Schnittke's teacher and his teacher's teacher."

Skempton: "Tolib *Shahidi* used these sorts of things, a *Tajik* composer." Skempton remembers something rather amazing. "I *tuned* in the BBC at half six and heard my music as *background* for a commercial for Pat *Barker's* latest novel." He wears a funny, potentially pleased expression.

Turin: "The thing I like about Schnittke is that he has these amazing lapses into appalling taste. It's something he shares with Shostakovich."

The A chimes again at 440 vibrations per second. The mass of bodies filling the atrium starts to reverse-flow back into the concert hall, sucked gently through the doors as if someone had unplugged a small drain in the floor of the stage.

The Skempton, "Concertante for Violin and Strings," when it leaps quivering into the air, sounds at moments like a machine someone forgot to turn off, running down to end its cycle, at other moments like a lush, febrile spring ladder into some cloud tower, rising and falling arcs of notes. It is relatively brief and intensely structural. Turin is utterly rapt. He cocks his head slightly to the right. He cocks it to the left. He says "*Huh*" to himself and thinks about it, lips pursed.

Walking back to the Citroën parked on Waterloo Bridge over the dark Thames, Turin is exclaiming. He loves it. "Every note of it!" Philippi is slightly less enthusiastic. She finds it standard English pastorale. "Oh, *please,*" says Turin. His mind is racing. "You know who'll be one day a very well known composer?" he demands of the London night and then states definitively, nodding his head: "Einojuhani Rautavaara."

◆　　◆　　◆

TURIN IS IN one of London's big, boxy black cabs at 5:30 A.M., heading for Heathrow to get the plane to India. He is wearing his black jeans and black polo shirt, which he will wear more or less the entire trip. He has brought several pairs of each.

What excites him perhaps most is his postconference trip: he is going to make a pilgrimage to the Bombay Muslims, among the most famous makers of perfume raw materials in the world. The perfume stores are lined up, so he understands, along Mohamedali Road. He is going to try to find the *oudh*. Not synthetic, some of the real stuff.

The hands of the perfumer are tied by the economics of perfume raw materials. Thousands of ingredients, thousands of different prices. The prices of raw materials in perfumery can vary by a factor of ten thousand. There's stuff at £3 a kilo, like Iso E Super, a kind of nondescript woody-lemony. Then there's iris-root butter from Florence: £30,000 per kilo. Like the best Turkish rose extract. *Oudh* wood from India is in that stratospheric league. It costs around £33,000 (about $50,000) per kilo. It's the wood of a certain Indian tree that has been eaten by a fungus. You carve out the rotten wood that has taken on the smell of the fungus and extract the fragrance. There's only one supplier to the West. It's a drop-dead smell, very complex, honey, fresh tobacco, spices, amber, cream. You do not use a lot of this stuff in perfumes unless you are financially suicidal.

It's like a red wine. The first ten dollars goes a long way toward a decent wine, but the price difference between a very nice wine and a stupendous wine is exponential. You can still make a very boring perfume from very expensive materials, and you can also make a quite nice one cheaply. Take *Joy* by Jean Patou. *Joy* retails at about three times the price of most other perfumes. In general, perfume raw materials cost at most £100 per kilo, and because perfume is about 80 percent dilution—alcohol, which costs nothing—that real cost is 80 percent diluted too, down to about £20 per kilo of actual fragrance. A kilo has thirty-five ounces in it, so every ounce of perfume costs, generously, under £1 in raw materials to make and sells for at least £50, though of course you have to allow for costs of bottling, marketing, advertising, and so on. It is generally recognized that only about 3 to 5 percent of a perfume's price tag goes for its smell. *Joy* is £150 to £200 per kilo because it has 10 percent Bulgarian rose, the real thing. And an expensive jasmine. Rose is actually a huge problem for the simple reason that we all know what a rose smells like, so if you're going to do a rose perfume, you have to have a serious budget. Turin was designing a perfume for Fragonard and told John Stephen he wanted an animalic rose. "How much you got?" asked Stephen (i.e., "How much is Fragonard willing to put into it per kilo?"). Turin said he had £70 per kilo, and Stephen said, "Forget it. I'll do you one for £130 per kilo, and you'll see what it would actually cost." So Turin forgot it—though Firmenich then came out with a relatively cheap rose synthetic, "and blow me," said Turin happily, "if it isn't pretty good."

There are still some houses who, by philosophy, stick almost entirely to naturals. Annick Goutal is one (her flagship store is across from Guerlain, between the Ritz and the Inter-Con, just off the Place Vendôme). *Petite Chérie,* a lovely super-pear, contains one molecule that Goutal chose from pears (at least 150 molecules make the subtle difference between the scent of a William pear and other pear varieties; Goutal keeps this molecule secret). *Petite Chérie* also contains a natural South American musk rose, though again this means something you don't really expect: only *two* species of rose, Centifolia and Damascena, are actually distilled, basically because most other rose species don't have enough odorant to make distilling them pay. So all the scents of every other species of rose, including "natural South American musk rose," are actually re-creations, mixtures of molecules that give you that species' smell: 100 percent natural and 100 percent engineered at the same time. And then *Petite Chérie* has natural vanilla from the island of Réunion, several natural peach molecules, and natural cut grass, which is to say the molecule that you get the second after you cut the grass but which disappears immediately. And once again: the "cut grass smell" molecule is extracted from other plants. It's 100 percent natural, 100 percent not-exactly-as-advertised, and 100 percent biochemically true: it's the grass molecule, just not from grass.

But just because a natural is in the mix doesn't mean it is trumpeted. Sometimes they are simply too odd. Goutal notes that the startling, deeply entrancing fruity-floral *Folavril* contains mango and Tasmanian Boronia flowers, and Grasse jasmine, yes, yes, yes, but they do not tell you that what actually powers the fragrance is tomato leaves. (An utterly wonderful smell. These are also from Grasse, by Robertet.)

After passport control and security, Turin stops at the new Cerruti fragrance for men, *Image,* which the duty-free shop is pushing heavily. Sprays it on his hand. "Oh hell, that's, huh, that's—huh—yeah, fine—hmm, basic, boring, hairy-chested. Nothing too original but perfectly fine."

People wait blearily in the Air India departure lounge, a few American backpackers, lots of Indian women in saris whose teenagers wear T-shirts and gelled hair and argue with each other in strong East London accents. About twenty-five minutes later, as Air India is boarding those needing assistance and those with small children, Turin says, "OK, now this is nice." His nose is dabbing at his hand. "Dihydromyrcenol, ambrox, and aldehydes. There's thirty to sixty things in there. And masculine perfumery that doesn't turn foul after half an hour is a minor triumph. See, generally they put all the money up front, particularly for men, all hair and hormones, because men are supposed to have more teeth than neurons. And so it bites you, and you buy it, and then half an hour later the money runs out. Masculine perfumery is defined negatively, by what you don't put in it. You can't put in a big rose. You can't put in floral notes, sweet notes, no amber or vanilla. It's like that novel by Perec that was written without the letter *e.* You can still do a good one, though that's rare."

They call the rows in the middle of the plane. His eyes are on the cold gray London dawn outside. As he is handing his boarding card to the flight attendant, stepping onto the jetway's metal lip, he says sort of pensively, "*Bois de Lune,* red berries and smoked tea and souchong, is absolutely wonderful. No one's yet dared to use really big smoky notes up front *as smoke.*"

The Air India food turns out to be delicious. He talks about the

Concorde's aeronautics and engineering, the construction of refrigerators, how the Americans got hold of the Russian-designed anti-radar airplane design, and how to diagnose smallpox. He falls asleep and wakes up hours later as the seat-belt lights come on, a bell dinging. The Air India 747 hits Bombay's concrete runway, bounces up groggily, slams back down, the landing gear straining, the jet engines screaming in reverse. While the plane is still careening forward at 150 miles per hour, the Indians leap up to be the first to grab baggage out of the overhead bins, then fight each other through the aisles toward the front.

As the 747 noses up to the jetway, the Air India flight attendants walk down the aisles spraying something from cans. Passengers look apprehensive. Insecticide? A mesmerizingly lovely apricot fragrance washes the cabin. People's faces relax; they smile. "Easy." Turin shrugs. "Throw in a couple esters, some lactones, and you're laughing."

◆   ◆   ◆

THE CONNECTING FLIGHT from Bombay to Bangalore lands at 3:00 A.M. All of India is awake. The Bangalore airport is teeming. Outside the air is liquid dark, smoky, and thick. Turin and his bags are propelled outward, flotsam on the arriving human waves. The TIFR people call out, "Dr. Turin!" from behind the banged-up metal police barricades.

The little white van buzzes through the traffic on the city's main roads. The traffic consists mostly of three-wheeled taxis with deafening two-stroke engines, and the roads even at this hour are half filled. The van turns into the Raman Center. Turin's face lights up; C. V. Raman was the great Indian physicist who invented Raman spectroscopy, which uses intense visible light instead of electrons. The TIFR people deposit him in a concrete room. Turin takes his malaria pills, gets into the low, hard bed in the concrete room, and, excited, falls asleep.

◆   ◆   ◆

THE MAIN GATE of the University of Bangalore campus is down the road from the temple of the Hindu god of mechanical objects, where people stop to have the god bless their motor scooters and cars. The scientists filter in, arriving from various flights from Europe and the United States and Japan, looking slightly the worse for wear but cheerful. A group of Indian students takes Turin to the Coffee Board to ask him about his theory. The Coffee Board is a sort of university canteen run in the open air on a space of packed dirt by a concrete wall. Turin is expecting some polite questions. To his surprise and delight, they have not only read his Vibration paper, they are able to discuss its full implications, the biology *and* the chemistry *and* the physics, and they are not at all shy about peppering him sharply with criticism. Since this is TIFR, India's premier scientific academic center, these are among India's best science students, which is to say that they are among the most brilliant in the world. ("Your claim about the power source," says a young woman sharply, "where is your proof that NADPH binds?" Turin grins and launches into the response with gusto, citing molecules and partial charges and the odd habits of receptors. They lean forward to hear, eyes narrowed in concentration, leaping on him the moment he makes the slightest suspect statement. He loves it.)

The Coffee Board serves coffee and rich, sweet chai in stained and chipped porcelain cups of uncertain cleanliness, which they drink sitting on stools on the dirt. Almost December, and the temperature is balmy, sunny, and pleasant. A handmade sign on the concrete wall reads EATABLES FROM OUTSIDE NOT ALLOWED. The traffic roaring toward the temple of the Hindu god of mechanical objects pours out pollutants and kicks up dust. Turin says, "*God, I love* this place! I *hate* cleanliness and luxury. I think I was a bacteria in a former life. I take cleanliness as a personal affront."

For lunch, one of the students, an energetic, handsome young man named Aditya Kapil, takes Turin to Koshy's. Aditya may be a neuron jockey, a Ph.D. candidate in physiology, but he is hip if he is anything, and Koshy's is Bangalore's hip dining hangout among young Indian professionals, almost unbearably atmospheric, more redolent than redolent of the British era, the slowly turning fans, the expanse of venerable linoleum. Aditya has invited his fiancée, Manisha Nair, an exquisite, poised young woman who is an executive at the *Times* of India, and, in a bit of daring mealtime casting, a friend and fellow Ph.D. candidate named Arjun Guha. Arjun, sharp as hell and intellectually combative, has heard about Turin's theory and wants to interrogate him. "I have several serious reservations about this," he informs Turin aggressively. Turin grins.

The waiters, of whom there seem almost as many as customers in the packed restaurant, deliver menus. The menus say, "TOP people have something more in common than an entry in 'Who's Who.' They always think of KOSHY's Bar & Restaurant, St. Mark's Road, Bangalore, when they think of dining out." Arjun tosses the menu aside, squints at Turin. "You interested in homeopathy?"

"I'm a fan of oddball theories," Turin says evenly, "but this one is complete bullshit." They discuss beliefs, and he asks them about the god of mechanical objects, all those people bringing their motor scooters to be blessed. "And they truly believe in this." It's a question. He waits, interested.

The Indians look at each other briefly, educated professionals, scientists. Many, many people believe this, they say. Their smiles gently distance themselves from the belief in the Hindu god of mechanical objects and his busy motor-scooter cult. Turin starts a debate with Arjun and Aditya over the merits of having a god bless your motor scooter, which turns into a debate over whether or not the god could bless Arjun's Mac.

Arjun: "I'd say yes, he could. Computers have become virtual transportation."

Aditya: "I say no. It's not mechanical, there are no parts in motion, so how would the god know?"

"Well," objects Turin, "not mechanical in a *classical* sense."

Arjun: "Unless we consider quantum mechanics classical at this point."

On second thought, Turin dismisses this: "Would the god of mechanical objects accept a particle as a mechanical 'part'? *Doubtful*."

Arjun looks unconvinced. He clearly thinks any god of mechanical objects worth his salt could accept a particle as a mechanical part, but the waiters are circling like sharks, and Manisha corrals them. "Listen, you order for us," Turin says to her, surveying the eighteen thousand or so items available at Koshy's Bar & Restaurant. Arjun starts studying the menu like a general mapping an invasion. Manisha, ignoring Arjun, gives a waiter efficient instructions, dispatches him. Are there other examples of electron tunneling in biology? Arjun asks Turin.

"Oh, electron tunneling in biology is very common," says Turin. "It's well known in mitochondria and electron-transport chains. Remember, it's really just electricity."

"Hmm," says Arjun, frowning. Rather amazing. Turin's is a rather amazing theory, he says, and he means it as a challenge. Receptors of flesh shooting electrons at molecules and measuring the way they jangle. Hmm! So Turin, calmly, starts telling them a story. "Rupert Sheldrake, the former botanist from Cambridge, asks a very interesting question. There is an animal that has a virtually absolute ability to locate a place no matter where it is on the planet. How in the world does this work? We have no idea."

Arjun: "Homing pigeons."

Turin: "Of course."

Arjun objects: "But we do have an idea—magnetic dip! They know from that."

Turin, flatly: "Doesn't work."

Arjun, one eyebrow shooting up: "Why not?"

Turin: "Simple." He reviews: "Take a compass. It oscillates on the horizontal plane, right? And it points north, so it actually tells you something, four things, to be specific—north, south, east, and west—which tells you about where you are and where you're going. This compass gives you your longitude. Right?"

They nod: Right.

"But there's another kind of compass that oscillates on the vertical plane. And it turns out the vertical plane conveniently has a magnetic dip, which varies according to latitude, so if you have *this* compass, you can actually know your latitude." Yes, yes, Arjun knows all this. Turin delivers the problem: "But the dip has equal values along certain parts. So in order to get home, a compass is not enough; you have to a) know where you are and b) have a map, or the compass is meaningless."

Arjun counters. He talks about fly navigation. Flies can find their way back home from far away.

Great, says Turin, I can do that, too, if I go on foot from London to Barcelona and keep my eyes open. "You take a homing pigeon raised in London, England. You put it in a box so it can't see. Hell, you constantly rotate the box while you're transporting it, so it should have absolutely no reference points whatsoever. And you even put magnetic coils around the vehicle. All of this, they've done. You take that pigeon to Barcelona or Minsk or Tokyo or Singapore, you release it, the thing goes up in the air, does two circles and then—bam!—heads directly home for London." He says calmly: "I think pigeon homing is such an extraordinary phenomenon that people don't really understand that this is what is called a miracle."

"A miracle," says Arjun flatly.

Turin looks at him. He disagrees? Arjun is considering it. Turin: "Sheldrake thought up a truly amazing experiment. Suppose that you start from the point of view that this is not a navigation problem in the sense we're used to. That pigeons are somehow connected to their homes by an invisible elastic band whose nature we just don't understand. Now, you can stretch this elastic band by moving the pigeon . . . *or* by moving its home. So Sheldrake's question is, What happens if you move their home? Do they know where their home is? And I think that's a really nice idea." Turin pauses, glowers at his plate. "Shit, I should have thought of that question."

He returns to the point. "Sheldrake says he talked to the Dutch navy, which, strangely enough, still uses homing pigeons, about doing an experiment where pigeons would be born and reared in a loft on board a ship docked in one fixed place. You release them, and they go out, and they come back always to this ship docked in this place. And then one day when they're grown you release them on a very long flight, and while they're gone you move the ship far, far away out to sea. And then you ask the question, What is 'home'? Do they fly back to where the ship *was* at the dock, or do they fly to where the ship *is* in the middle of the ocean?" Turin says, "If they fly to where the ship is, it is perhaps the most important experiment in biology since forever."

The waiter puts down plates. They are plastic but look stone. They are very warm. Both Arjun and Aditya, as in a trance, like small boys, reflexively press their palms into the comforting smooth warmth of the plates as they listen.

Arjun: "So why haven't they done the experiment?" They are all leaning forward now.

Turin hardens. The BBC had actually asked him, he says, if he had any great ideas for experiments, and he told them about Sheldrake and suggested this one. They loved it. So Turin approached someone about getting the funding. He got it. He called Sheldrake. "I say, 'Great news, Rupert, we've got the funding to do your experiment.' Sheldrake says, 'I don't want to do it. These people are too negative.' I say, 'What are you talking about? If those pigeons fly to the ship, you don't give a damn.' But he wouldn't do it." Crisply: "He doesn't want to know the answer. He'd rather be a martyr." They think about this. Fear of doing the experiment. Fear of finding out.

Turin does not, clearly, overlook the connection between the wildly implausible ability of pigeons and the wildly implausible sense of smell. Nor does he overlook the scientist's fear of finding out whether he is wrong. Scientists, who live doing experiments, have reason to loathe experiments. A few more Indians in suits come in, sit down, put their cell phones on the table. Aditya looks at the phones, says, "The god of mechanical objects."

Turin sighs. "As a friend of mine says, the problem with God is that there's no new data."

The food arrives en masse. Trays and steaming platters of it, and much shifting about and many bowls and spoons and plates being set down all at once from all four sides like hail falling on the table. They pick up utensils and absorb the food as if by osmosis.

A woman walks by. Turin is distracted, his eyes unfocus. He sniffs the air and sighs, instantly despondent. "*L'Air du Temps!*" he laments to the fans in the ceiling. "It used to be so much more benzyl salicylate! They changed the formula!"

Chewing, Arjun regards Turin critically. It's time. And so, in between bites, he launches his attack on the Vibration theory. He goes
about it methodically, with no sense of ego, merely an implacable
determination to root out Turin's weaknesses and use them to destroy him as completely as possible. Turin finds this normal. It's science. Manisha and Aditya observe as if at a tennis match. Turin is
calm and pleasant, and equally aggressive. Arjun wields his own
weapons expertly, threshold stats and hydrophobicity data. His
mind leaps agilely through his mental arsenal, now snatching this
weapon, now that one. The brain, says Arjun, taking a swing, has to
put all this information together to get that specific smell point, and
Turin hasn't explained how the brain does it.

Turin loves this sharpness, this directness, so unlike British prick-
liness or American diffidence or French bluff. He responds crisply.
"It's not my problem."

"But surely you have to explain how my brain does this."

"Surely I don't. I don't know, at this point, and I don't care, for
the painfully simple reasons that a) the neuroanatomy doesn't interest me and b) I know that we *can* do it. We do it with vision. The
brain uses an algorithm to sort that incredibly complex information
out. We do it with hearing. The brain sorts that information out.
*And not a single one of the vision or hearing people can tell you how the
brain does it.*" He is emphatic, not smiling now. "And I can't tell you
with smell. But I can tell you what they can tell you: the computer
we use to do hearing and vision—a.k.a. the brain—can use the
same algorithms to do smell. My concern is with the receptors, not
with the processing. The brain can take care of figuring out what the
damn odor is. What does interest me with smell is the same thing
that interests the vision and hearing people: how do we receive it?"

Arjun sits back to think about this. Aditya looks at Manisha and
grins. Turin sits back and looks around with interest. The waiters
clear some things from the table but don't clear others, with no apparent logic. Manisha wonders aloud who is really pushing Shape.
"No one," says Turin, "which means everyone. It's just intellectual
me-too-ism." He rolls his eyes.

She talks about the smells she enjoys, the difference between common smells in India versus Europe. "Well," interjects Arjun, "smell is, of course, about sex."

"Smell is, of course, *not* about sex at all," replies Turin severely, and then, with equanimity (the dispositive point): "If you lose your sense of smell, sex will still be terrific and food will taste like crap. I rest my case."

They talk about why blacks smell different from Asians, who smell different from Caucasians. Could simply be dietary differences making for different body chemistry, or different cosmetics and soaps, or it could be that Negroes and Asians and Caucasians all have different AMHC types, immune-system proteins, and that this is why people of different races smell different. East Asians used to say that whites stank of butter. "Diacetyl," says Turin. "What gives the butter smell. A very small molecule with two ketone groups."

"But," says Arjun, "what you smell is not necessarily what I smell."

Turin keeps his calm, then says in a painfully measured tone, "This is a very strange, perverse, and yet almost universal misconception. With color vision, the question of 'When I see cerulean blue, do you see cerulean blue?' is now relegated to philosophy departments, which is where it should be. Scientifically, unless you are Daltonian"—color-blind—"due to a genetic defect, it is a given that the blue you see is the blue other people see since it is the identical wavelength of photon. That's the sense called vision. Now the sense called touch. It is universally agreed that a flame held to the flesh of one hundred different people would be perceived by all one hundred as being hot. The sense called hearing: one hundred people hear a single tone at 440 hertz, and no one doubts that all one hundred of them hear an A. But for some bizarre reason—which I think has to do with the difficulty of correlating human language to odors, first, and second with the fact that we don't understand smell molecularly, whereas we know colors are a specific frequency—with the sense called smell, people don't believe that two things are perceived the same by two different people, despite the fact that if you take a thousand people and give each ten molecules and ask, 'OK, what do these smell like?' you quickly come to the conclusion, because you get consistent answers, that everyone smells mint as, surprise, minty."

Arjun has his opaque look. Turin presses the point. "Please. With color, no one would make this ridiculous argument."

Arjun begins nodding. He says, "Tigers mark their territory by urinating, and in zoos people smelled freshly boiled rice. It turned out to be the same molecule in both cases, so this may be simply a heterogeneity of perception—they call it rice or tiger piss, but they're talking about the same smell. It's a problem of the application of language to smell."

Turin is grinning, utterly pleased. "It's phthalate," he adds, "in both. As different as two descriptors can be, but we know it's the same smell because we now know it's the same molecule. Not subjective. Objective."

The waiters come and go in their crisp whites with sweet, milky coffee. Koshy's is nearly empty. The table is an island of midafternoon quiet in a sparse sea of what remains of the Bangalore business chat. Turin is thoughtful. "Cocteau," he says, "was interviewed in his house filled with fascinating, rare, exotic objects he'd spent his life collecting. They asked him, 'If this house were on fire and you could only take one thing with you, what would you take?' He replied instantly, 'The fire.'" He muses. "I was thinking that it's like science. We spend our lives trying to burn down all these wonderful ideas people have collected through their lives."

Aditya is thinking about the question of data. "George Bernard Shaw was asked," he says, "what was the one question he would pose to God. He said, 'Why have You given us such sparse evidence of Your existence?'"

"Did we order enough?" Arjun asks no one.

"My God," says Turin, "I think we did." Another woman walking by. His torso stiffens slightly, filtering the air through his nostrils. "Claude Montana's *Parfum d'Elle*," he says. "That's *so* strong, almost pure beta-damascone." The three Indians inhale, trying to capture some of the beta-damascone molecules, but they've vanished into the sunlit air.

✦   ✦   ✦

THE DEEPER YOU look at vision, a vibrational sense, the more you recognize smell. In vision, there's something called "sensory overload": get a sudden burst of car headlights in your eyes at night, and you're blinded for a moment. We always think of sensory burnout in visual terms. We take it for granted. But smell burns out just like vision: Smell a marigold (marigolds have hugely strong odor). Inhale the smell deeply. Now wait a second. Now try to smell it again. You can't. It's gone. You've burned out on it. You can smell anything else, but not marigold. You're "blinded." Walk into a bakery, and the smell of baking bread is overwhelming. Hang out a bit, and suddenly you realize you can't smell it even if you try. And you can't smell your own house. The sense of touch doesn't desensitize. (The reason, evolutionarily, seems pretty obvious: it mustn't—we have to get away from the thorns or fire.) But the sense of hearing does; try listening to your wristwatch after leaving a nightclub. And hearing is vibrational.

✦   ✦   ✦

EVERYONE IS PUT in buses and vans and driven south for hours. They talk to one another as the drivers rocket down the dusty road, avoiding bicyclists and goats and small children. The convoy threads through the hill station of Coorg, pulls up in front of a resort. The biologists and chemists and TIFR students pile out and, with a certain amount of controlled confusion, check in. There's a buffet dinner around the pool this evening, says the receptionist politely.

✦   ✦   ✦

A VERY WARM sunny day. The conference opens, in a large, fully darkened room just off the pool, with a talk by two postdocs. They both work in the lab of the great Richard Axel, wizard of the receptor-to-brain wiring of the smell system, master of the neurological universe, and thus their credentials are unquestionable.

Dr. Nirao Shah is a young, very thin, mild-mannered postdoc. His subject is "Receptors and Animal Response"; his delivery is reticent. (Could Dr. Shah speak up? Sorry, could he speak up a bit more?) "Mice have three noses." Shah's voice is further blurred by the slide projector's hum—he's speaking more to his slides on the wall than the audience arrayed at portable tables behind him. "The main nose, the vomeronasal nose, which receives phero-mones and thus governs mating, and the septal nose. In the pig, for example," he continues, "androstenone is a well-known phero-mone."

"Of course," interjects Eric Moyers from the dark on the side of the room, "it is well-known that if you plug up the vomeronasal organ, there's no effect on mating." Moyers is one of the world's major figures in smell. His factual bizarrity, which contradicts Shah, lands in silence. Everyone just stares ahead stiffly. Shah sidesteps it by clicking to the next slide. "So how does smell bind to the recep-tor?" he asks the wall. "Each neuron receives only one odor."

Turin: "That's wrong." He states this simply, from the second row, in a clear, pleasant tone of voice. Heads jerk guiltily toward Turin, then back to the slide, everyone holding their breath.

Shah stands with the slide changer in his hand. You just can't side-step Turin. "Oh," Shah finally says. (It's unclear whether "Oh" is a statement or a question.)

Turin: "With all due respect." Pleasantly.

Shah squints at the bright slide, clears his throat. "Well—"

"With all due respect, we don't know the number of molecules that bind to each receptor, nor the number of smellable molecules that exist. In fact, the number is infinite." The word goes around the room: *Infinite*. "Inasfar as we've never come across a molecule in the smellable size range that didn't smell, nor that didn't smell different from all the others."

A moment of uncomfortable silence. Turin sits patiently. Some-one asks those in the darkness—it is clear they are not asking Turin; they want someone else's opinion—if we can't figure out how many smells we can distinguish, but Turin answers. "As I said, as far as we know, the number is infinite. There is no number."

This precipitates Turin's first run-in with Eric Moyers. Several voices are murmuring, unpleasantly, "Infinite!" when Moyers, using a "let's be reasonable" tone, objects. "Well, *infinite,* Luca, is a big word."

Turin sets his jaw and repeats, slightly louder, "Infinite."

Moyers shifts in his chair. He is a friendly and bearded American, a highly respected biologist. He finds this a bit silly. "But," says Moyers, "you *can* do a calculation, and you *do* get a number. That's a number."

Murmuring: Yes, that's a number. *Infinite.* Turin, who never, ever backs down, no matter how extreme his statement, does not back down here, at which point somewhere in southern India a power plant has a digestive problem and the electrical power fails, the room is plunged into darkness, and the hotel's diesel generator just outside heaves itself on with a loud snort and groan. When the power sluggishly comes up and when they allow him, Shah continues: "The nipples of the dam are coated with a hormone that is necessary for mice to suckle. Wash the nipples, and the pups don't suck. . . ." Shah talks a lot, but he never talks about primary reception—*how,* or what, exactly, we smell in the molecule.

The next talk is by Susan Maas, a precise, supremely competent newly minted Ph.D., who gives a lecture entirely about making the smell receptors react to smells. She gives all sorts of details about how they act, what they do when you dab them with smelly molecules. And Turin squirms through the whole thing because she never talks about primary reception. For him, the receptors are just not interesting. He wants to know how they recognize the damn signals (i.e., vibrations or shapes). To him, Axel and his postdocs are a bunch of electricians obsessing over some wire simply used to carry a telephone signal while ignoring the mystery of how the telephone *generated* this amazing signal in the first place.

Maas also talks about the septal organ. Afterward, during the coffee break outside, Turin sighs, mutters, "I never heard of this damn septal organ in my life. But that just shows that I'm an idiot." He lifts the coffee to his mouth, sniffs, murmurs, "Wow, lots of pyrazine." Then drinks it. He squints. He says carefully, "When I say 'infinite,' I mean so far as we know. You assume it can't literally be infinite, but it is definitely not finite because we've never reached the smell system's limits. OK?" This is Turin, sort of backing down.

✦ ✦ ✦

MARCEL POSTAIN'S TURN. Another big name. He talks about the receptors and the wiring. Postain is an excellent speaker, perky and funny and energetic and clear. He is so thoroughly Shapist that not only does he not talk about primary reception (what Turin's theory is about) but he takes Shape as an ironclad given. He clicks up a slide of an ear, an eye, and a nose. The picture of the ear has sound waves going directly to it. The eye has light waves going directly to it. The nose is next to a rose and between them is a chaotic mess of random signals. "In the olfactory system," states Postain, "there is no spectral system. It's a fundamentally different problem from hearing or vision."

From Turin, now sitting in a chair in the dark at the back of the room by himself, nothing. He's biding his time.

✦ ✦ ✦

THE NEXT MORNING at breakfast, Turin says quietly, "I find it physically painful to listen to things that don't interest me."

In her presentation (on the receptors and their wiring), one of the Indian scientists, Uma Ladiwala, presents some surprising data. Her clinical trials, she reports with evident frustration, have shown that smokers actually smell better than nonsmokers. This is illogical.

Turin pipes up from the back in his lone chair: "Not at all." Pleasantly. They all look at him now. "Half the perfumers I've met have been smokers, and there's actually a good reason smoking would help people smell better."

Ladiwala's eyebrows are up her forehead. And what is that reason, she asks him.

"The carbon monoxide in the cigarettes totally blocks the enzyme cytochrome P_{450}, the enzyme in the nose that breaks things down. Block this enzyme with smoke, and you don't break down smell molecules, so they hang out in the nose longer than normal, and you smell better." He shrugs.

She sort of stands there for a moment, then returns to her talk.

✦   ✦   ✦

DURING THE BREAK, Turin talks beside the pool with Richard Doty, from Philadelphia. Doty is a cheerful American who looks like he golfs at some suburban country club. He edits *The Handbook of Olfaction and Gustation* (Turin calls it "the smell bible"). The only medically focused researcher at the conference, he works on things like "Why we sneeze" (his hypothesis: to shed viruses and things trying to get inside us).

Doty is creating a test for your smell health—the smell version of an optometrist's eye chart. "You may have noticed," he says, "that if you breathe through your nose, you tend to breathe through only one side of it for a while, then for a while through the other. This is the nasal cycle, and it is due to erectile tissue in your nose. The cycle in human mirrors the cycle in rat. When you smell information on the right side, you send it to the left side of the brain and vice versa, and you find a statistically significant increase in verbal scores when you breathe through the left side of your nose." He adds, "Much of this work was done by an American yoga expert."

Women, on average, have a better sense of smell than men, says Doty, and they keep this sense longer. As you get older, you start experiencing smell loss. Epileptics exhibit considerable smell loss. (In schizophrenics, incidentally, ten out of ten have a smaller right olfactory bulb than a left one. What does this mean? So far we have no idea.) Smell loss is one of the first symptoms of Parkinson's disease and, Doty adds, somewhat angrily, in fact olfactory loss is a *more* prevalent symptom in Parkinson's patients than trembling, yet it's generally ignored by their medical providers. The trembling, he says, we register in our all-important visual system, but smell loss is just *smell,* so, like, who cares?

Turin nods grimly. Yep.

People start moving inside. The next talk is Turin's. A few people glance at him. He is looking ahead, seems a little distracted. Across the pool, someone sneezes. "Ebola," says Turin dramatically.

"Gesundheit," says Doty to the blue sky.

✦   ✦   ✦

TURIN STANDS UP, walks to the front of the room, relaxed as a cat, friendly as an uncle, cool as a Hollywood producer at a pitch. He is actually, in a strange and indefinable way, "more himself" in front of an audience than he is in private. "I am going to be speaking on structure-odor relations," he says, simple as that, and he starts out by urging everyone to collect smelly chemicals from Aldrich to smell themselves. "You can get a very nice collection of molecules." Turin speaks very cleanly, briskly, and energetically, pacing a bit, using his body, and modulating his voice as necessary to place a point in just the right way.

He self-administers a concise bio, how he "got sucked into this," then enters the talk, sets up the central mystery for them, via per-fume. A few scientific eyebrows go up. Per-*fume?* He notes that there are seven big industrial fragrance firms in the world, that each one makes about two thousand compounds a year. And they do it "at random. It's manifest," he says, "from the way they work that they don't have a theory of odor." Moyers, the biologist Anne Houston, the biophysicist Upi Bhalla, Postain, Maas, Shah are all watching him, expressionless. Everyone, he says, figures it's shape. How, ex-actly? "Well, the chemists are convinced the biologists know that answer, and the biologists are convinced the chemists do, and when they get together they discover, to their horror, that no one does."

He clicks, the lights go out, a slide pops up on the screen, an an-tique notebook of rows and rows of exquisitely neat figures in dark India ink, carefully inscribed in a firm male European hand. This is the work of Jacques Vaillant, he tells them, a French chemist at Quest International. "He was looking for a good sandalwood that hadn't been patented. In this notebook he's tracking forty-five dif-ferent molecules, variations on the molecular theme of cam-pholenic acid." Turin points at the slide. "Each of the forty-five is about one week's work, and only one, number 4628, smells of san-dalwood. He's made a note in the margin." Turin points it out, translates into English: " '4628, interesting sandalwood note!' with an exclamation mark, and the exclamation mark comes from the fact that he's been working extremely hard for nearly a year before he got anything that resembles sandalwood. He gets all manner of fruity, woody, or bizarre things, but not a sandalwood. *This,*" says Turin, turning back around suddenly, "is what you do when you do not have a theory of structure-odor relations."

The wall of judges takes his measure, considers his burden of proof. Moyers is impassive. Obaid Siddiqi, the patrician TIFR scientist who organized this conference, peers at the screen, impassively weighing the evidence, leans sideways to slip a comment into the biologist Martin Heisenberg's ear. Heisenberg purses his lips with Germanic studiousness. Doty and the German-Italian biologist Giovanni Gallizia are both smiling, openly interested. The Indian students in back are devouring the screen.

"*However,*" says Turin pleasantly, "scientists who work in this field believe there must be a relationship between structure and odor." Houston is listening carefully. Maas is listening warily. "And I agree with them," says Turin to them. Moyers, at this, glances at him. So Turin smiles, starts the plot twist. "Now, a curious thing happens here. There appears to be a god of perfumery, and this god has a sense of humor. What happens is, every time someone publishes a theory of a particular correlation between shape and smell, someone else publishes a paper that demolishes it. So predictive rules have always failed. Take ambergris, which smells like a more finished, smoother version of isopropyl alcohol. Guenther Ohloff worked for years and years on ambergris, and he finally came up with his triaxial shape rule for molecules that smelled of ambergris. He said they'd all have three chemical groups in a certain spatial pattern. It appeared to be valid for *all* known ambergis-smelling molecules. Then the people at Quest discovered Karanal, which disproved Ohloff's rule.

"So then Vlad created another rule. Vlad said that ambergris had to be three atoms, a Hydrogen here, a Hydrogen there, at these distances." He pauses just an instant. "Timberol, found soon after, pulverized this rule.

"Take sandalwood. The theory was that every molecule that smells like sandalwood must have four things." He lists them, the first being that the molecule should be a monohydric alcohol, the second holding that there must be twelve to seventeen Carbon atoms, the third a very complex thing that he gives rapidly, and the fourth that there be precise distances between certain atoms. Fine. "These were the four rules," he says, and then he delivers the news: "Osyrol violates the last three of them. So Osyrol reset the clock once again to zero."

He bears down on the point. "Push fragrance chemists to the wall, and they'll tell you, 'Well, there's *one* structure-odor relationship which is totally solid, and that's camphoraceous smells.' What's the structure? All molecules that smell of camphor are, theoretically, round. Ferrocene—smells camphoraceous—is more or less round. But here's the problem: nickelocene—also round, in fact with virtually the identical shape of ferrocene—does *not* smell of camphor."

The biologist Emily Troemel speaks up. She wants to know (she rather clearly doesn't believe it) how what Turin is calling "camphoraceous" is objectively defined. Her quotation marks are audible; what you smell, they imply, is not necessarily what I smell. She asks: They use double-blind studies?

"Oh yes, absolutely," he confirms reassuringly. One on one, this "but smell isn't really 'real,' is it?" question can spark a backlash from him, but here on stage he responds with aplomb, Maurice Chevalier in black polo and black jeans. Solid empirical agreement, he informs her graciously, backed with rigorous double-blind studies. He glances around. They are eyeing his point. Onward.

"Another wonderful example of the *lack* of relationship"—he stresses the word *lack*—"between shape and smell is the converse phenomenon: a series of very *similarly* shaped molecules with very different smells." He brings up Wannagat ("some wonderful work," he says), tells the story of how they took a series of compounds with a tertiary butyl that hid inside it a central Carbon atom. How they replaced the Carbon with Silicon, Germanium, and Tin, "which are, as you know, tetrahedral and isosteric to Carbon." (Actually, most of them didn't know this.) And how that, of course, made molecules almost identically shaped but smelling radically different. To make the smell real—"real"—for them, he delivers the details. The one with Carbon smells ethereal with a fruity, red-currant note. The one with Silicon smells ethereal—sweet honey, floral, slightly camphoraceous. The one with the Germanium atoms smells sweet and aromatic, with an unpleasant chemical note. Tin has an unpleasant chlorinelike note. Four molecules. All same shapes. All different smells. And then he says: "And I have two examples right here." He holds up the two plastic vials he has care-fully carried from London, one red, one orange. People's eyes get slightly wider. Siddiqi murmurs to Heisenberg again. Someone shoots a look at Emily Troemel. "They are $1,1$-dimethyl cyclo-hexane"—he holds up the red—"and $1,1$-dimethyl sila cyclo-hexane"—he twirls the orange like a tiny bell—"and I ordered them from Aldrich. You'll see here their structure"—he points up at the screen, where an image has just appeared, and sure enough these two have the same shape—"and you'll smell a pretty clear dif-ference. One is camphoraceous, the other is unpleasant chemical green." He sets the vials aside, holding his weapons for the moment in careful reserve.

First strike successful. Time to retreat an inch or two. "Perhaps the most plausible form of the Shape theory—and I think this is the version of it that Eric Moyers would probably believe in"—a gen-tlemanly nod to Moyers, who nods back, slightly surprised—"would be that receptors feel *parts* of molecules, these functional groups many molecules have." This is Weak Shape. He refers to it as "Moyers's theory." (He's read Moyers's work.) But he then explains the problem with Weak Shape, which is that this only makes it harder for the receptor, now clinging only to pieces of the mole-cule, to recognize what it has in its hands. Even Michael Jordan—let him use only two fingers to hold on to the ball, and he'd have more trouble controlling it. And if you believe the receptors are feeling the odotopes' shapes, well, these small guys. . . . (He clicks the button and indicates several tiny molecules materializing behind him on the screen.) If you believe that, says Turin, then small mole-cules should bind weakly to large numbers of receptors, and thus, as with Jordan's weak, uncertain two-finger grip, you'd expect small odorants to have pretty weak, nondescript smells. "And they don't. These little guys have *extremely* strong, distinctive odors." He points at sulfur hexafluoride, SF_6, a tiny molecule. "I'm one of the few people who knows what this smells like. It smells of artichoke. *Strong.*"

A hand shoots up. Turin says, with the briskness of one who regrets not being able to stop, "Let me finish this up first."

Next point. "Another extraordinary thing about smell which everyone knows to be true but nobody talks about much is the fact that we can distinguish individual chemical groups in molecules. *Everyone* knows this is true with sulfurs, SHs. Every molecule with SH, no matter what else it might have, and no matter what other smells it has, has a sulfuraceous smell. They smell different." (He points at the series of sulfur-bearing molecules on the wall.) "This one is in grapefruit. This one is not used in perfumery, thank God! This one is methyl mercaptan, extremely unpleasant. They all have a different odor profile, but you know immediately that they all have sulfurs in them."

He now turns toward Moyers and Bhalla and the others, deftly gathers this data, and hones it to a sharp point: "How does a receptor know there's an SH group?" He looks at them. "How does it distinguish an SH from an OH with absolute reliability?" (Another jab at the Weak-Shape theory: "After all, S and O are above each other on the periodic table, they both stick out of molecules in similar ways." Come on, taunts the point. Explain this.) "And this business that a chemical group can be smelled doesn't just apply to SH. It applies to a large number of groups. The second best known is CN. A nitrile. Metallic smell. You can actually *smell these atoms.*" You go into a few molecules, rip out the aldehydes—an aldehyde that smells of cucumber, an aldehyde of cumin, an aldehyde of lemon—and replace them with nitriles. "What do you get? A metallic cucumber, a metallic cumin, and a metallic lemon. So the nitrile does just what the sulfur does. I have never heard this explained by any receptor theory."

He clicks his button. The first page of Dyson's original 1938 paper appears. "Malcolm Dyson, in a paper *modestly* titled 'The Scientific Basis of Odor,' published in 1938, proposed spectroscopic recognition of odors. It being Britain, the idea was received politely, and if you read the gentlemanly discussion after his presentation, in which he really didn't give much of any evidence for anything, you have excellent proof that Britain is a fine country in which to live if you're going to propose really crazy ideas. And then it was entirely forgotten. But it was revived in the 1950s by the Canadian R. H. Wright, who took the idea and elaborated on it. How many of you do infrared spectroscopy?" He glances around at the one or two raised hands, almost sighs. "Not a lot, no, I didn't imagine so. OK, let me explain this." He now begins his standard remedial lecture, "Physics for Biologists." He walks them through the fact that atoms are bound up into molecules by electron bonds, that the bonds vibrate, that if you use an optical spectroscope to shoot photons at the bonds and make them vibrate you can read the unique chord they play and identify the molecule. OK? A hand shoots up and then quickly back down. He pretends not to notice, sprints to the end. And that's spectroscopy, he says. He takes a quick breath.

"The problem with proposing that some huge optical spectroscope is how we smell," he says, "is, how do you get one up your nose?" They laugh at this, as everyone always does. The absurdity fresh as ever. He smiles along with them and at the instant before the laugh dies, smooth as silk, slips it in like a stiletto: "There's a way of doing spectroscopy that actually doesn't use optics." Very cool. "It's called inelastic electron tunneling. This is the original paper." Click. Behind him, a serious-looking paper jumps to the screen. "A couple of guys at Ford Motor Company discovered it by accident." They stare at it. No one is laughing.

"Electrons," he explains, "are quantum objects that wander around. They're adventuresome, curious creatures. When they come to an edge, an abyss in their path, they stick little fingers out to see if there's something they can jump to on the other side." Turin uses cute assimilable phrases—"Electrons stick out fingers"— acts things out to get the audience to follow, dances, jumps, moves back and forth. He's an electron, rushing to the edge of a gaping chasm, slamming on the breaks: What the hell is *this?* Looks around, scowling: How to get across? "Well, say you put something *in* that abyss. Say it's, oh, some molecule that has vibrations corresponding to the vibrations of the electrons waiting to tunnel. Then those electrons will be able to tunnel through this molecule to the other side." They're listening, many frowning, some stressing on overload with questions, a few obviously lost, but all listening. "It won't be hugely accurate, because thermal agitation will blur everything; it won't be as precise as a human-made spectroscope, but it will be able to tell you within three hundred wave numbers what vibrations that molecule has. And, so, what it is." He pauses and adds, "It's called tunneling because the electrons *tunnel* through the space in the gap." And then he adds casually, though it's not casual at all, that what is most remarkable about *this* spectroscope is that it's easy to build with tiny proteins. Like, say, the smell receptors in your nose. Eyebrows go up. A few whispers.

He knows he's over his time limit, tries not to let it hurry his delivery. "Now," says Turin, "I want you to cast your mind back to color vision." A glance at Postain, explicit denier of any analogy with color vision. "What if we still didn't know how color vision worked. We know we can distinguish ten thousand colors. So we might think there were ten thousand color receptors, one for *each color.* And of course we'd be totally wrong. Because there are three color receptors. Three. And they make ten thousand colors. So my point is this: if you had an array of smell receptors—let's say, ten smell receptors—tuned to different parts of the vibrational spectrum, you could do with smell what color vision does. You'd be doing a sort of infrared color vision."

But the hands are rocketing up now, there is murmuring and shifting around. Siddiqi and Heisenberg are deeply immersed in analyzing some point. The hands are demanding. He puts the end on hold, points, just to release a bit of pressure.

Moyers gets pointed at, asks the question, and it's bizarre. When you got right down to it, OK, says Moyers, is Turin's theory really *any different* from the Shape theory? With binding, that is, how the receptor grabs the molecule. What Moyers is saying, put bluntly, is that Turin's theory, which proposes an electron machine gun in the nose, isn't anything new.

Turin stops dead for an instant. Takes a breath. Keeps his temper, starts slowly. Well, he begins, the receptor grips the molecule by its shape, which is about as interesting as saying we grip a book by its cover. (We have to hold the thing somehow.) But we don't read the information in the book by our hands feeling its shape; our *eyes* need to read the words. That's where the info is. The receptor holds the molecule but *reads* its *vibrations*. With tiny electron spectroscopes inside nasal receptors.

Moyers (politely countering): "Well, except for your mechanism"—he means electron tunneling—"it's the same."

"There's a huge difference!" Turin says. It is astonishing, stunning really. Essentially Moyers is saying, Fine, so you've discovered that the stomach digests food with tiny nuclear reactors hidden inside digestive cells. So what? You're still eating through your mouth.

Moyers (politely countering): "Well, but it doesn't preclude that the receptors are reading shapes." Which ignores everything Turin has just said about Shape's disastrous rules.

Turin (politely disagreeing): "Well, yes, but then unless you just *dispose* of chemistry entirely, you go back to all the things I talked about, which is that you can't explain cyanates, thiols, nitriles, et cetera." Was Moyers even listening?

Moyers says somewhat impatiently: "Well, OK, let's get back to it later."

Click. Turin makes a run for it now, a sprint down the final stretch, throws his slide comparing the color spectrum of vision to his proposed vibrational spectrum of smell. But Maas, her voice distasteful with frustration, motions at the screen. "I don't know what this represents."

Turin: "It's comparing smell wave numbers with color vision."

Maas (confused): "This is actual data on the wave numbers?"

Turin: "No, no, this is *completely* hypothetical." He's just saying, "Hey, the spectrum of vibrations in vision might work like the spectrum of vibrations in smell," but judging from other looks, she's not the only one confused.

Turin (on to the next item): "OK. Well, you may say, What's the evidence *for* this. My next—"

Gallizia immediately asks, in his Italian-German accent, a very complex, lengthy question that boils down to: But what about shape? Here we go again. . . . Turin explains that a molecule's *shape* is just going to determine how it will be gripped by the receptor; its *vibrations* are what contain its smell information. The *vibrations*. . . . But this isn't penetrating, people are murmuring to each other, pointing at the screen. He takes a deep, quick breath: "Can I just—I should finish the—go on a bit? Thanks.

"So you say, What's the evidence for this theory." Click: the boranes and Sulfur at 2500. "I used a keyboard to illustrate it." They stare with curiosity at his keyboard slide, each key representing a wave number. "I had to ask a guy if I could smell his rocket fuel. He probably thought it was a new form of drug abuse." Some of them laugh. "After some searching, I found a stable borane, decaborane. As predicted," he says calmly, not overplaying it, "it turns out to smell like Sulfur." And then, calmly, he puts the point before them: "Borane and Sulfur are not in the same column of the periodic table. They have no shape and no chemistry in common. None."

He looks around at the audience. No one is moving. "Except they both have a 2500 vibration." Still no one moving.

"When I published my paper, a retired chemist called me up and scared the hell out of me. He said, 'Well, there is a borane, triethyl-amine borane, that doesn't smell at all of Sulfur.' I asked how did he know, and he said, 'Oh, I've been smelling them all my life.'" A beat. "He took early retirement, so there may be a problem there." More of them laugh. "I went and smelled it. It smells camphoraceous. I thought, 'Uh-oh . . .'" A beat. "And then I did the wave-number calculation. It turns out that *alone* among the boranes, this one's vibrations are shifted down to 2380." Which means, of course, that its non-Sulfur smell is proof for Vibration.

They're all listening. Eyes on him. The eyes move to the slide, then back to him. Maas clears her throat and asks, logically, if camphor then vibrates at 2380, and he replies that a camphor *smell* has no specific vibration, unlike Sulfur, which is an atom, and she says, so then the Vibration theory falls apart for camphor, and he says immediately no, and she says immediately, Why not? and he says, smiling, Because camphor (again) is not an atom, it's a smell that arises from a complex collection of vibrations in the lower register, not a single, simple, identifiable vibration in the upper register like SH's sulfur smell (and there's only one way to achieve a 2500 vibration, which is SH, but that in the lower register you could get a vibration through any number of combinations), and she says (heads are swiveling as at a tennis match), "Oh, so then the theory works for simple molecules but falls apart for complex ones," and he says— very, very patiently—that no, and that he would show her how it works if, he implies, she would let him. She sits back and folds her arms and waits. Turin breathes in, breathes out.

"The ultimate test is isotopes." Click. The eyes swivel. "You'd predict isotopes would smell different. Substitute, say, Deuterium for Hydrogen, and you've got a major shift in CH's vibration, from 3000 to 2200. To test this I compared acetophenone with acetophenone-D8." He tells the story, then says, "When I told my friends at Quest the isotopes smelled different, they said it must be impurities, and it's true that when you synthesize Deuterium compounds, you use a different synthesis route than with a normal Hydrogen one. So I went to Quest and put it through a gas chromatograph smeller." A beat. "And they smelled different." At this news, Martin Heisenberg laughs out loud with glee and sits back to gaze at the screen, his face filled with pure delight. Doty is grinning. Siddiqi and Bhalla are both actively processing it. Moyers wears no expression at all. Postain is frowning and taking a note.

Turin gives them facts, slides in anecdotes. "What I'm saying is that an odor—camphoraceous, black currant, and so on—depends not on a single wave number but on the exact relative amplitudes of all the peaks. Just like a color. Like when you see burnt orange, you're actually seeing some red, some yellow, and some blue." Maas's hand is resting on her chin, her eyes on him. OK, she's listening. Moyers and Houston are sitting with their arms crossed, stoic. Shah is opaque. Siddiqi's hands are crossed as if in prayer. Doty is still loving it. Heisenberg jots a few words, neatly replaces the pen cap, leans forward again.

Houston asks about alkanes, and Turin says that alkanes have weak odors because they lack charged groups. Charged groups? So he begins a disquisition on chemistry until it becomes apparent he's losing many of the biologists, to whom chemistry is a foreign tongue. He aborts this, returns to the ambergris smells he mentioned earlier, shows them the tunneling spectra he got from the twins. "They're programs called MOPAC and CAChe. Karanal—a molecule named after Karen Rossiter, its discoverer—demolished Ohloff's rule, and Timberol demolished the rule after that." And—click! "Here are MOPAC's plotted vibrational intensities of each one."

Maas (somewhat grimly): "Could you stop for one second? Somehow I'm lost as to how these calculations are done." She hazards a guess. "Is this—spectroscopy?"

No, says Turin politely, you take this quantum mechanics program, MOPAC, and—

"Oh." Her voice has instantly hardened. "So it's computer modeling." There is something very dismissive, deprecatory about the way she says it.

He hardens too. "I'm calculating vibrations here." They face each other. "Quantum mechanics," he elaborates. Almost cruelly, he marches into algorithms and particles, but this is quantum physics and software, and she is a biologist, and her jaw merely becomes more and more set. Bhalla asks a question about the infrared spectrum, and Turin tries switching over to it, talking physics, which Bhalla, because his training included engineering, mostly understands but pretty much everyone else does not. People strain to follow, bewildered. So he has aborted the chemistry lesson and, now, his explanation of the physics. He takes a breath, heads doggedly back to the central narrative and the four ambergris smells. "You show these molecules to fragrance chemists," he says, "and they tend to sit up." Why? Because they all smell of ambergris, are shaped differently, and . . . all have the same vibrations. But parts of the audience are still frowning over IETS. And he's way, way past his time limit.

He pauses. The room, tense, holds its breath. "I think I'm going to stop here." A bit uncertain. It's a strange ending. Outside it's dark

by now, a humid Indian night. The palm trees are swaying gently beyond the pool. The elephants are wandering around in their forest.
He adds, supportively, "Although this all may seem extremely
strange to you, it only requires a minor modification of a receptor
mechanism."

Finished. The lights come on. They applaud. Some frantically,
some bewildered, some pro forma, chopping their hands together
like threshing machines. Richard Doty, who has been thoroughly
enjoying this throughout, is just grinning ear to ear. The instant the
applause stops, the questions start coming in like tracer bullets.

Moyers opens fire on MOPAC's calculations. Gallizia attacks
Turin's flank on spectral curves. From left field, Doty tosses him a
slow ball, "Would enantiomers smell different?" Turin snags it
deftly from the air, talks about his enantiomer triumph, but Moyers
drums his fingers, jaw firming: "Luca, I think that's overstating it."
It's a warning.

Turin: "You're wrong, Eric." Irresistible force, immovable object. Into the face-off, Ito drops a question about how nematode
worms might feel about SH, and Siddiqi bursts out with a surprising
show of emotion: "But this is not about feeling! This is about the
brain! That is the problem I have with this!" By the time Turin really
understands Siddiqi's objection, it turns out to be simple: Siddiqi
just does not believe that smell is objectively real. Smell is just subjective. Turin is tiring now, his guard slipping, and someone else
piles on behind, agreeing that smells have no objective existence,
so he snaps, "What you're suggesting is untrue! Three-quarters of
audiophysiology and visuophysiology are based on perceptual tests.
The reason that people started looking at rods and cones was color
blindness! An entirely perceptual thing! And they confirmed the
perceptions with neurophysiological experiments and found that
colors are *real*."

Siddiqi just shakes his leonine head, untouched. They're throwing questions at Turin, threads and things that go off in various di-
rections, curl back on things he's said, biological points that are
missing chemistry, which he now starts reacting to by simply saying,
"You're wrong" and giving the chemistry. When they repeat ques-

tions others have asked, he says, "We've gone over this," and then goes over it again. He stands his ground. "The *only* thing I'm saying absolutely for sure is that it is more than just Shape. If it were only Shape, *isotopes would not smell different.* That's all there is to it!"

Bhalla (very measured): "I disagree with that. There are significant differences in chemical properties between isotopes. Heavy water is poisonous."

Turin (very quiet, tensed): "Hang on. Heavy water is poisonous because protons undergo reactions, *protonate* and *deprotonate* things——"

From the left flank, Houston moves in pointedly to support Bhalla: "Yes," she says, "and they *bind* as well."

Turin, with narrowed eyes: "If you can give a *single* reason that acetophenone and its isotope bind differently because of their *Shape,* I would be most grateful."

Bhalla: "No, no, I'm not invoking Shape, I'm invoking a chemical dissociation action."

Turin, frowns: "You mean, the molecule is broken down in the receptor?" But——(he almost laughs) Bhalla is, out of nowhere, suddenly proposing a completely new theory of smell!

Bhalla (blandly): "Yes."

At this, finally, Turin has had it. "Oh!" he says. The word is very loud. He's not smiling anymore. His face is furious. "Well, in *that* case, *all* of this is wrong!" He sweeps a large, violent arm at the wall to encompass everything he has presented, Vibration, and Shape, and everything else, his voice metal-hard and strengthening. At this point, they're just starting to pull theories out of thin air to combat him. "If these things are undergoing chemical reactions in the receptors, then all bets are off——*including Shape.* All of this is bullshit"—— he waves his hand at his own vibration slides—"*and everything else too.*"

Silence for a moment. Bhalla says nothing; he is perhaps having second thoughts about launching his own entirely new theory of smell.

Maas clears her throat. "Are there odorless compounds, and why are they odorless?"

Turin: "Yes, and several reasons. One. Compounds which do not have partial charges are odorless. Homonuclear diatonic gases like oxygen, for instance."

She glimpses something and thrusts: "So you're saying you can smell serotonin."

Turin frowns, goes into a defensive mental crouch (where is she going with this?). "Well, serotonin is water soluble," he parries, hesitantly, "and no water-soluble compounds—"

But she cuts him off, aborts her new tack even before he's understood it with a quick, grudging, "I guess you're right, I guess I'm wrong on that, but . . ." She sits back, lips pursed, arms crossed defensively in anger.

But Turin isn't going to let her get away with this mysterious attack-retreat. "*What?*" he demands, more at her than to her. Everyone is watching. No one is breathing. *"What!"* It's a challenge. It's all body language between them.

She is staring at the slide. "I just don't . . ." she says.

Moyers is looking at the screen. "You could apply serotonin in the aqueous phase," he suggests pensively. Turin's eyes widen with surprise. OK, *this* is bizarre: Eric Moyers is now helping Luca Turin think up tests to support the Vibration theory? Moyers clears his throat and says that, well, what we're really smelling according to the Weak-Shape theory isn't well defined.

Turin says, "OK . . ." very cautiously.

"I think," Moyers says, "I tend to agree with you that Shape per se is not a good predictor."

A beat. Turin starts breathing again, says heartily, "I agree," and half the room goes into nervous laughter because, OK, but then if it's not Shape, *what the hell is it?*

"I think," says Moyers to Turin, "that it's still incumbent on you to show it's Vibration."

"Oh, indeed!" says Turin. And it's a nice place to end the questions. Turin is looking at Moyers with wary gratitude.

They applaud. Over the applause Turin says, "I'd like to urge everyone to come up and smell these two guys." Holding up his little plastic containers. "The red is Carbon, orange is Silicon." A buzz of debate surges to life as people get up, compare notes on what he said, disagree about it, wander up, or just stand and look at him. Doty comes up with a huge grin, shakes his hand, says, "You blew my mind. That was fantastic." He is utterly lit up. Maas takes a deep breath and goes up to congratulate him. She too is grinning. "Can I smell the compounds?" she asks, somewhat shyly. "Sure!" says Turin, and escorts her over to them. He watches as she picks them up and smells each, her eyes going unfocused the way people's eyes do when they smell, the molecules entering her system. "Yep," she says, "they smell different." Turin feels happy. She says, "I hope you didn't take the criticism too badly. We really gave you a hard time." Turin, who took it very badly, lies through his teeth and assures her that he didn't. Moyers has been hovering just outside the group. He comes in now and smells the Carbon and the Silicon. Well. He passes them to Bhalla and Houston. Well, they say, holding the plastic vials up to their noses and looking at each other for confirmation. Three critics at a wine tasting. Well, they're different, yes, but they're not *very* different. "They don't have to be *very* different," says Turin. "They just have to be different."

Moyers says heartily, "So now you'll have to come up with some evidence, huh!" and grins.

When he leaves, Turin turns around bewildered and shakes his head, looking at the two molecules with the same shapes and different smells. With gritted teeth he mutters, "What the fuck is *this*, skywriting?"

◆　　◆　　◆

AS USUAL, THE hotel spreads an elaborate Indian dinner before them beside the pool. Gallizia is having chicken tandoori put on his plate; Maas is surveying the various steaming, succulent things. "Vegetarian?" asks someone, and the hotel's waiter points out several options.

Turin and Bhalla are sitting together, arguing about spectroscopy until they start arguing about the validity of theories in general, which evolves into a discussion of things people used to believe that were then proved untrue. "Look at the Steady-State theory of the universe," says Bhalla. "Everyone thought it was the answer for years, until the background microwave radiation brought us the Big Bang and it got put in the trash can." Turin nods. They start discussing wrong Nobel Prizes. Bhalla, thoughtfully: "Actually I think most of the screwups in Stockholm have not been for wrong things but to the wrong people. Jocelyn Bell actually did all the work for discovering pulsars. She didn't get it. Hewish did." This, he says grimly. "And at least he's a good scientist. Some of the others . . ."

Over at Heisenberg's table, a few feet away, Siddiqi is again making it clear he doesn't believe in the objective reality of smells. You may smell Sulfur differently from the way I smell Sulfur, he says in his patrician tones. Smell is subjective. A folder is lying on the table, a yellow one. Does he, someone asks, see yellow? Siddiqi shakes his head at this logic. "You cannot compare vision and smell," he says. "Vision is objective." One of the students hears this comment, comes over to Turin, recounts it. Turin listens. "If everyone perceived odors differently," replies Turin simply, "we couldn't have perfume." Full stop. He shrugs, rolls his eyes. "If everyone perceived a major third differently, we couldn't have tonal music. If everyone perceived red differently, we couldn't have painting, fashion, interior decoration . . ."

Turin and Bhalla return to arguing about spectroscopy.

✦   ✦   ✦

THE NEXT DAY, everyone gets in vans to see a local Indian tourist attraction, a waterfall, and as the van ascends increasingly steep and curving roads, Eric Moyers opens diplomatic channels. "You should come and present to us," says Moyers with a concertedly jovial, open, American approach. He's talking about the prestigious U.S. Association of Chemoreceptor Sciences meeting, where the senior scientists in smell gather. "Submit an abstract, and we'll take it from there." Turin, in his window seat, controls his reaction and replies that his theory is not some smallish incremental step, that you can't really fit it on a poster. "Oh," says Moyers genially, "I'm sure you can put down the basic point. Submit an abstract to reserve a place, and then we'll talk to you."

Turin manages to be pleasant during the exchange, and afterward, when they are walking down a narrow path of ancient stone steps crowded with women in neon saris and men in sandals and lots of children, the sound of rushing water becoming louder through the jungle, he is happily livid. "So they want me to come with my tail between my legs, ears flattened, so the big ridgebacks can smell my butthole and see me in the submission position." The more livid and outraged he gets, the more animated and vocal he becomes. "I haven't paid my dues. Eric Moyers organized a Gordon conference"—another of the prestigious scientific conferences—"on smell this past summer in the U.S. He didn't ask me to come. Now he wants me to come and clean the toilets in Sarasota. I've got better things to do. Eric 'suggests' that I should submit an *abstract*—a little tiny abstract." He holds up the tips of his index fingers squared against the tips of his thumbs to make a tiny little square. Squints through it sardonically. "Anyone can submit an abstract—the hotel *waiter* can submit an abstract, because abstracts are not *refereed*. And then he suggests that I go and *stand next to it*"—Turin strikes a dramatic pose à la Oscar Wilde, suggesting a Babylonian slave girl—"like some prostitute hawking my wares while the ridgebacks come and sniff me at their convenience." The sound of water is loud now. "These people have these pathetic lives where they go from one meeting, one conference, to another, trading postdocs and trading gossip and figuring out what the next microscopic little step is going to be. I'm not planning on pitching my tent and hawking my wares to them. The worst thing now for Eric Moyers is for smell to be solved, because then what does the guy do? He's bet his whole life on the wrong theory, and he's in so deep he doesn't even realize the implications. They say, 'Oh, come to the AchemS meeting and present to us because some aspects of your theory may be unfamiliar.' They can't read a twenty-page published paper that's sitting on the Internet staring them in the face? Frankly, they can take their AchemS conference and shove it up their asses. Why should I go? Why the fuck should I go?"

What more could he have done to convince them? He is standing now on a precipice overlooking a waterfall that towers above him, hundreds of gallons per second plunging off a cliff into the void. Below in the ravine, where the water crashes into a pool, the Indians are swimming in their saris and their clothing, shouting happily. He watches this and thinks about the acetophenone and its deuterated version, but at the memory he looks disgusted. "You're talking to people who can't smell the difference between diacetyl and 2, 3-pentane dione. Please. No use presenting them *those*. These people couldn't tell the difference if their lives depended on it."

◆　　　◆　　　◆

THAT AFTERNOON, WHILE Postain, Maas, and Shah hang out by the pool and Siddiqi and Heisenberg chat, and Turin talks physics with the Indian students, and Moyers and Houston walk the elephant paths, Gaetri Bannerjee, a young Yale biologist from Delhi, and Michael Strout, a brand-new postdoc in Randy Reed's lab, rent an ancient automobile and its owner to visit a nearby power plant, more or less just because it's there, because it's a destination. Bannerjee is sitting in the well-worn back seat. What, she asks from the back, did Strout think of Turin's theory? The windows are open, letting in light and wind and dust.

"He was so defensive, it was a little hard to say," says Strout. "A large part of the problem is trust: we have to trust that what he's giving us—his characterization of the smells, what he claims about the shapes of these molecules—is true." Strout works on smell, but, first, he is a biologist, not a chemist, and second, he doesn't smell things.

"That's the problem with being interdisciplinary," Bannerjee concedes. "No one understands what you're doing. In this case," she says forthrightly, "the physics are the problem for us biologists."

Strout: "He shows us a mock-up of a molecule. But we don't know if it's accurate."

Bannerjee: "Yes, if he's not just citing what's convenient and forgetting the rest."

They exchange a significant look.

Strout: "And at the end, he started admitting his theory wasn't everything. Well, at least admitting that Shape is part of it." (Actually, Turin said that Shape is virtually no part at all, but they are fixated and have misinterpreted his words.)

Young scientists, they talk about the big guns in the field: Firestein, Reed, Axel, Buck, Shepherd. As a postdoc, Strout has read their names on a hundred papers in a hundred grad school courses, but, he says with a little bit of awe, "I'd never met Moyers before. It's pretty funny to actually *meet* him, like, *as the person.*" But the awe turns to something else. "It's good because if you come and talk to them in respectful tones, they don't resent you as much." Rolls his eyes. Strout and Bannerjee have a strictly bifurcated view of the smell community: people are either Old Guard or New Wave. They themselves, molecular biologists, are New Wave. "I've never met Gordon [Shepherd]," says Strout, his tone indicating he doesn't really want to.

Bannerjee, placatingly: "Gordon's a good guy. The problem with the elder statesmen is that they feel unappreciated and resentful."

Strout nods. "Moyers's put in years of good old-fashioned benchwork on this, but now *we're* here, molecular gene jockeys crashing the gate."

Bannerjee: "Well, we should crash the gate." She says this vehemently. "The field was stagnant. Gordon Shepherd has been in smell forever, and the questions he's asking and his methodology in asking them are legit, but he's been asking them for years. Time for some new blood."

She pauses a moment. The elderly car rattles along the dirt road. The driver scowls at a goat. Of course, she murmurs, everyone hates change, even scientists, who are supposed to seek it out and embrace it.

Look at Moyers. Richard Axel is one of the biggest molecular barbarians around, and Strout says with vicarious resentment, "When Richard came along with all Richard's progeny"—he means Axel's molecular biology postdocs—"and found the actual neural wiring for smell, Moyers's response was, 'Oh, they've found the axons that extend from the olfactory bulb to the neurons? That's not new, we predicted that.'" Headline: Eric Moyers says, "Nothing new."

They talk about Axel, who is one of these molecular new barbarians. Strout (grinning): "Of course Richard's personality hasn't helped." Axel is notorious for abrasiveness and arrogance.

Bannerjee (crisply): "True. He has no use for the Old Guard, and since he has no worries about his grants he tells them, in no uncertain terms, that they're fools and assholes, and for some reason they don't seem to appreciate this." She looks out the window at the palm trees going by and says simply, "But what does someone like Richard Axel care?"

Is Firestein Old Guard? Strout asks her idly.

"No," she says, gazing at a small child beside the road looking back at her with black eyes, "he's one of the ones making the transition."

◆   ◆   ◆

THE CONFERENCE IS over. In the meantime, during a quiet moment between talks, Doty has asked Turin to contribute the chapter on structure-odor relations in his next edition of the *Handbook of Olfaction*. This is on Doty's part a daring and generous move, and Turin is thrilled. The next morning, everyone leaves Coorg in a small flotilla of oddly shaped buses and vans and cars, neurologists and molecular biologists and their TIFR handlers and the Indian Ph.D. students packed into assorted vehicles for the dusty retreat to Bangalore, a scientific *Grapes of Wrath*.

◆   ◆   ◆

TURIN'S PLANE LANDS in Bombay. The next morning, he gets up early and leaves on his pilgrimage to Mohamedali Road, famous for perfume, firecracker shops, and *muglai* food snack joints. He is looking for the rare and expensive perfume ingredient *oudh*.

Perfume shops are everywhere. Peer into their dim interiors, and most look like old, dusty apothecaries, lined with large metal containers and huge glass jars of things. There is Arabic writing—virtually the entire immense perfumery business in Bombay is Muslim—and English, and Hindi and Gujarati script in some places. He walks slowly, selecting the right store. He enters one and asks, "Do you have *oudh?*" Yes, yes, they do, and they get it and he smells it, very excited, and he frowns and there's some discussion and it turns out that no, this is a synthetic. "You don't have the real thing." No, sir, don't have real thing, very sorry. He leaves politely.

Beggar kids are collecting like a cloud of flies, buzzing in odd orbits around him as he walks, demanding money and dancing daringly close. He sort of ponders their existence, mostly ignores them and examines the stores.

He tries another place. This time they just say: No. No have *oudh.*

On the street he purses his lips. Sighs gently. "Damn. This stuff is going to be hard to find."

He tries another place, they say, Have, have! Synthetic have!

He walks along the dusty road, cars and trucks grinding along noisily, people streaming. Stops before Abdul Aklur, 107 C. Mohamedali Road, 400 003, then goes in.

A few old men and a boy, a teenager. All Muslim—the hats, the clothes differentiate them from the Hindus. The beggar kids make a pro forma effort to follow him in, retreat immediately to the street at a glare from one of the men. The boy approaches like a cat, silently, not hostile, not helpful. Turin, perusing the bottles behind the counters with great interest, appears not to notice the boy's opaqueness. He points at amber 320. "Could I smell that?" The boy gets down amber 320, dips in the strip, hands it to Turin silently. Turin blinks at it. The smell strip has "Robertet" printed on it. Turin laughs out loud. "Here in the middle of India, smelling things with Robertet"—he gives it the French pronunciation—"smelling strips. Robertet is one of the two or three truly great Grasse firms still producing naturals." He smells the amber 320, asks for another amber to compare, which the boy wordlessly delivers. "Hmm. Hmm."

He narrows his eyes, visually strafes bottles on top of bottles, stops on a rose. The boy moves toward it, hands over the smell strip. "*Very* peculiar. *Very* peculiar." The boy gives him a few more. "Now *here's* an interesting one. This is why Susan Maas, who works on smell, is so ignorant. 'You mean you can *smell* seratonin?'" He mimics her. "Little does she know, silly cow, that if you remove the amino group from serotonin you get indole, one of the strongest odors around. We smell indoles all day, especially when we crap. Fecal matter is filled with indoles."

He starts questioning the boy about the ingredients. Gets the boy to talk, a bit. Kannauj, it turns out, is where everything is made. He sniffs the amber 320 again. "When it settles down, it's actually a very nice, earthy amber." But he is restless. His eyes scan the rows of glass bottles. He says, more to himself, "But you don't have *oudh*." The young Muslim watches him and then says, emotionless, "Have *oudh*."

Turin's eyebrows shoot up. "Natural?"

"Yes. Natural."

Turin's eyebrows go up farther. "You have natural *oudh*?"

The boy just looks at him, impassive. Then he says: "You want smell."

"*Yes*, I want to smell it." Turin waits, holding his breath. The boy starts moving, catlike. He gets down a large glass bottle with a particularly ornate, garishly painted flower exterior, topped with a round glass plug. He dips in the smell strip, holds it out. Turin accepts it with reverence and skepticism. Holds it to his nose like a lit and trembling match flame licking at the tip of a finger. He breathes in. His eyes are open, but he is seeing nothing. He breathes out. He breathes in.

The *oudh* is unbelievable. Incredibly strong, first of all. It knocks you over, clubs you like a falling stone. But its vast dimension is what astonishes: a huge smell, spatially immense, and incredibly complex, a buttery layer as deep as a quarry, entirely animalic in impact, and yet the *oudh* itself is not actually an animalic, spicy without being a spice. The fungus—the tiny organic bugs that have eaten, digested, and defecated this sensual wood—have left behind their fragrance, and *oudh* is the smell of this rotten, priceless wood and billions of tiny dead animals. How much? The boy points first at the amber, the best-quality amber, gives the price for one *dohla,* or eleven grams, in rupees. Turin does the calculation rapidly in U.S. dollars. About $33.80 for eleven grams of the amber. "Huh!" says Turin, "The Ruhkhus A/Y, this absolutely incredible cucumber, only costs about, ah"—he calculates—"five dollars and thirty cents for eleven grams." He turns to the boy. "And the *oudh*?"

"*Oudh*," says the boy, "one *dohla*," and gives the price in rupees. Turin does a lightning calculation, looks at the boy, smiles. One *dohla*, eleven grams, of *oudh* is $309.

Turin leaves both thoughtful and elated. He takes a turn down a side street, walks maybe forty yards, the child swarm following, pushing and yelling a bit, and on his left he sees a store that has, over it, a sign reading AQUA AROMA. It is almost literally a hole in the wall, a room that is more a very large five-sided box. Red and tan coir carpets. Just enough room for a guest or two to sit on the six-by-six-foot floor amid bottles atop bottles. From his seat in the big box, Quraysh Aziz Attarwalla is watching him, expressionless. (*Attarwalla* means "perfume seller" and functions as both family name and occupational designation, like Smith.) Turin looks up at him. "Hello," says Turin, stopping. The *attarwalla* nods his head, once. His hand indicates the coir carpet. Turin takes off his shoes, climbs up on the carpeting, and sits cross-legged.

"Are you interested in perfumes?" asks the *attarwalla*.

"Yes," says Turin.

An assistant is dispatched scurrying for tea, and the *attarwalla* begins with a sandalwood from Mysore, a natural. "Very nice," says Turin, "it's good stuff." One *dohla* for three hundred rupees, about six dollars. They talk. Turin mentions perfume ingredients, flowers, gives the provenance of a classic perfume. The *attarwalla* takes it in impassively but shifts into a different—collegial, now—demeanor. He proposes a geranium. It is one hundred rupees for one *dohla*, two dollars. Turin inhales it, and his face automatically turns upward. The movement means nothing but that he is processing the smell. "Minty, aromatic." He is gazing up, not seeing the light blue Indian sky, his focus interior. He smells again. "Oh! Of course. The stalk is prominent, that's the greenhouse–flower shop note." Looks down, says crisply: "People don't realize that geranium is heavily mint."

The Muslim *attarwalla* considers this. "Call me Quraysh," he says. He evaluates Turin. Then he has his assistant bring out some ingredients. He makes these smells himself, he says. He takes his own raw materials, macerates them, processes the smells, puts them in the bottles. He is the manufacturer for and proprietor of this tiny little store. He says this matter-of-factly. Offers his *chameli*—tiny white Indian flowers—and then a jasmine. Turin notes, quite frankly, that the jasmine starts wonderfully and then descends into pure aldehyde soap. He doesn't try to be polite about it, he simply states it, but Quraysh acknowledges it with perfect equanimity. It's true. It does. Some are better than others.

He says, "I also create my own perfumes."

"Oh, really," says Turin with interest.

He hands Turin a business card:

Quraysh Aziz Attarwalla

Aqua Aroma

47 Bhajipala Street, Near Crawford Market, Mumbai 400 003, India

Tel (91-22-3443432)

mail@AquaAroma.com

"I would like to present you my own perfume creation," he says.

"Great," says Turin.

Quraysh motions to the assistant, who quickly reaches up the wall of boxes and hands down something. The smelling strip. "I call it *Rebecca*."

Turin smells *Rebecca*. "Nice. Like *Trésor*. A peony-and-jasmine effect." He smells. "Opopanax?"

Quraysh: "No. Mostly C_{11}, C_{10} aldehydes."

Turin: "Ah, that's it, *Chanel No. 5*!"

Quaraysh (laughs): "OK, yes."

Turin realizes something. He's alerted: there's an experiment to do here. But how to do this. . . . He tries not to startle his quarry, works toward it elliptically. "So," he enters casually, "what do you think of C_{10}?"

Quraysh likes it. "Smooth, fruity."

Turin: "And C_{11}?"

Quraysh says, "Coconut oil." Harsher.

Turin: "C_{12}?"

Quraysh says, Yes, fruitier again.

Turin is grinning, swinging in on it now. "Really? So you think C_{10} is like C_{12}?"

And then it comes: "Yes," says the *attarwalla*. "The even numbers are softer and fruitier. The odd numbers are harsh."

Turin looks at him, grinning like the Mad Hatter. It is the observation his Vibration theory predicts.

The beggar kids hover outside in the invisible no-fly zone that surrounds all commercial establishments. When they start to clamor, the assistant snaps at them and they hush. Quraysh shows Turin a synthetic rose, then *khus,* a sort of supergreen made, Quraysh tells him, of vetiver.

Turin goes through sandalwoods as Indian scooters honk piercingly, each shattering blast on the upper edge of the human auditory spectrum, ringing bells, kicking up dust from the baked asphalt. He asks if Quraysh has created a truly expensive perfume. Quraysh brings out one he calls *Novalia*. "Somewhat close to *Rebecca,*" says Turin, thinking about it. "A little more heart." Quraysh: "Yes. Like *Charlie,* don't you think?" Turin thinks about it. "It's fruitier than *Charlie*. That's a more classic chypre. This has a powdery, fruity note. Sugary, with a spice. I find this more modern." He inhales. "Really nice. *Really* nice. What's it like in drydown?"

The Indian is pleased as punch. He laughs, but there is a reticence. He says, "Don't just say that to be polite. It's encouraging to me, and I feel——"

Turin: "No, no! Not at all! Believe me!"

Quraysh (wistfully): "——because you in the West have a more scientific way of doing this." (Turin makes a face that conveys utter contempt for the West.) "Here we create perfumes only hit or miss."

Turin (snorts): "How the hell do you think they do it in the West?"

Quraysh: "What perfumes do you like?" Turin recommends *Tocade*. "It's for women?" asks Quraysh. "Yes," says Turin. "I wear it occasionally." The *attarwalla* hands him another of his own compositions. He enunciates the name: *Musk Tea*. Turin puts it on his hand. The Indian raises an eyebrow. "You're smelling it on your hand?

That's not the right way, is it?" "I do it this way often," says Turin, "because it makes it move faster." "Hm!" says Quraysh, delighted. Turin smells the elixir on his hand. A dark, intoxicating mix of the mild South Asian narcotic *pan, sopari* (the flavoring that comes from the drug betel nut), tobacco, musky and animalic. "An absolutely classic base, the animalic," says Turin, "very 1900s Paris. They were all like this. I think the person who figures out how to make this smell modern is worth millions."

A band of beggars and women with babies have joined the children just below the box and are floating daringly just inside the no-fly zone. The assistant gives them a dark look. Back. They demur, warily. They are patient and, every time Turin glances toward them, encouraging. We're here. A few coins afterward?

They talk about *Brut.* "Now, the old *Brut,*" says Turin, "the first one, that had a lot of nitro musks in it. It gave that tremendous sweetness."

Quraysh: "So what do they use now?"

Turin scrunches up his face, thinking. "If they have the money, they have macrocyclics."

Quraysh: "Ah! Yes. We get some very good musk xylol here."

Turin: "Really! They have a *fantastic* effect in composition. These are the musks that came from TNT. The explosive, trinitro toluene. These things just have a couple more methyls and an aldehyde group."

Quraysh hands him another home brew. Turin's eyes narrow. Almost warily: "Dihydromyrcenol?"

Quraysh's head goes back: "*Yes!*"

Turin laughs as well. "*I'm* impressed I got that one." He explains, "It's the nutmeg effect." He lauds the lack of vanilla. "Vanilla has been used so much; every time people run out of ideas they put in vanillin. It's become completely banal, and unless you get the very top, the Guerlains, *Shalimar,* arguably *the* great Big Vanilla . . . Otherwise, well, it's the usual suspects, ethyl vanillin, maltol . . ." He rolls his eyes. He says, "Someone once criticized Jacques Guerlain to Ernest Beaux for using vanilla. Beaux retorted, 'When I use vanilla, I get crème caramel. When Jacques uses vanilla, he gets *Shalimar.*"

This reminds him. "Guerlain," he recounts, "used to buy his

vanillin from de l'Aire, whose first vanillins were all yellow with rubbish, infected with all sorts of things, smelt of guaiacol and everything. Then de l'Aire improved the extraction method, and suddenly he was producing a very nice, pure vanillin. And Guerlain didn't want it. He actually paid *more* money for the dirty vanillin infected with crap. It was more interesting, and de l'Aire thus carried on making dirty vanillin for years."

Quraysh: "We do that. We actually get the best labdanum we can and then distort it."

Suddenly, Turin changes the subject eagerly. If he might? *Oudh.* If the *attarwalla* has some? Natural? (This is his standard procedure. Try the smell, try it again, get a fix on it, imprint it in memory, figure it out.)

Ah, says Quraysh, *oudh* . . . He motions briskly with a hand, and the assistant scurries out for some *oudh.* He says that the name *oudh* comes from the Arabic word *udder,* which means "wood."

Hmm, says Turin. It's a sweet, honey amber, says Quraysh, not animalic. Turin frowns. "Right next door to you, we got this stuff here." He takes out the *oudh* smelling strip from Abdul Aklur, glares bemusedly at it. "*Hugely* animalic. Like castoreum!" The assistant pops back with an almost microscopic bottle in his palm. "This is immensely expensive," says Quraysh, needlessly, given the size of the bottle. He has to fold the smell strip in half lengthwise to force it through the tiny opening. "A woody," says Quraysh, extracting a few of the precious molecules on the strip of paper. He hands it over.

Turin leans into the scent. In lotus position, he holds himself over it. Then: "You don't call this animalic?" At Abdul Aklur, Turin reveled in the smell. Here he is analyzing it. This one is slightly different.

Quraysh: "I call it woody."

Turin (grudging): "Weeeellll. . . . OK, *woody* a bit, but animalic."

Quraysh: "In the Middle East, they say civet."

Turin: "It has a slight civet note, but really more castoreum."

Quraysh: "Castoreum, yes, but castoreum giving it a woody effect."

They jab and feint. Quraysh says cedar, and Turin finally does get that. "Ye-es, *yes,* now I see the wood angle." He is rolling the scent around, twitching the strip through the air with thumb and forefinger, sending shots through his neural wiring every which way he can. "When you said cedarwood, that did it. Fascinating! Of course, with the prices we're talking about, maybe three perfume houses are going to buy this stuff. And Chanel may want to have a tiny bit just for reference. But it's like natural iris butter. No firm can afford it because no customers can afford to buy perfumes made with it."

Quraysh: "Ten thousand dollars per kilo?" In the West, he means.

Turin: "Oh, more than that." Turin is familiar with the Agony of *oudh* among perfumers in the West. "By the time it gets to them we're talking forty thousand. There's a firm called Laboratoire Monique Remy—they do absolutely the best. They have a *stupendous* narcissus. And one . . . I forget the name, a tiny flower that only grows, wild, in central France, they pick it by hand, I smelled it once." He has to stop talking at the devastating memory of the scent. Then he snaps back: "Then the accountants start demanding substitutions, and the quality goes down, down, down, down."

Quraysh has a synthetic *oudh* at eleven grams for eight hundred rupees, or seventeen dollars, so it's one-eighteenth the price of Abdul Aklur's, but it's also one-eighteenth the smell. No comparison. Quraysh says he can't figure out what they're putting in this thing. He studied three years of chemistry in Bombay, "but it's not enough for this," he says, regretful.

"A *lot* of perfumers know no chemistry at all," says Turin, supportively.

"I make my perfumes by trial and error," admits Quraysh somewhat forlornly.

"That's how they *all* do it," Turin yells. The Indian looks at him sharply, wonderingly. Turin raises both eyebrows, grins, nods. "Those guys in their big gleaming expensive labs in Switzerland and France, they gas-chromatograph everything, and then in the end they just try sticking everything with everything else and smell it all. And that's it." Quraysh thinks about it. He feels better. He turns around with interest, selects, hands Turin another bottle. Turin inhales. "You really have the nitro as your base note in that one."

"Yes, I love it. I put in a tree moss," the *attarwalla* says, slightly doubtful, "because here, you see, you have a real spicy turmeric smell. And that will clean it. But . . ." He asks for Turin's advice on how to improve it.

Ah. Turin settles into this seriously. His whole body both relaxes and stiffens, preparing. His eyes go not exactly soft-focus but rather hard-focus on the smell, which looks similar. The bottle levitates under his nose. He frowns. "There's a beta-damascone, a single molecule with a clean floral-woody wittiness that would help you achieve the woodiness with a seventy-five percent oak moss. It's a great note to balance, a wry presence, a dried-fruit note—very clean—at high concentration." The Indian is sitting absolutely stock-still. Not writing it, absorbing it. The bottle still hovers, vision lasering nothing. "I would start with a woody moss base, and then I would add emoxyfurone until you get just that spicy effect that you don't have with the moss. And then I'd sweeten it with maltol." Turin lowers the bottle. Eyes snap back. Some mechanics now: "Maceration is at room temperature. You put your whatever it is in pure ethanol, forget it for six months, come back, filter it, and that's it. You get whatever dissolves in alcohol. Problem is, the quality's not constant."

Quraysh: "What do you use to dilute?"

Turin: "Oh, well, normally *I* use dipropylene glycol."

The perfumer pauses slightly. Up on Mohamedali Road, an immense truck lumbers anciently past, demurely covering itself with a veil of thick black diesel smoke. The beggar children have lowered their hands. They're just watching now. The *attarwalla* frowns, pleasantly. "What do you do, incidentally? Professionally."

"I'm a scientist," says Turin. "At University College London. I research smell."

❖   ❖   ❖

WHEN TURIN ARRIVED home in London, he debriefed Dearborn and Stewart in the United States on the reception his theory got in India before the bigwigs, then sat back to see if anything would now happen. Contacts from scientists, interest in his theory. Nothing happened.

VII

◆

RUSSIA

*J*UST AFTER INDIA, Turin drove down to Paris to the launch of the perfumes he and John Stephen had created for Fragonard. The event was to unfold on the seriously chic main level of Fragonard's Paris office, 39 boulevard des Capucines, a spectacular 1930s theater around the corner from Chanel's barracks on rue Cambon. Fragonard was calling the fragrances the Absolus. Turin circled the block a few times, found a place to park the blue Citroën, and showed up to find things in full swing. He greeted Agnès Costa warmly and shook hands with her mother, a handsome Frenchwoman wearing a mink raincoat and diamonds. Everything bubbled like molten metal. The lighting was Martian, and it intimidated.

There were a few different languages moving around the air, French and English and something Russian-like and Italian, and Turin cocked his head at them. "The French like luxury," he said, looking thoughtful and sipping something, "but what the French call luxury is actually call-girl chic. Put it this way. After finishing secondary school in Milan at sixteen, I went back to Paris to go to university, Paris XII, Pierre et Marie Curie. I rented a room from Madame Clouzot, the sister of the film director Henri-Georges

Clouzot, right near the Champs Elysées. She explained that there were only really two great French perfume makers. Guerlain and Caron. Guerlain, she said, was for *cocottes*—kept women. Caron was for the *duchesse*. But in fact it is 1880s cocotte style that today passes for chic in France. What the French consider 'chic' is actually a sort of kept-woman vulgarity." He looked very grim, then permitted himself to pronounce "Hermès" and then "Vuitton." "Caron, on the other hand," he said, brightening, "is absolutely proper, proper chic." And what is that? He laughed, thought about it, said "um" and "oh God." "Chic is, first, when you don't have to prove you have money, either because you have a lot and it doesn't matter or because you don't have any and it doesn't matter. Chic is not aspirational." He sighed, despondent. "Chic is the most impossible thing to define. Luxury is a humorless thing, largely, and when humor happens in luxury it happens involuntarily. Chic is all about humor. Which means chic is about intelligence. And there has to be oddness—most luxury is conformist, and chic cannot be. Chic must be polite and not incommode others, but within that it can be as weird as it wants.

"The Italian perfume aesthetic is, of course, completely different. What I call cashmere indigestion. They like floral Orientals, spice, and flowers together, that sort of warm, uniform, suntanned beauty with no chic whatsoever. Middle-class taste writ large. There's a couple of really great Italian fragrances, mind you. *Helietta* by Princess Helietta Caracciolo. I actually tracked her down at her shop in Rome recently to ask her if she still had any of the fragrance. She's a sweetheart. Orange-peel chypre with a woody angle. And *Teorema* by Fendi. But in general, Italian perfumery—I essentially look down on it. It's boring. Nothing is more nauseating than good taste in high doses.

"The British have floral dresses, which are pale, and leathered libraries, which are better. They've done some great masculines, since Englishmen really do care. The dandy was an English creation. Monogrammed-slippers-and-monocles like *No. 89* by Floris or *Lords* by Penhaligons. America is generally big and beautiful, the perfume interpretation of the Hoover Dam. Americans are hygienic and athletic. *Cabochard*—not the piss sold under the name today, the real stuff that you can't get anymore—you have to be into soiled underwear for that. It is a *fucking* wonderful fragrance. *Not* for Americans. But having said this, Americans have done some really great fragrances. Estée Lauder's *Youth Dew, Aliage, White Linen.* Among the truly greats. *Tommy Girl,* which is *quintessentially* American and one of the greatest twenty perfumes of all time. It was done by Calice Becker. She's French. Actually, she's one hundred percent Russian.

"Obviously, perfume culture itself is to a great degree gay culture, though some people think you're not supposed to say it. Gay guys were bored with all these stupid hairy-chested male fragrances and went out and bought *Alpona,* by Caron, which is wonderful. Actually, there aren't many gay perfumers. It's weird. Jean Guerlain said, 'I composed *Chamade* for my then girlfriend,' and I thought, 'Right.' Turned out it was true. I mean, it's not weird in that the Grasse milieu is still completely homophobic—I know one young guy who was not taken in perfume school simply because he was gay. Mind you, he was also a raging pain in the ass, but so what? The thing is, all their customers are gay, and you'd think it would be to their advantage to have a few around 'in house.' But instead they get Englishmen. Fashion is gay. We're living under a gay dictatorship; I'm sick of it. Look at that vile Gaultier's *Le Male,* what do I care about that stuff? Put it this way: I love *Old Spice*—you go back to the time of freshly shaven Daddy. What's wrong with that?"

At Fragonard candles incinerated fragrant molecules into the dark electrical air. Powerful speakers at one-hundredth their capacity were pumping a beat into the floor. The new four Absolus lined the swank walls in oils and soaps and sprays, which the Fragonard employees—young women like caryatids, slender as insects, sheathed in black—were handing out to guests in immense shopping bags. The guests peered inside, turning the bags this way and that.

Turin went back to the French. "If you consider *Shalimar* by Guerlain, lovely, with a marvelous little black *sillage,* the trail of perfume you leave behind you, *Shalimar* is nice the way the Paris

Opéra is nice, lots of plush velvet and gold. This is not to say, by the way, that Guerlain hasn't done some chic perfumes. *Mitsouko* is infinitely chic. But look at *Tabac Blond* by Caron. There's something dykey and angular and dark and totally unpresentable about that. It's a phenolic fragrance. If you bring the girl home and she's wearing that, your mom's going to be alarmed. Unless your mom's chic, in which case she'll say, 'I really like that girl who wears *Tabac Blond.*' *Tabac Blond* is a woman smoking cigars and driving—not being driven—*way* too fast."

◆   ◆   ◆

THE UPSHOT OF the reaction in India, or the lack of it, had convinced Turin that he needed a definitive punch people just couldn't sidestep. He had thought one up. This was a new version of the ultimate test—the isotope experiment—except that (here was the brain wave) instead of pale acetophenones or light-scented sila compounds, he'd use a super-powerful, revolting smell: boranes. Now *that* was a smell. He'd thought about it and decided to use his decaborane, the first borane he'd smelled in his lab with Tibor Krenacs—"It smells like boiled onion, Luca!," which meant it smelled like Sulfur. He'd make an isotope version of *that*—wrench out all the Hydrogen atoms and screw in Deuteriums instead. That would massively shift the molecule's vibrations, which would, or should, give you a massive difference in smell, not like the puny delicate orangy scent of the acetophenone that you had to strain to pick up.

If he was right, the isotope version of this stinking, Sulfur-smelling beast shouldn't smell of Sulfur at all: that was his prediction. It was a New and Improved Isotope Test, the definitive, killer isotope test. One he could really push in people's faces so they couldn't stand there and say, Well, they're different, yes, but they're not *very* different."

As always, of course, if the test went against him, it would destroy everything.

Once again, he started trying to find his beasts. Locating a lab that would make an isotope of the nasty decaborane was not, he knew, an easy task. He called Aldrich. Aldrich told him that yes, they could make it, but it would only cost him a small fortune. So that was out. He went to his computer and typed the word *decaborane* into the Northern Light search engine, hit "Enter," and up popped a few labs, some people who'd published. He sent the question out as if fly-fishing. Got nothing. He heard there was "a lot of this stuff" coming out of Russia, and tracked down two labs who'd published recently on boranes and phoned both of them. One said they'd call back and never did. The other one, in Moscow, said, *Da, da,* most interested, please send information.

It was run by Dr. Elias Burshetsky, a professor of chemistry at the Moscow Scientific Institute. Burshetsky indicated that fully deuterated decaboranes had never been made, ever, but he would make them—decaborane-D_{14}, five grams of the stuff. The only five grams that had ever existed in the world. That would be $2,000, please. Delivery by Christmas. Turin actually felt a little sad. "Here's this poor starving scientist hiring himself out for cash. Ah, Russia." But he was happy to have found Burshetsky.

Turin was soon nervous as a cat. He called Moscow regularly to see if the decaborane was ready and heard no, no, no have, not ready. (Would the stuff smell different, as he'd predicted? And if disaster struck and it smelled the same, was there *any* possible way he could get out of this? No, there wasn't.) Next call: No, not made yet, no, wasn't ready. (Why was he putting himself through this again?) And suddenly the voice from Russia replied that yes, the deuterated decaborane is ready. Turin's colleague Tonia Dunina-Barkovskaya was making the call for him in Russian from his UCL office, and he asked her to *beg* Burshetsky to smell the decaborane isotopes. She turned back to the receiver: Please, Elias Alexandrovich, what does it smell like? From Moscow, a startled Burshetsky barked down the telephone line, *What? Smell* like?

Burshetsky replied forcefully that he believed decaborane to be as toxic as World War I nerve gas. He said, It smells like the normal decaborane! (It was the same shape, after all.) Why should I smell nerve gas! to which Turin, not entirely sotto voce, joked darkly, "Tell him to have his student smell it then," which horrified Dunina-

Barkovskaya. Finally Burshetsky said heavily, OK, call me back at seven minutes to three. Already in a semidelirious state of tension, Turin found this truly weird. *Seven minutes to three.* Good God. They sat there in silence, Dunina-Barkovskaya placid, Turin's pulse fast and erratic. Exactly fourteen minutes went by. At *seven minutes to three* she looked at the clock, picked up the receiver, slowly dialed the number, and waited as the signals wheezed through the Russian circuits. Turin sat there, the veins taut in his neck. She said into the receiver, "*Da* . . . ? *Da.* . . . *Da.* . . . *Da.* . . . " Yes. . . . Yes. . . . Yes. . . . She turned to Turin, placid. She said: "He says they smell completely different. The entire lab is amazed."

He had to swallow a few times and get up and walk around before his pulse started dropping.

✦ ✦ ✦

IN EARLY FEBRUARY 1999, he got on a plane to Vilnius, Lithuania, and from there he departed for Russia in a rickety old Tupolev 134A. He loved it. "Wonderful aircraft, Tupolevs are gorgeous, typical Aeroflot, banged up to shit." It was twenty degrees below zero centigrade in Vilnius. They took off in a snowstorm.

Burshetsky met him at the airport. He looked, to Turin, like a boar hunter. His daughter was there; she spoke good English. Burshetsky was slightly edgy. They drove interminably through the vile muddy slush of Moscow, mud all over the windscreen, and Turin was gulping it in because he loved Moscow and hadn't been back for years, not since the wall and the change. He found Moscow even more insane and weirder than ever, because along with all the sad cars there were now rich people everywhere in mink coats. Burshetsky's office was on Leninskii Prospekt in the huge Institute of Inorganic Chemistry. As they were entering, Burshetsky told Turin what Russians always told him, which was "Don't speak English until we get to my office." They silently passed the two old Soviet ladies guarding the door like trolls.

The office was clean, spartan, spare, with what Turin called the "typical shitty little drawings of molecules tacked on the wall. The legends are never printed and they're always hand drawn, so they

look like relics from the 1930s." Burshetsky served a little tea because Moscow was, said Turin, the Orient, Syria with snow, you
couldn't go straight to the point, which was all he wanted to do.
Smell the damn things and pay and get the hell out.

Finally they went down to the lab. Incredibly cluttered, two
men, one fat and awake, one thin and asleep. The thin one woke up.
Everyone was uncomfortable. Everyone had something hidden
going on. He couldn't figure it out. They put the deuterated decaborane in front of him, the isotope that shouldn't smell of Sulfur. It
was poison. He lifted it and, very briefly, took a sniff. It didn't smell
of Sulfur. He started breathing again. They began negotiating the
price, and instead of Burshetsky, Turin found himself bargaining
with the quote unquote president of the fictional company that had
billed him. Turin pointed out that they'd made only four grams, not
five, and they hadn't converted every last Hydrogen to Deuterium.
By the time they'd agreed on $1,200, the man was arguing that
Turin should pay all of it now, and Turin was arguing he shouldn't,
and he finally gave them $800, took two grams, and left the other
two to have their Deuterium purified. Fine. Everyone sat down to
take a little celebratory picture, which Burshetsky refused to be in
for his own mysterious reasons. Everything was sort of sad. Turin
felt he should invite them to dinner. They went to an Indian restaurant. It was indescribably awful, and they hated it. Burshetsky finally
warmed up, though, toward the end of the little meal.

✦   ✦   ✦

TURIN GOT BACK to London. He walked outdoors feeling light
and refreshed. He touched the two tiny grams of isotope in his
pocket and looked up at the sky.

✦   ✦   ✦

"YOU KNOW WHAT'S funny?" Turin said. "I'm finding that truth is
actually a developing quantity. I mean, I always believed this was
true, but I now discover that I always have room for more belief. No
matter how absolutely dead certain I was that this theory was right,
every time I smell more proof, I believe in it even more. I mean, I
slept *so well.*"

He e-mailed a message to Nick Short at *Nature*.

> Date: Tue, 9 Feb 1999
> To: nickshort@nature.com
> From: l.turin@ucl.ac.uk (luca turin)
> Subject: smells!

Dear Nick,

I have just returned from Moscow with a small sample of a molecule that was custom-synthesized for me by researchers at the Institute of Inorganic Chemistry. It is the fully deuterated equivalent of decaborane ($B_{10}H_{14}$), i.e., $B_{10}D_{14}$. One of the salient predictions of my vibrational smell theory which so exercised your referees was that boranes should smell of Sulfur because of their virtually identical vibrational frequencies, Å2550 cm-1.

The strongest possible test of such a theory is isotope replacement of Deuterium for Hydrogen, which should take Boron-Hydrogen vibes from 2500 down to about 1800. Boron-Deuterium happens to be very stable. K. A. Solntsev and his colleagues made several grams of deuterodecaborane for me. NMR shows it to be chemically pure and isotopically >95% pure. It smells _very_ different from decaborane. Thus we _can_ smell isotope replacement, in which Shape remains identical but Vibration changes. Only two things need be ascertained by Vibration doubters: the nature of the molecules (NMR, mass spec) and their smells (easily done!). I plan to make the decaborane and its isotope available to anyone who needs them. Would *Nature* be interested in making this astonishing fact known?

all the best,
luca

✦   ✦   ✦

Short said no.

VIII

✦

END

Most laypeople," says Luca Turin, "subscribe devoutly to this lovely little fiction that science is a perfect intellectual market." And indeed, most of us do. We want to believe that science is dispassionate, objective, and (for those who don't have use for a theological god), omniscient. We want to believe that every idea that merits attention is given it. That the good ideas are kept, the bad ones discarded, the industrious rise, the lazy sink, and that hard work and honest data are rewarded.

This isn't real. Perhaps unfortunately, perhaps not. Scientists are human. Vested interests beat out new ideas. Egos smother creativity. Personalities clash. Corruption is as common as the survival instinct.

Turin is today involved in studying energy storage in cells. His theory on energy storage in cells is based on a highly unlikely possibility. He'll be walking down a street and take a call from Leonor Cruzeiro-Hansson, his new collaborator, on his cell phone, and talk passionately about a membrane-ion pump. "Can you hear me? Yeah, so I call this guy, he says, 'Oh, you can just replace a Hydrogen ion with a Sodium ion with only a small increase in energy.'" Turin snorts. "Yeah, like *a billion kilocalories per mole*. I mean, the guy is *sniffing glue*, you know?"

He continues to write about perfume. There, he always appreci-ates the truly weird. He noted that the small firm L'Artisan Par-fumeur was first to associate vanilla and the candy-floss note of ethylmaltol in *Vanilia,* first to use coffee in *L'Eau du Navigateur,* and now they'd gone and done something else: "*Dzing!* is a fragrance of superlative oddness. For the first twenty minutes, it simply smells of cardboard. For those prosaic souls who would question a press-ing need to smell of cardboard, a few words. One of the most sur-prising things about smell is the fact that complex combinations often give simple results, if simplicity is defined by our ability to name things unambiguously. Conversely, despite its workaday ori-gins, cardboard is actually a rich, warm, woody smell with a spicy angle. Much in the way that a great painter like Giorgio Morandi can transfigure for our benefit the homeliest of objects, a great per-fumer can reveal to us beauty where it is often most safely hidden: right under our noses. *Dzing!* Weird. A must-have."

He and Philippi have two young children now, a boy and a girl, Tazio and Adela. The children's last name is Philippi because Luca and Desa agreed that if the first child was a girl, the kids would have his name, and if a boy, hers. The first was a boy. What about carry-ing on his family name? "Oh," says Turin, glancing out the window, "I couldn't care less."

He changes the subject. "The postgrads here asked me to give them a lecture on 'The greatest scientific discoveries of the past thousand years.'" He is thinking about his strange experience with his smell theory, what it could possibly mean. "And I said, 'Oh, yeah, well that's nice, that's fun, you could talk about this or that, gravity or whatever.' And then I realized there's really only one great scientific discovery: the scientific endeavor itself, the idea that there is a way of generating knowledge that, objectively, irre-versibly modifies our view of the world. And the discovery is not over. We haven't elucidated science itself. We are still in a state of great conflict. The scientific question is, What is the best way to or-ganize science so it delivers the maximum amount of what we want it to deliver? My lecture will be about yes, there's been amazing scientific progress, but we really haven't answered this question. Peer review when it manifestly doesn't work. This veneration of publishing when everyone knows one great paper is enough for one lifetime. The organization of science into a rigid, hierarchical *corporation,* like General Motors with punch clocks and test tubes and memos from superiors. A friend of mine said, 'Science is turning into a command economy.' And this completely contradicts a fundamental political reality: science is inherently a libertarian enterprise. As Feyerabend, the philosopher of science, put it, the only governing principle you can have for scientific research is 'There can be no government.' Anything goes. *À bas le système.* All these internal contradictions, as Lenin would say. A few nights ago I was saying to Desa that what the BBC should do is *The Trouble with Science.*"

The trouble with science is that, as a rule, oddity among scientists—perfume obsessions, strange work habits—is often indistinguishable from inefficiency. What appears ludicrous and implausible and outrageous usually is. And then, sometimes it's not, the problem being telling the difference. "I really do not," says Turin, "think that a 'balanced view' is derived from tepid opinions. It comes from having extreme opinions and seeing the most extreme sides. In a lecture on Cervantes's *Quixote* Vaclav Czerny said, 'Forgive us our madmen, and we will forgive you your idiots.' The thing is, the problem of smell wasn't that hard to crack. The catch was that to crack it, you had to know a huge number of disparate facts. It was simply a question of probability. How many people would be aware simultaneously of the recipe for *Chanel No. 5,* the vibrational numbers of boranes, Blitz, and Malcolm Dyson. And also have my particular approach, which was: if I smell it to be true, it is true. I had complete self-confidence because I had written a perfume guide, I'd written smells into the metaphors of language, and I trusted what I smelled. Which most people don't. And I loved writing that thing. I'd never written a word in my life, and it just flowed.

"Metaphor is the currency of knowledge. I have spent my life learning incredible amounts of disparate, disconnected, obscure, useless pieces of knowledge, and they have turned out to be, almost all of them, extremely useful. Why. Because there is no such thing as disconnected facts. There is only complex structure. And both to explain complex structure to others and, perhaps more important——this is forgotten, usually——to understand them oneself, one needs better metaphors. If I was able to understand this, it was because my chaotic accrual of information simply gave me better metaphors than anyone else.

"My father always said if you translate a proverb from one language into another, you pass for a poet. The same for science. Work strictly within one area, and it's diminishing returns, hard to make progress. But translate a concept from its field for use where it is unknown, and it is always fresh and powerful. In buying outside, you are doing intellectual arbitrage. The rate limiting step in this is your willingness to continuously translate, to force strange languages to be yours, to live in between, to be everywhere and nowhere."

INDEX

Page numbers in *italics* refer to illustrations.

THE

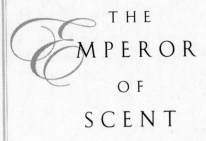

MPEROR

OF

SCENT

CHANDLER BURR

A READER'S GUIDE

To print out copies of this or other
Random House Reader's Guides, visit us at
www.atrandom.com/rgg

A CONVERSATION WITH
CHANDLER BURR

Can you tell us a bit about yourself as a writer? I guess that's a way of asking, simply enough, how you became one.

Well, I'm a journalist normally based in New York, though I've lived for the past two years in Paris. I'm thirty-nine, born in Chicago and raised in Washington, D.C. I studied at a Chinese University in Beijing, got a certificate of political studies from l'Institut d'Etude Politiques in Paris, did an internship in Tokyo with a huge Japanese corporation, Mitsui Bussan, while getting my masters in international economics and Japanese. And sort of in the middle of things, a bit by accident, I started my career as a journalist at age twenty-three when a friend who was working at *The Christian Science Monitor* happened to call (I was living in Japan at the time) and mentioned that their Southeast Asian correspondent was looking for a stringer. I called the guy in the Philippines, and two months later I'd started my career in Manila, interviewing senators and the archbishop and reporting on a coup d'état with the sound of machine guns in the background. It was an unforgettable time for me, both wonderful and terrifying. I sometimes thought I was going to drown, but I learned an enormous amount enormously fast.

How did *The Emperor of Scent* begin?

As the result of pure chance. On January 5, 1998, I was waiting in line to board the Eurostar in Paris's Gare du Nord to go to London when the loudspeakers announced there'd be a twenty minute delay. So I started talking to the guy next to me, around forty, nice, open, with what I thought was a very Italian face (Luca has an astonishing physical resemblance to Gianni Versace). We talked about the scene in the first *Mission: Impossible* where Tom Cruise flies the helicopter into the Eurostar tunnel. "But of course," said the guy, "that's impossible according to the laws of physics," and he explained why in detail. I said, You know a lot of physics. "I'm a biophysicist." Oh yeah? What do you work on? "Smell. I created a new theory of smell." We talked during the entire trip, and at Waterloo I said to Luca Turin, I want to write about you.

So you started writing it, but often we don't complete projects we start. What made you finish?

It's funny, but unlike with other projects, I never once—not once—had the thought that this wasn't absolutely worth telling. The further I got into it, the more I found this story both mesmerizing and, actually, important. Perfumes with their unforgettable beauty, the huge secretive corporations that manufacture them, a man with an extraordinary, almost supernatural power. And though I've written about science, the profoundly dysfunctional, corrupt, backbiting aspects of it were to me both new and astounding.

How did you discover the world of perfume?

Entirely through Luca's experience as a passionate, obsessive, devoted genius of perfume. I'd never thought about perfume before. I didn't even find out about his perfume collection and his book, *Parfums: La Guide,* this bestseller in France, until weeks into our conversations on smell, when he casually said, almost as an aside, "By the way, did I tell you how I got into this question of a theory of smell?" The stories of him at age five, analyzing and describing odors and perfumes, perceiving the world of smells that usually we don't even notice, took me completely by surprise. One moment that really drove home to me the art and craftsmanship of perfume was in the conversation in Bombay with Quraysh, the *attarwallah,* a seller of *attar,* perfume. Although it takes about four minutes to read the parts I put into the book, the conversation actually lasted several hours, Luca talking to Quraysh, Quraysh showing him fragrance after fragrance, and Luca could (I'd never really seen this before), just from smelling them, not only give the fragrances' names (and their creators and the stories of their origins) but, for the perfumes the *attarwallah* had himself created, name the molecules and atoms the guy had put in.

What's a "good perfume"?

People ask me this a lot now. I'll respond very specifically. A good perfume is one that doesn't deteriorate in an hour, one that is a work of art during its entire journey and not just the first ten minutes, one that doesn't start in a field of tuberose next to an azure sea only to finish in a laboratory. These things are absolutely necessary. As for the aesthetics, I could give you my opinions, but everyone decides for themself what they love.

For you, is a perfume a work of art the same way that a painting is?

The specific nature of each biological sense—smell, sight, hearing, touch, taste—leads us to create an art that speaks to that sense, and each sense's art is profoundly different. Someone once said that all art aspires to the state of music, because the nature of the sense of hearing demands that hearing's art, music, take an entirely ephemeral form; you stop playing the instruments, the art disappears, whereas a painting is always there on the wall. But at the same time, a sublime meal is also an art (for the sense of taste) born to die immediately, and yet fine cuisine is no less physically real than a painting. The biology of the sense of taste determines the form of the art made for the sense of taste. A perfume enclosed in a bottle and thus impossible to smell is not different from a painting in another room, impossible to see. But when it escapes, perfume changes. It ripens, flowers, rots with time. It decays and disappears, and a painting can't do all that. Smell, sight, and taste have biological commonalities. And significant differences. Just like the art we create to satisfy each of them.

Is the world of perfume open or closed?

Closed. Absolutely. This is not to say they're nasty people, simply that their work is secret. What they do makes an enormous amount of money for Estée Lauder, Donna Karan, Gaultier, Mugler, and on and on, and these guys demand absolute loyalty and confidentiality, which creates a culture wary of outsiders.

Do smells have secret powers?

Secret? I don't think so. Just astonishing powers: you walk into a florist's shop, take a breath. . . .

Finally, what are your ten favorite perfumes?

Well, I'll give you a list of my ten favorites as of today, right now. But the list could go on and on. And it changes all the time. You have to, I think, start out understanding that there is no such thing as a "masculine" or "feminine" fragrance. Luca once said to me that masculine perfumery is (unfortunately for it) defined negatively, which is to say by what you "can't" put in it, flowers, bright notes, et cetera. And the marketers straitjacket feminine fragrances, simply in the opposite direction, no "masculine" notes, whatever that's supposed to be. Don't listen to them. Luca has always worn whatever he's liked, and so have I. So the following list (in no particular order, I should add) has a mix of masculines and feminines, and you should feel free to wear any perfume you like.

1) *Angel* by Thierry Mugler. Marketed as a feminine, in reality as unique as a person, this utterly marvelous scent is, to quote Luca, "brilliant, at once edible (chocolate) and refreshingly toxic (caspirene, coumarin)." Created by the legendary parfumeur Yves de Chiris, *Angel* doesn't bother even pretending to pay lip service to categories. Don't let its initial personality startle you; wearing it is like having a conversation, because this thing will talk to you for hours on various subjects, sometimes chocolate / cinnamon, sometimes fresh ginger and spices in cream, and

sometimes the heady, symphonic interior of a Greenwich Village flower shop (irises, lilies, roses, their cut stems and leaves) mixed in with the scent of the concrete and car exhaust of the New York street that enters with every customer. I have dined in fine restaurants with *Angel* on, and it was the most delicious thing about the entire evening. Wear it and see.

2) *Vera Wang* by Vera Wang. There are some fragrances that are good in any circumstances and some that lend themselves to certain times and places. Wearing anything Guerlain to play tennis would be weird (while wearing *Tommy Girl* to play tennis would be perfect). It depends on what the perfume evokes and how you want to use it. Vera Wang has created a fragrance that is simply elegance in a bottle. Smelling it is like watching a beautiful woman in an evening gown walk leisurely past and give you a radiant smile. Since this is a self-assured, quiet American elegance, it's relaxed, and you could use it at the office if you wanted. But I'd hold it in reserve for evening. You smell this, you stand up a little straighter, your eyes a little brighter in the smooth air, the jazz combo sound flows a little richer. Gorgeous.

3) *Quartz* by Molyneux. When I was seventeen, I used to make pocket money by selling perfumes at a little French perfumery in Georgetown, in Washington D.C., where I grew up. One of the scents I loved was *Quartz,* which I bought (and still buy) for my mom. This is not grandiose perfumery; *Quartz* is a fragrance of simple loveliness and grace marked by a quality of absolute clarity. If you like those things, you will like *Quartz*. Its heart is orange blossom (I'm told), Molyneux markets it as a feminine, and it is a classic female fragrance. And I can tell you that a football player jock high school roommate of mine sprayed some on one morning as a joke (this was at boarding school, I had a bottle of it) and that afternoon hunted me down and, gripping my arm, demanded, "Hey, where can I *get* this shit?" In our AP English class alone he'd had five girls nuzzle him as they leaned in, astonished and delighted, to smell his neck.

4) *Hanae Mori for Men* by Hanae Mori. What amazes about Hanae Mori's creation is that it manages to be at once elegant, enticing, understated, and (crucially) just ever so slightly odd (the citrus, which you only perceive from time to time). This is not a showy fragrance. It is calm and classic and subtle, a scent that both bathes you in soothing limes and cloaks you in the most tasteful charcoal suit you've ever worn. *Hanae Mori for Men* will always be correct. It will always "work." It's arguably a perfect fragrance. I would say that it is also arguably much better on women than on men, but I don't believe that; it's for anyone who appreciates its superb qualities.

5) *Paris* by Yves Saint Laurent. Someone once said to me that of all the perfumes they know, the perfume brief in which YSL described to the perfumer what they hoped to get out of *Paris* must have been the shortest brief ever written: "Make us the most gorgeous rose perfume in the world, over and out." In my view, they've done it. *Paris* is a gigantically wonderful rose. In fact, what I like about it is that it is not anything else. It pretty much dispenses with top notes and bottom notes, just explodes onto the scene and envelopes you and starts radiating unabashed luxury. (Jo Malone's got an absolutely terrific rose created by Maurice Roucel that is sort of *Paris* in the sleek modern Waterloo station.) *Paris* has, to my mind, the most class in the YSL lineup. And it stakes out another position too: contrast *Paris* to, for example, YSL's *Baby Doll*; almost strange that YSL would decide to market a perfume that is essentially a millimeter away from Fiorucci's supersweet olfactory joke (and I like *Baby Doll,* but it *is,* in part, with it's supersweet pinkness, meant to make you laugh). Clearly the YSL people simply wanted to give us two terrific characters playing two utterly different roles. *Baby Doll* defines its delightful Betty Boop territory. And *Paris* reigns over the perfume terrain of powerful, bold, glorious, heady, rosy grandeur.

6) *The Dreamer* by Versace. After all those goddamn, tired out, hairy chested, cliché macho, standardized masculine fragrances,

you have to wonder: who the hell at Versace was the genius who came up with *The Dreamer*? First, this is so not your father's aftershave that it smells like it fell to earth from the strange, powdery stellar globulous pictured on its box. Like *Angel, The Dreamer* startles you. Smell *Eau Sauvage,* and you think, "Oh, men's cologne." (Ho hum.) You smell this thing, and not only do you *not* think men's cologne (because you can't possibly), you think, "What *is* it?!" "It" is, first, absolutely mouthwatering. It is walking through a French pastry shop next to a spice market in southern Thailand. Then there's ice cream, gun powder, fruit candy, hot cocoa, marshmallows, blood-orange peel, and probably some DDT. It is the most mesmeric fragrance I know.

7) *Coco Mademoiselle* by Chanel. I offended a perfumer in Paris by describing *Coco Mademoiselle*. What I said was that Chanel had clearly decided to create a perfume that American teenage girls would immediately want. His eyebrows arched; "Well, it's a bit more than *that,*" he said. Yes, I agree. It was an entirely forehand compliment: As with *Ralph* by Ralph Lauren, which was obviously created for the same purpose, *Coco Mademoiselle* is both an entry level Chanel fragrance and a very smart marketing decision, and there's nothing wrong with either, at all. God knows *Nos 19* and *22* can be tough to appreciate immediately. If you like nice scents, you like this perfume, instantly. Period, end of discussion. It is lovely, flowery, a fresh-faced seventeen-year-old in a summer dress, of excellent quality so the fragrance lasts, and, behind the seeming sweet simplicity, something much more compelling than might at first appear. That something is simply that when you come across someone wearing it, you want to lean closer to them.

8) *Happy for Men* by Clinique. A rare example of the marketing and creative people working together, *Happy for Men* is exactly what it says it is. This is (let's be clear) a feminine fragrance being sold to men, and every man, and lots of women, should own it. Wake up *Happy,* work *Happy,* go to the barbeque *Happy;* a guy

who smells like this is sunshine and cool, summer beach and intelligence, snowboarding and sexiness. I'd describe the scent, but nah, track it down and try it. *Damn,* this stuff is nice.

9) Pure extract of hay by Laboratoires Monique Remy. This is not a perfume. It is a perfume ingredient. I smelled it once or twice in a tiny glass vial. It smells like absolutely pure sunshine that has puddled on a barn floor in summer. It is astonishing.

10) *Bigarade* by Jean-Claude Ellena and *En Passant* by Olivia Giacobetti for Frédéric Malle/ Editions de Parfums. I only put these two together because they were both created for Frédéric Malle's uniquely strange and difficult-to-find perfume outfit, which produces fragrances made like no others, rather expensive, and appallingly good. Malle got an idea in his head, went to individual great perfumers, and offered a deal: Make me a perfume. Your ideal perfume. Put whatever the hell you want in it, the most expensive, fabulous stuff around. Create it *exactly* as you think it should be. And I'll bottle and sell it. In the little Malle boutique at Barneys, which is the only place in New York City you can smell these things, they make a big deal out of their central metaphor, that these perfumes are written by individual authors given full authorial integrity and simply published by Malle, who may edit a bit here and there but basically just puts out the work. (It's why it's called "Editions de Parfums," which is also the website: www.editionsdeparfums.com; a *maison d'edition* in French is a publishing house.)

Weird Concept. The result is outrageous. All eleven fragrances in the current lineup range from very good to truly superb; two strike me as outrageously superb, *Bigarade* and *En Passant,* though they are utterly different. The best way to describe Jean-Claude Ellena's *Bigarade* is to say, first, that it is a vast smell. And second, that it smells like a human being in the summer in a complex weather system; whoever this person is, we can smell them, they're showered and clean but it's warm and they have a smell all the same, and the lovely, complex smells of summer are all around and clinging to their skin, and also it seems to have just rained because there's the scent of rainwater on pavement and perhaps a bit of ozone, plus some flower petals and grass that got washed into the puddle they're stepping in. As for *En Passant,* Giacobetti has done a perfect flower, but the scent is so fascinating that what this woman has crafted isn't just a smell; the damn thing *transports you with loveliness.* I would say that it's magic, but I know it's simply molecules. Still, your retinas shrink from the pure pleasure of this scent.

QUESTIONS FOR DISCUSSION

1. Perfumes are made by commission (as much great art has historically been) from a recognized palette of materials (like a painting) that strike different notes (like music) in a specific medium (like sculpture). They are also made by giant corporations according to marketing research for the purpose of making profits. Is a perfume a work of art or a commercial product?

2. Given Luca Turin's experience, how close is "the scientific endeavor" in its largest and most philosophical sense—objectivity, complete sharing of data, openness and transparency, and the unbiased testing of new ideas and data—to the actual practice of science? To what degree does *Emperor* challenge your beliefs about or trust in science?

3. What do each of the following words evoke for you positively, negatively, viscerally, symbolically: *smell, scent, fragrance, odor, nose.* Do you use your sense of smell?

4. Have a friend or someone in your book group take five to ten common items from your home—talcum powder, toothpaste, Coca-Cola, vitamin B pills—and then close your eyes, ask your friend to hold them up to your nose, and see if you can identify them.

5. List the five senses in descending order of importance to you. Then list what you consider the top art forms that speak to each sense (e.g., architecture for vision, R&B for hearing, velvet for touch) and explain your order.

6. Bring a perfume to your group (make sure each of you brings a different fragrance). Have everyone smell all of the fragrances. Now you and the other members do two things. First, choose your favorite and write a description of it without using any adjectives or

boring old categories ("floral," "woody," "musky," et cetera) but instead only nouns, similes, and metaphors/images. Read your descriptions aloud. Second, defend to the group your choice for best perfume; this will mean that each of you will have to have a theory of what makes a perfume good or bad.